Study Guide for

Wong's Nursing Care of Infants and Children

Ninth Edition

Marilyn J. Hockenberry, PhD, RN, PNP-BC, FAAN
David Wilson, MS, RNC

By

Anne Rath Rentfro, PhD, RN
Associate Professor of Nursing
The University of Texas at Brownsville in partnership with Texas Southmost College
Brownsville, Texas

Linda Sawyer McCampbell, MSN, APRN, BC
Family Nurse Practitioner
Rural Clinics of South Texas
Port Isabel Health Clinic
Port Isabel, Texas

ELSEVIER
MOSBY

3251 Riverport Lane
St. Louis, Missouri 63043

STUDY GUIDE FOR
WONG'S NURSING CARE OF INFANTS AND CHILDREN
Ninth Edition

ISBN: 978-0-323-07123-9

Notices

Knowledge and best practice in this field are constantly changing. As new research and experience broaden our understanding, changes in research methods, professional practices, or medical treatment may become necessary.

Practitioners and researchers must always rely on their own experience and knowledge in evaluating and using any information, methods, compounds, or experiments described herein. In using such information or methods they should be mindful of their own safety and the safety of others, including parties for whom they have a professional responsibility.

With respect to any drug or pharmaceutical products identified, readers are advised to check the most current information provided (i) on procedures featured or (ii) by the manufacturer of each product to be administered, to verify the recommended dose or formula, the method and duration of administration, and contraindications. It is the responsibility of practitioners, relying on their own experience and knowledge of their patients, to make diagnoses, to determine dosages and the best treatment for each individual patient, and to take all appropriate safety precautions.

To the fullest extent of the law, neither the Publisher nor the authors, contributors, or editors, assume any liability for any injury and/or damage to persons or property as a matter of products liability, negligence or otherwise, or from any use or operation of any methods, products, instructions, or ideas contained in the material herein.

Managing Editor: Michele D. Hayden
Developmental Editor: Heather Bays
Publishing Services Manager: Deborah Vogel
Project Managers: Deon Lee and Bridget Healy
Senior Book Designer: Kimberly Denando

Working together to grow
libraries in developing countries

www.elsevier.com | www.bookaid.org | www.sabre.org

ELSEVIER   BOOK AID International   Sabre Foundation

Printed in the United States of America
Last digit is the print number: 9 8 7 6 5 4 3 2 1

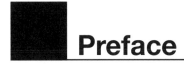

Preface

This Study Guide accompanies the ninth edition of ***Wong's Nursing Care of Infants and Children***. Students may use the Study Guide not only to review content but also to enhance their learning through critical thinking. The Study Guide is designed to assist students in mastering the content presented in the text, developing problem-solving skills, and applying their knowledge to nursing practice.

Each chapter in the Study Guide includes questions that will assist students to meet the objectives of each corresponding textbook chapter. Because most students using this Study Guide will also be preparing to pass the nursing examination (NCLEX), we have primarily used a multiple-choice format. Features to help students learn and retain pediatric terminology are included in each chapter. A Critical Thinking section is also included for each chapter, with questions designed to help students analyze the chapter's content and address their own attitudes about pediatric nursing practice. Case Studies are used in many of the Critical Thinking sections to give students experience in addressing specific practice issues. All case presentations are fictitious but designed to address situations frequently encountered by the nurse in practice.

HOW TO USE THE STUDY GUIDE

We intend for students to use this Study Guide as they study a chapter in the textbook, processing the material chapter by chapter and section by section. For this reason, we chose to present the questions in an order that generally follows the textbook's content. Students will find the answers to the questions for each chapter at the end of the Study Guide. Page numbers from the textbook have been included to facilitate finding content related to the answers.

It is our hope that this Study Guide will function as both an aid to learning and a means for measuring progress in the mastery of pediatric nursing practice.

Anne Rath Rentfro
Linda Sawyer McCampbell

Contents

1 Perspectives of Pediatric Nursing

1. Lillian Wald, a nurse who had far-reaching effects on child health and nursing:
   a. founded the Henry Street Settlement.
   b. founded public health/community nursing.
   c. established the role of the full-time school nurse.
   d. all of the above.

2. Risk-taking behaviors:
   a. do not generally begin until adolescence.
   b. have declined since 2002.
   c. are not influenced by education or parental disapproval.
   d. all of the above.

3. Mental health problems in children:
   a. affect 1 in 20 school-age children.
   b. make the children less likely to drop out of school than those with other disabilities.
   c. include attention deficit hyperactivity disorder (ADHD).
   d. all of the above.

4. According to *Healthy People 2020,* strategies that address leading health indicators for the nation would include all of the following areas except:
   a. decreasing tobacco use.
   b. increasing innovative treatments for cancer.
   c. decreasing substance abuse.
   d. increasing immunization.

5. Which of the following statements is true about infant mortality in the United States?
   a. There has been a recent dramatic increase in infant mortality in the United States.
   b. The United States is currently a world leader in reducing infant mortality.
   c. In 2001 the United States ranked last in infant mortality rate among nations with similarly sized populations
   d. The United States has lower infant mortality rates than most other developed countries.

6. The major determinant of neonatal death in technologically developed countries is:
   a. birth weight.
   b. short gestation.
   c. long gestation.
   d. human immunodeficiency virus (HIV) infection.

7. Which of the following causes of death account for the most deaths in infants under 1 year of age?
   a. Pneumonia and influenza
   b. Infections specific to the perinatal period
   c. Accidents and adverse effects
   d. Congenital anomalies

8. Infant mortality decreased significantly in the 1990s for:
   a. low birth weight.
   b. congenital heart defects.
   c. human immunodeficiency virus (HIV) infection.
   d. sudden infant death syndrome (SIDS).

9. Which of the following differences is seen when infant death rates are categorized according to race?
    a. Disparities among races have continued to increase dramatically in the United States.
    b. Infant mortality for Hispanic infants is much higher than for any other group.
    c. Infant mortality for African-Americans is twice the rate of Caucasians.
    d. Infant mortality for Caucasian infants is the same as for other races.

10. After a child reaches the age of 1 year, the leading cause of death is from:
    a. human immunodeficiency virus (HIV).
    b. congenital anomalies.
    c. cancer.
    d. unintentional injuries.

11. Children 12 years of age and older who are victims of homicide tend to be killed by:
    a. firearms.
    b. family members.
    c. stabbing.
    d. poor safety devices on firearms.

12. The disease that continues to be a leading cause of death in all age-groups of children is:
    a. diabetes.
    b. acquired immunodeficiency syndrome (AIDS).
    c. cancer.
    d. infectious disease.

13. Morbidity statistics that depict the prevalence of a specific illness in the population are:
    a. presented as rates per 100 population.
    b. difficult to define.
    c. denoting acute illness only.
    d. denoting chronic disease only.

14. Fifty percent of all acute conditions of childhood can be accounted for by:
    a. injuries and accidents.
    b. bacterial infections.
    c. parasitic disease.
    d. respiratory illness.

15. Identify one major category of disease that children tend to contract in infancy and early childhood.

16. List three factors that contribute to increasing morbidity of any disorder in children.

17. Along with clean drinking water, what other public health intervention has great impact?

18. Another term for "the new morbidity" is:
    a. pediatric social illness.
    b. pediatric noncompliance.
    c. learning disorder.
    d. dyslexia.

19. Which of the following statements about injuries in childhood is false?
    a. Developmental stage partially determines the prevalence of injuries at a given age.
    b. Most fatal injuries occur in children under the age of 9 years.
    c. Developmental stage helps to direct preventive measures.
    d. Children ages 5 to 9 years are at greatest risk for bicycle fatalities.

20. The current trend toward evidence-based practice involves:
    a. questioning whether a better approach exists.
    b. analyzing published clinical research.
    c. increased emphasis on measurable outcomes.
    d. all of the above.

21. _____ refers to the best approach to prevention that uses teaching and counseling of parents and others about developmental expectations and that alerts parents to the issues that are most likely to arise at a given age.

22. Match each federal program with the impact it has on maternal and child health.

    a. Education of the Handicapped Act Amendments of 1986 (P.L. 99-457)
    b. Social Services Block Grant
    c. Alcohol, Drug Abuse, and Mental Health Block Grants
    d. Education for All Handicapped Children Act (P.L. 94-142)
    e. Medicaid
    f. Family and Medical Leave Act (FMLA)
    g. Aid to Families with Dependent Children (AFDC)
    h. MCH Service Block Grant
    i. Women, Infants, and Children (WIC)
    j. Omnibus Budget Reconciliation Act of 1990

    _____ Created in 1965, the largest maternal-child health program; program under which the Child Health Assessment Program (CHAP) provides services for children and pregnant women, with eligibility varying from state to state

    _____ Created in 1935 as a cash grant to aid needy children without fathers

    _____ Provides services to reduce infant mortality, disease, and disabilities and to increase access to care

    _____ Established in 1981 to fund projects related to substance abuse and treatment of mentally disturbed children

    _____ Provides funds for child protective services, family planning, and foster care

    _____ Started in 1974 to provide nutritious food and education to low-income childbearing women, infants, and children up to age 5 years

    _____ Passed in 1975 to provide free public education to disabled children

    _____ Provides funding for multidisciplinary programs for disabled infants and toddlers

    _____ Allows employees to take unpaid leave (1993)

    _____ Requires states to extend Medicaid coverage to children 6 to 18 years of age with family incomes below 133% of poverty level

23. List three barriers to health care in the United States and give an example of each.

24. Define the following components of prospective payment.
    a. Prospective payment system based on diagnosis-related groups

    b. Health maintenance organizations

    c. Managed health care

25. Two basic concepts in the philosophy of family-centered pediatric nursing care are:
    a. enabling and empowerment.
    b. empowerment and bias.
    c. enabling and curing.
    d. empowerment and self-control.

26. The role of the nurse in the parent-professional partnership is to:
    a. decide what is most important for the family.
    b. decide what is most important for the child.
    c. strengthen the family's ability to nurture.
    d. manipulate the available resources.

27. An example of atraumatic care would be to:
    a. eliminate all traumatic procedures.
    b. restrict visiting hours to adults only.
    c. perform invasive procedures only in the treatment room.
    d. remove parents from the room during painful procedures.

28. _____ _____ _____ involves questioning why something is effective and whether a better approach exists. The concept also involves analyzing and translating published clinical research into the everyday practice of nursing.

29. As the movement for providing care based on evidence continues, nurses will be using methods to evaluate research such as:
    a. Agency for Health Care Policy and Research (AHCPR) guidelines in place of guidelines developed locally.
    b. guidelines that are based on traditional practice.
    c. the GRADE criteria.
    d. guidelines that reflect current research but decrease job satisfaction.

30. Match each role of the pediatric nurse with its description.

    a. Family advocacy and caring
    b. Disease prevention and health promotion
    c. Health teaching
    d. Support
    e. Counseling
    f. Therapeutic relationship
    g. Coordination and collaboration
    h. Ethical decision making
    i. Research and evidence-based practice

_____ A mutual exchange of ideas and opinions

_____ Health maintenance strategies

_____ Working together as a member of the health team

_____ Establishing relationships with children and families yet remaining separate

_____ Systematically recording and analyzing observations

_____ Attention to emotional needs (listening, physical presence)

_____ Transmitting information

_____ Using patient, family, and societal values in care

_____ Acting in the child's best interest

CRITICAL THINKING—CASE STUDY

Marisa Gutierrez arrives with her infant, Sara, in the well-baby clinic. Sara, who is 14 months old, is the youngest of three children. Her mother has brought her to the clinic for well-child care. Sara's two brothers, who are 7 and 8 years old, have come along. As the nurse interviews the mother, Sara explores the examination room. She reaches for her older brothers' marbles and puts one in her mouth.

31. After organizing the data into similar categories, the nurse correctly decides that:
    a. no dysfunctional health problems are evident.
    b. high risk for dysfunctional health problems exists.
    c. actual dysfunctional health problems are evident.
    d. potential complications are evident.

32. The nurse then identifies a possible human response pattern to further classify the data. Which of the following functional health patterns would be best for the nurse to select?
    a. Role-relationship pattern
    b. Nutritional-metabolic pattern
    c. Coping-stress tolerance pattern
    d. Self-perception/self-concept pattern

33. Based on the data collected, which of the following nursing diagnoses would be most appropriate?
    a. Altered Family Process
    b. Altered Family Coping
    c. Altered Individual Coping
    d. Altered Parenting

34. Which of the following patient outcomes is individualized for Sara?
    a. Sara will receive her immunizations on time.
    b. Sara will demonstrate adherence to the nurse's recommendations.
    c. Marisa Gutierrez will verbalize the need to keep small objects away from Sara to avoid aspiration.
    d. Sara's brothers will verbalize the need to stop playing with small objects.

35. During the evaluation phase, which of the following responses by Sara's mother would indicate that the expected outcomes have been met?
    a. "I will have to go through all of the boys' things when we get home to be sure there aren't any other small objects that could hurt Sara."
    b. "I had forgotten how curious babies are. It has been many years since the boys were babies, and they didn't have an older child's toys around."
    c. "I will have to start to discipline Sara now so that she knows not to play with the older children's belongings."
    d. "I am afraid she cannot receive her immunizations. She had a fever after her last one."

36. At Sara's next well-baby visit, what information will be most important to document in the chart?
    a. Written evidence of progress toward outcomes
    b. The standard care plan
    c. Broad-based goals
    d. Interventions applicable to patients like Sara

1. Match each term with its definition or description.

a. Transcultural nursing orientation
b. Culture
c. Race
d. Socialization
e. Material overt culture or manifest culture
f. Nonmaterial covert culture

g. Subculture influences
h. Social roles
i. Primary group
j. Secondary group
k. Ethnic stereotyping
l. Absolute standard of poverty
m. Visible poverty

n. Invisible poverty
o. Relative standard of poverty
p. Working poor
q. Uninsured children
r. Parens patriae
s. Homeless individual

_____ Characterized by limited intermittent contact; generally less concern for conformity except in rigidly limited areas

_____ A biologic term distinguishing variety in humans by physical traits

_____ A holistic view of care that provides a theoretical intellectual framework and research methodology for providing culturally congruent patient care that involves an awareness that every family, child, and health care provider comes to a clinical encounter with a cultural lens through which they see and interpret the world

_____ The process by which society communicates its competencies, values, and expectations to children

_____ Examples are ethnicity and social class

_____ One of the major reasons for the growth in the number of poor children over the past decade

_____ Refers to those aspects that cannot be observed directly, such as ideas, beliefs, customs, and feelings of a culture

_____ Refers to social and cultural deprivation; for example, limited employment opportunities; inferior educational opportunities; lack of, or inferior, medical services or health care facilities; and absence of public services

_____ Labeling that stems from ethnocentric views

_____ Characterized by intimate, continued, face-to-face contact; mutual support of members; and the ability to order or constrain a considerable proportion of individual members' behavior and role assumption; for example, the family and the peer group

_____ The rich context through which people view and respond to their world and that provides the lens through which all facets of human behavior can be interpreted

_____ Cultural creations that define patterns of behavior for persons in a variety of social positions

_____ Delineates a basic set of resources needed for adequate existence

_____ Reflects the median standard of living in a society; refers to childhood poverty in the United States

_____ Legal principle that says the state has an overriding interest in the health and welfare of its citizens

_____ Refers to a lack of money or material resources; for example, insufficient clothing, poor sanitation, and deteriorating housing

_____ Describes approximately 11.6% of all children in the United States; members of this group are more likely to miss school, thus jeopardizing their health and their education

_____ Refers to the observable components of a culture, such as material objects (dress, art, utensils, and other artifacts) and actions

_____ Those persons who lack resources and community ties necessary to provide for their own adequate shelter

2. Match each cultural term with its definition or description.

a. Biculturation
b. Cultural shock
c. Cultural sensitivity
d. Culturally competent care

e. Acculturation
f. Assimilation
g. Cultural relativity

_____ Care that goes beyond the awareness of similarities and differences to implement care that is empathetic while maintaining an openness to gain more understanding

_____ The process of developing a new cultural identity

_____ An awareness of cultural similarities and differences

_____ The concept that any behavior must be judged first in relation to the context of the culture in which it occurs

_____ Characterized by the inability to respond to or function within a new or strange situation

_____ Gradual changes produced in a culture by the influence of another culture, causing one or both cultures to be more similar to the other

_____ The straddling of two cultures; involves the ability to efficiently bridge the gap between an individual culture of origin and the dominant culture

3. The following terms are related to cultural/religious influences on health care. Match each term with its definition or description.

a. Miseries
b. Locked bowels
c. Caída de la mollera
d. Susto
e. Dolor, duels, lele

f. La diarrhea
g. Chi
h. Yin-yang
i. Curandero/curandera
j. Acupuncture

k. Acupressure
l. Moxibustion
m. Kahunas
n. Ho'oponopono

_____ The term for *diarrhea* used by some Hispanic people

_____ The term used by some Hispanic people for a fallen fontanel resulting from dehydration

_____ The term for *pain* used by some Hispanic people

_____ The term for *pain* used by some African-Americans

_____ Application of pressure to cure maladies

_____ The Chinese term for the innate energy that leaves the body through the mouth, nose, and ears and flows through the body in definite pathways, or meridians, at specific times and locations

_____ Hawaiian folk healers

_____ The term for *fright* used by some Hispanic people

_____ Insertion of needles to cure maladies

_____ The practice of healing family imbalances or disputes among Native Hawaiians

_____ The Chinese terms for the forces of hot and cold that are believed to be out of balance when a person is ill

_____ The term for *constipation* used by some African-Americans

_____ Application of heat to cure maladies

_____ The Mexican-American folk healer

4. The following terms are related to folk medicine practices that may be harmful. Match each term with its definition or description.

   a. Coining
   b. Forced kneeling
   c. Female genital mutilation (female circumcision)
   d. Topical garlic application

   e. Greta, azarcon, paylooah, surma
   f. Azogue
   g. Paylooah

   _____ Traditional remedies that contain lead

   _____ Traditional remedy used for rash and fever in Southeast Asia

   _____ Removal of, or injury to, any part of the female genital organ; practiced in Africa, the Middle East, Latin America, India, the Far East, North America, Australia, and Western Europe

   _____ Child discipline measure of some Caribbean groups

   _____ A practice of Yemenite Jews; applied to the wrist to treat infectious disease; can result in blisters or burns

   _____ Vietnamese practice; may produce weltlike lesions on the child's back

   _____ A mercury compound commonly used in Mexico and sometimes sold illegally to low-income Hispanic families in the United States as a remedy for diarrhea; can cause permanent central nervous system damage

5. When considering the impact of culture on the pediatric patient, the nurse recognizes that culture:
   a. is synonymous with race.
   b. affects the development of health beliefs.
   c. refers to a group of people with similar physical characteristics.
   d. refers to the universal manner and sequence of growth and development.

6. Which of the following social groups is an example of a primary group?
   a. Six inseparable teenagers
   b. A second-grade class
   c. The members of a national church
   d. The city garden club

7. Societal fostering and reinforcement of certain behaviors help to establish:
   a. feelings of comfort about wrongdoing.
   b. an outlet following wrongdoing.
   c. rewards for culturally acceptable social behavior.
   d. internalization of the cultural norms.

8. Match each of the following subcultural influences with its description or its influence on a child's cultural development.

   a. Ethnicity
   b. Ethnocentrism
   c. Socioeconomic status
   d. Poverty
   e. Homelessness

   f. Migrant families
   g. Biculture
   h. Religious orientation

   _____ A subcultural group in which children face less conflict when their language and culture are supported, even if the dominant language is used

   _____ Occurs when there is a lack of resources for adequate shelter

   _____ Differentiation within a population that is determined by similar distinguishing factors such as customs, characteristics, and/or language

   _____ Limit of resources needed for adequate existence

_____ Belief that one's own ethnic group is superior to others

_____ Three of every five of these families live below the federally designated poverty line

_____ Dictates the code of morality

_____ Determined by one's economic and educational level; not to be confused with cultural or ethnic diversity

9. Currently in North America there is less reliance on tradition, families are fragmented, and transmission of customs is limited because of:
   a. a growing proportion of ethnic minorities.
   b. more emphasis on ethnic diversity.
   c. the frontier background of the American culture.
   d. increasing geographic and economic mobility.

10. Most children in North America grow up in some form of:
    a. nuclear family.
    b. extended family.
    c. blended family.
    d. None of the above

11. Which of the following is the fastest-growing minority group in the United States?
    a. Spanish/Hispanic
    b. African-American
    c. Asian
    d. Native American

12. A child has become acculturated when:
    a. a gradual process of ethnic blending occurs.
    b. the child identifies with traditional heritage.
    c. ethnic and racial pride emerges.
    d. counteraggressive behavior is eliminated.

13. Which of the following strategies is likely to produce the most conflict when considering the concept of cultural shock?
    a. Teaching the family some of the dominant culture's customs
    b. Having an older son or daughter translate a health history
    c. Identifying some of the usual family customs
    d. Learning tolerance of others' values and beliefs

14. To understand and deal effectively with families in a multicultural community, nurses should:
    a. be aware of their own attitudes and values.
    b. learn about different cultural beliefs to manipulate them.
    c. learn how to change longstanding health beliefs.
    d. recognize that all cultures are very similar to one another.

15. Innate susceptibility is developed through:
    a. the child's general physical status.
    b. exposure to environmental factors.
    c. long-term proximity to disease.
    d. generations of evolutionary changes.

16. Match each disease or disorder with the racial or ethnic group with which it is associated.

a. Tay-Sachs disease
b. Cystic fibrosis
c. Sickle cell disease
d. Phenylketonuria
e. Cleft lip/palate

f. β-Thalassemia
g. Clubfoot
h. Ear anomalies
i. Werdnig-Hoffman disease

_____ Greek
_____ Middle Eastern
_____ Japanese
_____ Jewish
_____ Irish
_____ Polynesian
_____ Navajo American Indian
_____ African-American
_____ White American

17. In which of the following ethnic groups is the finding of sickle cell disease most common?
a. Scandinavian
b. Scottish/Irish
c. African-American
d. Native American

18. Which of the following statements about mass media is true?
a. Clear evidence documents a relationship between television viewing and increased risk behaviors in adolescents.
b. Educational television programming teaches the habits of mind to be a good leader.
c. Reading ability and intelligence are linked to the number and type of comic books read.
d. Mass media and increased use of tobacco by adolescents have been linked.

19. Of those factors listed below, which is the most influential for the North American child's health?
a. Genetic background
b. Proximity to the disease
c. Social class
d. Health beliefs and practices

20. The concept that any behavior must be judged first in relation to the context of the culture in which it occurs is called:
a. cultural relativity.
b. cultural stereotyping.
c. nonverbal communication.
d. culturally sensitive interaction.

21. Match each custom or belief with the ethnic group with which it is associated.

    a. Japanese
    b. U.S. dominant culture
    c. Hispanic
    d. Asian
    e. Native American

    _____ Eye contact is considered a sign of hostility.
    _____ Nonverbal communication is a practiced art.
    _____ Focus is on time; the expression "time flies" is commonly used.
    _____ To "lose face," or to feel ashamed, is highly undesirable.
    _____ Infants are particularly vulnerable to the "evil eye."

22. Which of the following strategies is not considered culturally sensitive?
    a. Active listening
    b. Slow and careful speaking
    c. Loud and clear speaking
    d. Repetition and clarification

23. Cultural food practices may have a:
    a. physiologic origin.
    b. religious significance.
    c. nurturing purpose.
    d. All of the above

24. To integrate spiritual care into practice, the nurse should:
    a. demonstrate respect.
    b. support visitation of spiritual leaders.
    c. listen to ensure understanding.
    d. do all of the above.

25. To transmit an attitude of respect for a family's ethnic or religious heritage, the nurse should:
    a. have the dietitian explain why the hospital diet must be followed.
    b. maintain good eye contact.
    c. help the patient by interjecting the correct terms during the interview.
    d. acknowledge concern for differences in food preferences.

26. Voodoo is an example of an influence that is considered:
    a. a supernatural force.
    b. a natural force.
    c. an imbalance of the forces.
    d. an imbalance of the four humors.

27. Adopting a multicultural perspective means that the nurse:
    a. explains that biomedical measures are usually more effective.
    b. uses the patient's traditional health cultural beliefs.
    c. realizes that most folk remedies have a scientific basis.
    d. uses aspects of the cultural beliefs to develop a plan.

28. Which of the following terms is not used to describe a kind of folk healer?
    a. Azogue
    b. Curandera
    c. Curandero
    d. Kahuna

29. Which of the following health practices may compromise the health and well-being of either mother or fetus?
    a. The mother reaching her arms above her head
    b. The practice of eating clay
    c. The use of asafetida
    d. The practice of ho'oponopono

30. To provide culturally sensitive care to children and their families, the nurse should:
    a. disregard one's own cultural values.
    b. identify behavior that is abnormal.
    c. recognize characteristic behaviors of certain cultures.
    d. rely on one's own feelings and experiences for guidance.

31. In planning and implementing transcultural patient care, nurses need to strive to:
    a. adapt the family's ethnic practices to the health need.
    b. change the family's longstanding beliefs.
    c. use traditional ethnic practices in every patient's care.
    d. teach the family only how to treat the health problem.

32. Awareness of generalizations about cultural groups is important, because this information helps the nurse to:
    a. learn the similarities among all cultures.
    b. learn the unique practices of various groups.
    c. stereotype groups' characteristics.
    d. categorize groups according to their similarities.

CRITICAL THINKING

33. During assessment the patient reveals that her family uses an acupuncturist occasionally. Based on this information, the nurse realizes that another health practice commonly practiced by the same cultural group is:
    a. voodoo.
    b. moxibustion.
    c. Santeria.
    d. kampo.

34. Consideration of cultural assessment data is most important for which of the following nursing diagnoses?
    a. Decreased Cardiac Output
    b. Impaired Skin Integrity
    c. Ineffective Airway Clearance
    d. Altered Nutrition

35. In planning any meal for a patient whose family holds beliefs of Islam, the nurse would exclude which of the following foods?
    a. Pork
    b. Corn bread
    c. Rice
    d. Collard greens

36. Using a framework to evaluate transcultural nursing care, which of the following health practices is typical?
    a. A Japanese family cares for a disabled family member in their home.
    b. An African-American family uses amulets as a shield from witchcraft.
    c. A Puerto Rican family seeks help from a curandera.
    d. A Mexican-American family seeks help from santeros.

3 Family Influences on Child Health Promotion

1. Match each term with its description or characteristics.

   a. Family
   b. Structure
   c. Consanguineous
   d. Coping strategies
   e. Discipline
   f. Limit-setting

   g. Time-out
   h. Divided or split custody
   i. Joint custody
   j. Function
   k. Adoption
   l. Blended family

   m. Household
   n. Family of origin
   o. Open family
   p. Closed family
   q. Behavior modification

   _____ Establishment of the rules or guidelines for behavior

   _____ Family interaction

   _____ Persons sharing a common dwelling

   _____ A group of people, living together or in close contact, who take care of one another and provide guidance for their dependent members

   _____ Blood relationships

   _____ A system of rules governing conduct

   _____ Family situation in which each parent is awarded custody of one or more of the children, thereby separating siblings

   _____ Resources for dealing with stress, such as community services, social support, and the adoption of a future orientation

   _____ Family unit into which a person is born

   _____ Composition of the family

   _____ Refinement of the practice of "sending the child to his or her room"; based on the premise of removing the reinforcer and using the strategy of unrelated consequences

   _____ Accepting of new ideas, resources, and opportunities

   _____ Family situation in which the children reside with one parent, although both parents act as legal guardians and both participate in childrearing

   _____ Resists input; views change as threatening and suspicious

   _____ Establishment of a legal relationship of parent and child between persons not related by birth

   _____ Family situation that includes at least one stepparent, stepsibling, or half sibling.

   _____ Practice based on the belief that behavior, if rewarded, will be repeated and behavior not rewarded will be eliminated

2. Which of the following is not a correct definition of the term *family* as it is viewed today?
   a. The family is what the patient considers it to be.
   b. The family may be related or unrelated.
   c. The family is always related by legal ties or genetic relationships, and members live in the same household.
   d. The family members share a sense of belonging to their own family.

3. Match each family theory with its description. (Some theories may be used more than once.)

   a. Family systems theory
   b. Family stress theory
   c. Developmental theory

   _____ Crisis intervention strategies are used, with the focus on helping members cope with the challenging event.

   _____ Continual interaction occurs between family members and the environment.

   _____ Focus is on the interactions of family members rather than on an individual member. A problem or dysfunction is not viewed as lying in any one family member but rather in the interactions within the family.

   _____ Concepts of basic attributes, resources, perception, and coping behaviors or strategies are used in assessing family crisis management.

   _____ Changes in the family over time are addressed, based on the predictable changes in the structure, function, and roles of the family, with the age of the oldest child as the marker for stage transition.

   _____ The family and each individual member must achieve developmental tasks as part of each family life-cycle stage.

4. In working with children, nurses include family members in the care plan. Which of the following statements does the nurse recognize as false when planning nursing interventions for the family?
   a. A complete family assessment is needed to discover family dynamics, family strengths, and family weaknesses.
   b. There is no expectation for parents to participate in their child's care when using the systems theory.
   c. The intervention used with families depends on the nurse's view of the theoretic model of the family.
   d. The level of assistance a family needs depends on the type of crisis, factors affecting family adjustment, and the family's level of functioning.

5. Debbie is 2 years old and lives with her brother, Mark; her sister, Mary; and her mother. Her father and mother recently divorced, and now her father lives 1 hour away. Debbie sees her father once a month for a day's visit. Her mother retains custody of Debbie. Debbie's grandparents live in a different state, but she visits them each year. Debbie's family represents which of the following?
   a. Binuclear family
   b. Extended family
   c. Single-parent family
   d. Blended family

6. Identify determinants often used as measurements for parenting infants and young children.

7. Identify the following statements as true or false.

   _____ Roles are learned through the socialization process.

   _____ *Role continuity* is defined as role behavior that is expected of children conflicting with desirable adult behavior.

   _____ All families have strengths and vulnerabilities.

   _____ Each family has its own standards for interaction within and outside the family.

   _____ Role definitions are changing as a result of the changing economy and increased opportunities for women. Marital roles, however, are still most stereotyped among the middle classes.

   _____ One quality of a strong family is the flexibility and adaptability of the roles necessary to obtain resources needed for the family.

8. Children learn role behavior and to perform in an expected way within the family at a very early age. One factor that influences the role each sibling is assigned within the family structure is the _____ _____.

9. Parenting practices differ in small and large families. Which of the following characteristics is not found in small families?
   a. Emphasis is placed on the individual development of the child, with constant pressure to measure up to family expectations.
   b. Adolescents identify more strongly with their parents and rely more on their parents for advice.
   c. Emphasis is placed on the group and less on the individual.
   d. Children's development and achievement are measured against those of children in the same neighborhood and social class.

10. Because age differences between siblings affect the childhood environment, the nurse recognizes that there is more affection and less rivalry and hostility between children whose ages are:
    a. 4 or more years apart.
    b. 4 or fewer years apart.
    c. 3 or fewer years apart.
    d. 2 or fewer years apart.

11. Johnny has always been viewed by his parents as being less dependent than his brother, Tommy, or his sister, Julie. Johnny is described as affectionate, good-natured, and flexible in his thinking. He identifies with his peer group and is popular with classmates. His parents tend to place fewer demands on Johnny for household help. From this description, the nurse would expect Johnny to have what birth position within the family?
    a. Firstborn child
    b. Middle child
    c. Youngest child
    d. Any of the above (birth position does not affect personality)

12. Monozygotic twins are:
    a. the result of fertilization of two ova.
    b. the result of fertilization of one ovum that became separated early in development.
    c. different physically and genetically.
    d. of dissimilar behaviors with greater sibling rivalry.

13. The most essential component of successful parenting is which of the following?
    a. Strong religious and cultural ties to the community
    b. Previous experience in having been nurtured as a child
    c. An understanding of childhood growth and development
    d. One person responsible for providing child care within the family structure

14. Which of the following does not identify a method to promote separation-individuation among twins?
    a. Parents discipline and praise twins as a unit.
    b. Parents foster feeling of separateness between twins.
    c. Parents avoid using the phrase "the twins."
    d. Parents foster opportunities to build one-to-one relationships with each twin.

15. List the three basic goals of parenting.

16. Limit setting and discipline are positive, necessary components of childrearing. Which of the following best describes how these functions help children?
    a. Reduce the need for children to have limits set
    b. Support children's ability to test their limits of control
    c. Allow unrestricted freedom to ensure children's growth potential
    d. Reassure children that they are able to protect themselves from harm

17. Identify the following as true or false.

    _____ A couple who has attended parenting classes before the birth of their infant can expect no disruption in the role transition to parenthood.
    _____ The time between the ages of 18 and 35 years is the best childbearing period.
    _____ The father's role has become less significant to the family's health and well-being as the age of the mother has increased.
    _____ Parent education classes taken in high school are more effective in relieving parental transitional stress than are classes taken closer to the childbearing period.

18. Which of the following is not a successful adaptation to the stress of transition to parenthood?
    a. Maintaining activities with friends
    b. Maintaining rigid schedules
    c. Appreciating the importance of the husband-wife relationship
    d. Using family, friends, and community for information and advice

19. Match each parenting style with its description.

    a. Authoritarian or dictatorial
    b. Permissive
    c. Authoritative or democratic

    _____ Allows children to regulate their own activity; sees the parenting role as a resource rather than a role model
    _____ Establishes rules, regulations, and standards of conduct for children that are to be followed without question
    _____ Respects each child's individuality; directs the child's behavior by emphasizing the reason for rules

20. Child misbehavior requires parental implementation of appropriate disciplinary action. Identify which of the following would not be an appropriate guideline for implementing discipline.
    a. Focus on the child and the misbehavior by using "you" messages rather than "I" messages.
    b. Maintain consistency with disciplinary action.
    c. Make sure all caregivers maintain unity by agreeing on the plan and being familiar with details before implementation.
    d. Maintain flexibility by planning disciplinary actions appropriate to the child's age, temperament, and severity of misbehavior.

21. Which of the following is a correct interpretation in the use of reasoning as a form of discipline?
    a. Used for older children when moral issues are involved
    b. Used for younger children to "see the other side" of an issue
    c. Used only in combination with scolding and criticism
    d. Used to allow children to obtain lengthy explanations and a greater degree of attention from parents

22. Which of the following is not a description of the use of time-out as a discipline?
    a. Allows the reinforcer to be maintained
    b. Involves no physical punishment
    c. Offers both parents and child "cooling off" time
    d. Facilitates the parent's ability to consistently apply the punishment

23. Johnny spills his milk on the living room rug. His mother smacks him on the bottom and says, "You are a messy, bad boy, Johnny." Which of the following discipline strategies are used?
    - i. Consequence
    - ii. Corporal punishment
    - iii. Scolding
    - iv. Behavior modification
    - v. Ignoring

    a. i, ii, and iii
    b. ii and iii
    c. iii and v
    d. ii, iii, and iv

24. Mike and Beverly Parker are adopting a 3-year-old girl from Russia. They have approached you for preadoptive counseling. What would you include in the counseling?
    a. Instruct them to have the child checked at their pediatrician's office for a thorough examination and review of immunizations and laboratory screening on return home from Russia.
    b. Reassure them that because they are adopting the child at an early age, the child is less likely to remember previous parenting persons.
    c. Reassure them that the health information they receive about their new daughter will be complete.
    d. Instruct them on how to form an early parent-infant attachment that will eliminate difficulties.

25. Areas of concern for parents of adoptive children include:
    a. the initial attachment process.
    b. telling the children that they are adopted.
    c. identity formation of children during adolescence.
    d. all of the above.

26. Which of the following statements about adoption is true?
    a. Adoptive children should be treated no differently than biologic children.
    b. The task of telling children that they are adopted should follow clear-cut timing guidelines.
    c. The sooner infants enter their adoptive home, the better the chances of parent-infant attachment.
    d. Older children display fewer behavioral changes after adoption disclosure than do younger children.

27. Identify the following statements about the impact of divorce on children as true or false.

    _____ Research has shown that children of divorce suffer no lasting psychologic and social difficulties.

    _____ Divorce constitutes a major disruption for children of all ages, and all children suffer stress second only to the stress produced by the death of a parent.

    _____ Children of divorce cope better with their feelings of abandonment when there is continuing conflict between parents.

    _____ Preschoolers assume themselves to be the cause of the divorce and interpret the separation as punishment.

    _____ Positive outcomes of divorce include a successful postdivorce family that can improve the quality of life for both adults and children.

    _____ Adolescents have feelings of anxiety, may withdraw from family and friends, and may have a disturbed concept of sexuality.

    _____ Even when a divorce is amicable and open, children recall parental separation with the same emotions felt by victims of a natural disaster: loss, grief, and vulnerability to forces beyond their control.

    _____ Child characteristics such as age or sex are more crucial to the child's well-being during divorce than are family characteristics.

28. Which of the following is not considered important by parents when telling their children about the decision to divorce?
    a. Initial disclosure should include both parents and siblings.
    b. Time should be allowed for discussion with each child individually.
    c. The initial disclosure should be kept simple, and reasons for divorce should not be included.
    d. Parents should physically hold or touch their child to provide feelings of warmth and reassurance.

29. Which of the following describes joint legal custody?
    a. Each parent is awarded custody of one or more of the children.
    b. The parents alternate the physical care and control of the children on an agreed-on basis while maintaining shared parenting responsibilities legally.
    c. The children reside with one parent but both parents are the legal guardians and both participate in childrearing.
    d. The children reside with the grandparents while both parents assume legal guardianship.

30. Single parenting, step-parenting, and dual-earner family parenting add stress to the parental role. Match each family type with an expected stressor or concern.

    a. Single parenting
    b. Step-parenting
    c. Dual-earner family parenting

    _____ Shortages of money, time, and energy are major concerns.

    _____ Overload is a common source of stress, and social activities are significantly curtailed, with time demands and scheduling seen as major problems.

    _____ Competition is a major area of concern among adults, with reduction of power conflicts a necessity.

CRITICAL THINKING—CASE STUDY

Ester and Roberto Garcia are the proud new parents of twin boys, Timothy and Thomas. Ester and Roberto have been married less than 1 year. Ester is 17 years old and plans to return to finish school next year. Roberto finished high school and works with his father in a local auto repair shop. He is taking a week off from work to help Ester at home with the boys. Neither Ester nor Roberto attended child parenting classes. You are making a home visit to the couple on the day after they have brought Timothy and Thomas home from the hospital. As you arrive at the house, you see that both boys are crying. Ester is trying to give Timothy his bath while Roberto is busy trying to get Thomas to take his formula. Both new parents appear tired, and Roberto admits they have been up all night with the infants and that either Timothy or Thomas seems to be crying "all the time" and that "something must be terribly wrong with them."

31. As you begin your assessment of the family, you know that the Garcias are in stage II, families with infants, according to Duvall's developmental stages of the family. Which of the following is a developmental task of this stage?
    a. Reestablishing couple identity
    b. Socializing children
    c. Making decisions regarding parenthood
    d. Accommodating to parenting role

32. Which of the following is a priority nursing diagnosis for this family?
    a. Altered Family Process related to gain of family members
    b. Altered Growth and Development related to inadequate caretaking
    c. Fear related to new parental role
    d. High Risk for Injury related to unsafe environment

33. As the nurse developing the plan for this new family, which of the following would you choose as the priority intervention?
    a. Teach the parents about Duvall's developmental stages, explaining that what they are experiencing is normal transition into parenthood.
    b. Reassure the parents that you will examine both infants but that they appear to be healthy and that the parents are doing a good job.
    c. Take over the feeding and bathing of the infants, explaining to the parents the necessity of child parenting classes.
    d. Check the infant supplies and environment to make sure the home has been made safe for children.

34. Both Thomas and Timothy are now sleeping, and you have completed your family assessment with Roberto and Ester. As a nurse, you decide to use the family stress theory to promote adaptation to the family's new role. Which of the following is not a capability the family can use to manage the crisis?
    a. Basic attributes of the family
    b. Resources within the family
    c. The family's perception of the situation
    d. Closed boundary within the family system

35. Identify a long-term goal for the Garcia family, and discuss nursing interventions that will foster achievement of this long-term goal.

36. Compare and contrast the following types of consequences, and give an example of a discipline technique for each type.
    a. Natural
    b. Logical
    c. Unrelated

37. Discuss the use of corporal punishment and the concerns of using this form of discipline to stop or decrease certain behaviors.

4 Community-Based Nursing Care of the Child and Family

1. The following terms are related to community health concepts. Match each term with its description.

a. Community
b. Population
c. Stakeholders
d. Community care

e. Community health nursing
f. Roles and functions
g. Core functions

_____ A list developed by the Institute of Medicine that guides the work of public health professionals and is directed at providing population-wide services, personal services, and home services for people at risk

_____ Individuals in the community who contribute resources, services, and financial support; implement interventions; or are the recipients of services

_____ A group of individuals with shared characteristics or interests who relate to one another

_____ A collaboration of individuals and groups within a specific community, including health care providers, advocates, governments, managed care organizations, businesses, children, and families, whose goal is the provision of services that promote health initiatives

_____ A group of people who live in a community (e.g., school-age children)

_____ Examples: caregiver, advocate, case manager, case finder, counselor, educator, epidemiologist, group process leader, health planner, and manager

_____ Focuses on promoting and maintaining the health of individuals, families, and groups in the community setting

2. The following terms are related to community health research and measurement. Match each term with its description or function.

a. Demography
b. Demographic characteristics
c. Risk
d. Epidemiology
e. Morbidity rates
f. Natality and mortality rates

g. Incidence
h. Prevalence
i. Agent
j. Host factors
k. Environmental factors
l. Primary prevention

m. Secondary prevention
n. Tertiary prevention
o. Screening
p. Economics
q. Cost-effectiveness analysis

_____ Factors such as age, gender, race, ethnicity, socioeconomic status, and education

_____ Level of prevention that focuses on screening and early diagnosis of disease

_____ The science of population health applied to the detection of morbidity and mortality in a population

_____ Factor that is responsible for causing a disease (e.g., *Mycobacterium tuberculosis*)

_____ Used to measure disease and injury

_____ The probability of developing a disease, injury, or illness

_____ The most common type of economic evaluation

_____ Measures the occurrence of new events in a population during a period of time

_____ Variables that provide the setting for the disease or condition, including conditions related to climate, home, neighborhood, and school

_____ Measures existing events in a population during a period of time

_____ The level of prevention that focuses on health promotion and prevention of disease or injury

_____ The rates of birth and death in neonates and individuals, respectively

_____ Characteristics of a disease or condition that are specific to an individual or a group

_____ In health, the measure of the amount of resources individuals and communities are willing to pay for health; allocation of health care dollars and methods for estimating cost of health

_____ A secondary prevention activity used to detect and treat disease early

_____ The level of prevention that focuses on optimizing function for individuals with disabilities or chronic diseases

_____ The study of population characteristics

3. The following terms are related to community nursing process. Match each term with its description.

a. Community needs assessment
b. Community health diagnosis
c. Community health programs

d. Community interventions
e. Community evaluation
f. Goals

_____ Based on three classic levels of prevention

_____ Outcomes that give direction to interventions and provide a measure of the change the interventions produced

_____ Collection of subjective and objective information about the target population or community

_____ Analysis to determine whether community goals were met

_____ The reflection of health status, risks, or needs in relation to a causative agent

_____ Frequently take the form of health programs for improving the health status of the target population

4. A community that is considered healthy would typically:
   a. have high-quality medical care.
   b. provide a safe place to live.
   c. provide a nurturing place to grow.
   d. do all of the above.

5. Describe the characteristics of a healthy community.

6. When community health nursing is successful, it is because:
   a. the nurse provides what the community needs.
   b. the community is empowered.
   c. acute care services are at their best.
   d. the community is the nurse's personal responsibility.

7. Settings for traditional community health include:
   a. pediatric intensive care units.
   b. neonatal intensive care units.
   c. psychiatric intensive care units.
   d. emergency departments.

8. Which of the following are useful concepts to address community health concerns that have been identified in the Public Health Nursing's Scope and Standards of Practice established by the American Nurses Association and the Quad Council of Public Health Nursing Organizations?
   a. Assessment, collaboration, and resource utilization
   b. Demography, epidemiology, and data collection
   c. Surveillance, policy development, and assurance
   d. Data collection, policy development, and surveillance

9. According to the Institute of Medicine, a community health nurse must be able to:
   a. provide care to acutely ill patients.
   b. intervene in disputes with insurance companies.
   c. bring about change in organizations.
   d. administer immunizations.

10. There is an increased risk associated with race and ethnicity that is thought to be due to a complicated relationship between:
    a. genetic predisposition and class.
    b. minority status and socioeconomic status.
    c. low level of education and class.
    d. genetic predisposition and socioeconomic status.

11. If asthma is more prevalent in School A than in School B, the nurse should expect that:
    a. there were more new cases of asthma this year than last year in School B.
    b. there were fewer new cases of asthma this year than last year in both schools.
    c. there are currently more cases of asthma in School A than in School B.
    d. there are currently more cases of asthma in School B than in School A.

12. Screening is an excellent tool to use to detect a disease:
    a. as a one-time program.
    b. that is not well understood.
    c. when treatment is too costly.
    d. with a latent symptomatic stage.

13. An understanding of economics is essential because it enables the nurse to:
    a. trade resources for patients needs.
    b. participate in discussions about the worth of health programs.
    c. develop new methods for estimating cost.
    d. do all of the above.

14. A cost-effectiveness analysis contains results expressed as a ratio, with the denominator as health units and the numerator as:
    a. health programs.
    b. the costs.
    c. risk programs.
    d. lives saved.

15. The end point of a cost-effectiveness analysis is calculated in:
    a. dollars.
    b. units of time.
    c. health units.
    d. cost-benefit terms.

16. In community nursing the focus of the nursing process shifts from:
    a. the community to the individual.
    b. the target population to the individual.
    c. the individual to the family.
    d. the individual to the target population.

17. The community health nurse collaborates with:
    a. other nurses.
    b. politicians.
    c. religious leaders.
    d. all of the above.

18. An example of a method to collect objective information in a community needs assessment is the:
    a. windshield tour.
    b. patient questionnaire.
    c. direct interview of a patient.
    d. telephone survey.

19. List the eight community systems that the nurse should examine as part of the community needs assessment.

20. An example of comparing the rates in a community with those of a standard population to evaluate a community needs assessment is to compare:
    a. tuberculosis rates with diabetes rates.
    b. county teen pregnancy rates with state rates.
    c. tuberculosis rates from one year with diabetes rates of another year.
    d. county teen pregnancy rates with tuberculosis rates.

21. Match each evaluation component with its focus.

    a. Structure
    b. Process
    c. Outcome

    _____ Focuses on whether program objectives and community goals were met

    _____ Focuses on the qualifications of personnel; the adequacy of building(s), offices, supplies, and equipment; and the characteristics of the target population

    _____ Focuses on the interaction between the patients and provider, using indicators such as the number of people who attend a program

22. Match each health program or intervention with the level of prevention it provides. (Levels of prevention may be used more than once.)

    a. Primary prevention
    b. Secondary prevention
    c. Tertiary prevention

    _____ Diabetes self-management clinic
    _____ Hepatitis B immunization program
    _____ Depression risk education
    _____ Diabetes screening
    _____ Support group for stroke victims

_____ Battered women's hotline

_____ Cardiac rehabilitation

_____ Papanicolaou smear testing

_____ Firearms safety program

Use Box 4-3 (textbook p. 70) to answer questions 23 through 26.

23. List the three disaster management stages.

24. The focus for family preparedness should be:
    a. determination of the lines of authority.
    b. first aid training, emergency supplies, and communication plans.
    c. coordination of personnel, supplies, and equipment.
    d. rescuing victims and care of the dead.

25. One important issue for community nurses to consider in disaster planning is:

26. The prevention management stage of disaster planning includes:
    a. first aid training, emergency supplies, and communication plans.
    b. coordination of personnel, supplies, and equipment.
    c. rescuing victims and care of the dead.
    d. identification of disaster risks and education about what actions to take.

CRITICAL THINKING—CASE STUDY

As the parish nurse for a small church, you see the need for a program that will address the obesity problem in the children of the parish.

27. Focusing on the core functions of population-wide service, you correctly decide to begin with:
    a. an interdisciplinary approach.
    b. quality improvement techniques.
    c. assessment of health status of the children.
    d. problem identification.

28. You decide to meet with a group of leaders in the parish. One of the primary reasons for this action is to:
    a. begin to determine how you will build capacity within the church community.
    b. find out who in the parish already has diabetes.
    c. determine the eating patterns of the members.
    d. do all of the above.

29. The parish members decide to hold a screening event to screen for overweight and obesity in the children. This screening would be classified as a:
    a. health promotion activity.
    b. primary prevention activity.
    c. secondary prevention activity.
    d. tertiary prevention activity.

30. To evaluate the program, you decide to examine whether the program had an impact on the health status of the parish members. Which of the following evaluation methods would be used?
    a. Structure
    b. Process
    c. Outcome
    d. None of the above

5 Hereditary Influences on Health Promotion of the Child and Family

1. The following terms are related to genetic influences on health. Match each term with its definition or description.

a. Genes
b. Chromosomes
c. Major structural abnormalities
d. Minor anomalies
e. Syndrome
f. Association
g. Congenital anomalies
h. Cytogenetics
i. Structural chromosome abnormalities
j. Ring chromosome
k. Euploid cell
l. Monosomy

m. Trisomy
n. Gamete formation
o. Mitosis
p. Nondisjunction
q. Alleles
r. Aneuploidy
s. Transcription
t. Contiguous gene syndromes
u. X inactivation
v. Consanguinity
w. Mutation
x. Variable expression
y. Telomere

z. Phenotype
aa. Genomic imprinting
bb. Prader-Willi syndrome
cc. Angelman syndrome
dd. Uniparental disomy
ee. Single-gene disorders
ff. Karyotype
gg. Fluorescence in situ hybridization
hh. Mapping
ii. Multifactorial disorders
jj. Teratogens

_____ Malformations that may result from genetic and/or prenatal environmental causes, resulting in serious medical, surgical, or quality-of-life consequences.

_____ A recognized pattern of malformations resulting from a single specific cause (e.g., Down syndrome or fetal alcholol syndrome).

_____ A segment of nucleic acid that contains genetic information necessary to control a certain function, such as the synthesis of a polypeptide (structural gene). This segment is often referred to as a site, or locus, on a chromosome.

_____ A nonrandom pattern of malformations for which a cause has not been determined, such as VATERL (vertebral defects, anal atresia, cardiac defect, tracheoesophageal fistula, and renal and limb defects) association.

_____ Filament-like nuclear structures that consist of chromatin, store genetic information as base sequences in DNA, and have a constant number for each species; found in pairs in somatic cells (homologous) and in single copies in germ cells. One member of a homologous pair is of paternal origin, the other of maternal origin.

_____ Birth defects; occur in 2% to 4% of all live-born children; often classified as deformations, disruptions, dyplasias, or malformations; deviations from that which is normal or typical; examples are Down syndrome and fetal alcohol syndrome.

_____ Anomolies or normal variants with no serious consequences, such as a sacral dimple, an extra nipple, or a café-au-lait spot.

_____ Chromosomal alterations resulting from breakage, deletion, or translocation and rearrangement of some of the genes of a chromosome.

_____ A cell with a chromosome number that is a multiple of 23.

_____ The study of chromosome disorders, started in 1952 with Lejeune's discovery of the genetic basis of Down syndrome. In recent times, molecular-based knowledge and technologies have been greatly accelerated by the Human Genome Project, which is rapidly identifying genes and DNA variations associated with disease.

_____ A relatively rare structural chromosome abnormality that can occur as a result of chromosomal "sticky ends." The ends, therefore, may fuse together, forming a circle. The clinical manifestations depend on which genes are affected.

_____ Failure of homologous chromosomes or chromatids to separate properly during anaphase meiosis I and II, or mitosis, resulting in daughter cells with unequal chromosome numbers. Meiotic nondisjunction may result in gametes with abnormal chromosome number. Mitotic nondisjunction in a developing embryo may result in mosaicism.

_____ Abnormal chromosome pattern; total number of chromosomes is not a multiple of the haploid number (n = 23); for example, 45 or 47 chromosomes.

_____ Meiosis; spermatogenesis in males, oogenesis in females.

_____ Describes mates who were selected based on geographic, ethnic, or religious restrictions; increases chances of rare genetic disease.

_____ Aneuploid condition; presence of an extra chromosome added to a pair; results in 47 chromosomes per cell; for example, Down syndrome.

_____ Disorders characterized by a microdeletion or microduplication of smaller chromosome segments, which may require special analysis techniques or molecular testing to detect.

_____ The aneuploid condition of having a chromosome represented by a single copy in a somatic cell; that is, the absence of a chromosome from a given pair. Generally compatible with life, except in the case of a missing X chromosome in Turner syndrome (45,XO).

_____ Type of equational cell division in which the resulting daughter cells have the same number of chromosomes as each other and the mother cell.

_____ One version of a gene at a given location (locus) along a chromosome. The most common version of a gene in a population is called the _wild type._

_____ Differences in the extent and/or severity of manifestations of genetic diseases.

_____ The process by which genetic information is copied from DNA to RNA.

_____ Any observable or measurable expression of gene function in an individual (eye color, hemoglobin type) may result from interaction of genotype and environment.

_____ Lyonization; the process by which, in a normal female, most genes on one of the X chromosomes are inactivated during early embryonic development, so that alleles on the active chromosome are allowed full expression.

_____ Structural or chemical alteration in genetic material that persists and is transmitted to future generations.

_____ The distal portion of a chromosome.

_____ Characterized by central hypotonia, cognitive dysfunction, dysmorphic appearance, behavioral disturbances, hypothalamic hypogonadism, short stature, obesity, abnormally low body temperature, an increased tolerance to pain, and diminished salivation.

_____ Modification, in some instances, of genetic material, resulting in phenotypic differences based on whether the genes and chromosomes were derived from the mother or the father. Exhibited during pregnancy, when paternally derived chromosomes seem to positively influence placental development and maternally derived chromosomes seem to positively influence fetal development. This phenomenon also occurs in some genetic disorders, such as Prader-Willi and Angelman syndromes.

_____ Diseases and defects that show an increased incidence in some families but have no clear-cut affected/unaffected classification and show no specific mode of inheritance; prenatal and environmental factors appear to play an important role; examples are neural tube defects, cleft lip, congenital hip dislocation, and pyloric stenosis.

_____ A disorder that includes severe cognitive impairment, characteristic facies, abnormal (puppetlike) gait, and paroxysms of inappropriate laughter. Children with this syndrome are usually nonverbal, although they may vocalize.

_____ FISH; process in which chromosomes or portions of chromosomes are "painted" with fluorescent molecules; useful for identifying chromosomal microdeletions.

_____ Caused by one gene.

_____ Situation in which both copies of a chromosome pair are determined to have come from one parent, instead of one from each.

_____ The chromosome constitution of an individual represented by a laboratory-made display in which chromosomes are arranged by size and centromere position.

_____ The ability to locate a gene on a specific chromosome or segment of a chromosome; reverse genetics.

_____ Agents that cause birth defects when present in the prenatal environment.

2. The following terms are related to the impact of hereditary disorders on the family. Match each term with its definition or description.

a. Predisposition testing
b. Sensitivity
c. Specificity
d. Screening test
e. Diagnostic test
f. Maternal prenatal screening tests
g. Fetal blood sampling

h. Fetal biopsy
i. Fetal echocardiography
j. In vitro fertilization
k. Preimplantation genetic diagnosis
l. Genetic counseling
m. Proband
n. Pedigree chart

_____ Ability to detect true positives; few false positives (test results indicating a problem when it in fact does not exist).

_____ Targeted to the population; ideally has high sensitivity and specificity. It must yield rapid results, be safe, and be cost-effective; it should cause minimum physical and emotional discomfort to all involved.

_____ Targeted to the individual; determines with a high degree of accuracy the presence or absence of a disorder.

_____ Blood drawn from the umbilical vein after 18 weeks of gestation; usually done for prenatal evaluation of fetal hematologic abnormalities, inborn errors of metabolism, fetal infection, and rapid chromosome analysis.

_____ May be performed for further diagnosis when a cardiac defect is noted on ultrasound.

_____ Ability to detect false negatives (test results indicating a problem does not exist when, in fact, it does).

_____ The identification of gene mutations associated with genetic disorders in asymptomatic individuals that has been made possible by the advent of molecular diagnostic techniques.

_____ Free β-human chorionic gonadotropin, pregnancy-associated plasma protein A, and α-fetoprotein is detectable.

_____ Sometimes used to diagnose certain genetic skin disorders and metabolic disorders when DNA studies are unavailable or are uninformative.

_____ The technique used to transfer the embryo after it has been tested for the presence of a specific genetic disorder. The unaffected carrier embryo or embryos are transferred. Used for Tay-Sachs disease, cystic fibrosis, and some X-linked disorders. Has also been used to provide a human lymphocyte antigen–matched birth for an affected sibling who needs stem cell transplantation.

_____ A communication process that deals with the human problems associated with the occurrence, or risk for occurrence, of a genetic disorder in a family. This process is necessary with carrier screening to ensure that individuals understand the limitations of testing and the implications of results. Even so, there may be significant misunderstanding or misuse of information.

_____ A relatively new in vitro process in which an embryo is tested at the six- to eight-cell stage for the presence of a genetic disorder before transfer.

_____ Family tree; genogram.

_____ The genetic counseling term for the affected person or index case.

3. Trisomy 21, or Down syndrome, is an example of a(n):
a. congenital chromosomal association.
b. sex chromosomal abnormality.
c. autoimmune aberration.
d. autosome aneuploidy.

4. All of the following chromosomal disorders are considered sex chromosomal abnormalities except:
   a. Turner syndrome.
   b. Klinefelter syndrome.
   c. cri du chat syndrome.
   d. triple X syndrome.

5. Lyonization refers to:
   a. X inactivation in females during embryonic development.
   b. children with shorter stature and poor coordination.
   c. chromosome abnormalities that are easily identified at birth.
   d. chromosome abnormalities that result in severe disabilities.

6. Match each disorder with its inheritance pattern. (Inheritance patterns may be used more than once.)

   a. Autosomal dominant
   b. Autosomal recessive
   c. Sex-linked (dominant or recessive)

   _____ Xeroderma

   _____ Tay-Sachs disease

   _____ Gardner syndrome

   _____ Neurofibromatosis

   _____ Duchenne muscular dystrophy

   _____ Adenosine deaminase deficiency

   _____ Hemophilia A

   _____ Fragile X syndrome

   _____ Ocular albinism type 1

   _____ Achondroplasia

   _____ Cystic fibrosis

   _____ Galactosemia

   _____ Friedreich ataxia

   _____ Marfan syndrome

   _____ Myotonic dystrophy

   _____ Huntington disease

   _____ Phenylketonuria

   _____ Thalassemia

7. A disease or defect encountered frequently in the population without a clear-cut inheritance pattern is classified as:
   a. a mutation.
   b. a mosaicism.
   c. a uniparental disomy.
   d. multifactorial.

8. Which of the following disorders is clearly teratogenic?
   a. Type 1 diabetes
   b. Rheumatoid arthritis
   c. Fetal alcohol syndrome
   d. Myasthenia gravis

9. One common use of fetal surgery that has been controversial is the treatment of:
   a. ambiguous genitalia.
   b. urinary tract abnormalities.
   c. facial and limb deformities.
   d. pyloric stenosis.

10. The deleterious effects of phenylketonuria are expressed with the ingestion of:
    a. milk.
    b. hormones.
    c. gluten.
    d. vitamin supplement.

11. The *Essential Nursing Competencies and Curricula Guidelines for Genetics and Genomics* delineates that the registered nurse:
    a. integrate genetic and genomic knowledge into assessment and planning.
    b. identify clients who may benefit from specific genetic and genomic information.
    c. interpret selective genetic and genomic information for clients.
    d. do all of the above.

12. Careful counseling is necessary when screening an individual for carrier status of hereditary disorders (e.g., cystic fibrosis) because:
    a. mass screening for these disorders is widely conducted.
    b. of possible ethical dilemmas.
    c. this type of screening is expensive.
    d. the emotional threat for the child is always devastating.

13. Which of the following statements is not a part of the controversial aspect of mass genetic screening programs?
    a. Health professionals sometimes lack knowledge about the purpose of the testing.
    b. The public cost of testing does not always outweigh the benefits.
    c. Technology is advancing for routine mass screenings of numerous genetic disorders.
    d. The psychologic implications of the carrier states may not be handled properly.

14. Match each type of prenatal genetic test with its purpose.

    a. Biochemical maternal serum testing   c. Amniocentesis
    b. Ultrasonography   d. Chorionic villi sampling

    _____ To perform chromosomal and biochemical analysis
    _____ To estimate gestational age and identify structural abnormalities
    _____ To perform chromosomal analysis at the earliest possible point during pregnancy
    _____ To screen for chromosome anomalies (aneuploidy) and neural tube defects

15. Preimplantation genetic diagnosis has been used for parents at risk for having a child with:
    a. Down syndrome.
    b. a neural tube defect.
    c. a congenital heart defect.
    d. cystic fibrosis.

16. Which of the following actions is not considered an appropriate nursing responsibility in genetic counseling?
    a. Choose the best course of action for the family.
    b. Identify families who would benefit from genetic evaluation.
    c. Become familiar with community resources for genetic evaluation.
    d. Learn basic genetic principles.

17. The most efficient genetic counseling service provided by a group of genetic screening specialists may:
    a. predict the outcome of the disease.
    b. take less than 2 hours.
    c. evaluate the affected child only.
    d. be inaccessible to the people who need it most.

18. *Proband* is the term used in genetic counseling to mean the:
    a. affected person.
    b. genetic history.
    c. clinical manifestations.
    d. mode of inheritance.

19. When teaching families about genetic risks and probabilities, the nurse may need to:
    a. make specific recommendations.
    b. use the example of games such as flipping coins and horse racing.
    c. realize that most people have a basic understanding of biology.
    d. recognize that each pregnancy's probabilities build on the previous pregnancy's probabilities.

20. Which of the following assessment findings should alert the nurse to the need for genetic counseling?
    a. Individuals with a family history of tuberculosis
    b. Parents who had an infant born at 42 weeks of gestation
    c. Couples with a history of infertility
    d. Pregnant adolescents

21. Which of the following assessment findings in an infant should indicate to the nurse that there is a need for genetic referral?
    a. Vernix caseosa
    b. Acrocyanosis
    c. Mongolian spots
    d. Unusual breath odor

22. In a drawing of a pedigree genogram for genetic purposes, which of the following facts is least significant?
    a. The proband's paternal grandmother had two stillbirth pregnancies.
    b. The proband's sibling died as an infant in a motor vehicle accident.
    c. The proband's paternal grandfather was a carrier for sickle cell disease.
    d. The proband's half brother carries the sickle cell trait.

23. In regard to genetic counseling, which of the following statements is false?
    a. Families have a tendency to be more ashamed of a hereditary disorder than other illnesses.
    b. The nurse's role in genetic counseling involves sympathy and supportive listening.
    c. The nurse ensures that patients have accurate and complete information to make decisions.
    d. Once the family understands the situation intellectually, they will be able to cope.

CRITICAL THINKING—CASE STUDY

Mr. and Mrs. Jones are waiting in the obstetrician's office for a routine prenatal checkup. They are Roman Catholic and do not view abortion as a feasible option. The obstetrician has recommended a screening test to rule out neural tube defects. Mrs. Jones does not see any benefit from this testing procedure and does not want to undergo the procedure.

24. Which of the following factors is the least important consideration during the assessment phase of this visit?
    a. The nurse is not Roman Catholic.
    b. The test is a venipuncture and carries little risk.
    c. Most couples receive normal results from prenatal tests.
    d. Results of the tests will be provided before the delivery date.

25. Which of the following considerations should the nurse deal with first?
    a. The couple believes that testing is used to identify anomalies in order to terminate pregnancies.
    b. The couple's clear-cut beliefs about pregnancy termination are different from the reality of raising an abnormal child.
    c. The nurse believes that pregnancy termination for fetal abnormalities is often the best option.
    d. The nurse believes that raising a child with a terminal illness is extremely difficult.

26. Which of the following goals is most appropriate for the nurse in this situation?
    a. To provide nonjudgmental supportive counseling
    b. To help Mr. and Mrs. Jones make their decision
    c. To provide follow-up care to the couple
    d. To educate the couple about neural tube defects

27. Which of the following statements by Mrs. Jones indicates that the nurse's goal was met?
    a. "I had no idea what was involved in raising a disabled child."
    b. "Your ideas have been very helpful. I think one of them will work."
    c. "We will discuss this and call you tomorrow with our decision."
    d. "I had no idea what neural tube defects were."

6 Communication and Physical Assessment of the Child

1. Match each term with its definition or description.

a. Interview process	f. Triage	k. Skinfold thickness
b. Listening	g. Empathy	l. Arm circumference
c. Sympathy	h. Family function	m. Family structure
d. Egocentric	i. Anthropometry	
e. First-degree relatives	j. Orthostatic hypotension	

_____ See things only in relation to oneself and own point of view

_____ An essential parameter of nutritional status; the measurement of height, weight, head circumference, proportions, skinfold thickness, and arm circumference

_____ The capacity to understand what another person is experiencing from within that person's frame of reference

_____ Refers to the composition of the family; to those living in the home; and to the social, cultural, religious, and economic characteristics that influence the child's and family's overall psychobiologic health

_____ Not therapeutic in the helping relationship because it leads to feelings of emotional overinvolvement and possible professional burnout

_____ Most important component of effective communication

_____ Parents, siblings, grandparents, and immediate aunts and uncles

_____ Measurement of body fat

_____ Specific form of goal-directed communication

_____ Concerned with how family members behave toward one another and with the quality of the relationship

_____ Indirect measurement of muscle mass

_____ Involves assessing symptoms and forming clinical judgment for further medical care

_____ Often manifests as dizziness or syncope

2. Which of the following would negatively affect the communication process between the nurse and the patient?
   a. The nurse allows the child to express his or her concerns and fears.
   b. The nurse includes the child, as well as the parents, in the communication process.
   c. The nurse uses verbal and nonverbal communication to reflect approval of the patient's statement.
   d. The nurse uses a slow, even, steady voice to convey instruction.

3. Mrs. Green has brought her daughter Karen to the clinic where you work as a nurse. Karen, age 12 years, is a new patient and needs a physical examination so that she can play volleyball. Which of the following techniques would not be helpful to establish effective communication during the interview process?
   a. You introduce yourself and ask the name of all family members present.
   b. After the introduction, you are careful to direct questions about Karen to Mrs. Green, because she is the best source of information.
   c. After the introduction and explanation of your role, you begin the interview by saying to Karen, "Tell me about your volleyball team."
   d. You choose to conduct the interview in a quiet area with few distractions.

4. The nurse says to 15-year-old Monique, "Tell me about your cough." This is an example of which type of communication technique?
   a. Direct
   b. Open ended
   c. Reflective
   d. Closed

5. While conducting an assessment of the child, the nurse communicates with the child's family. Which of the following does the nurse recognize as not productive in obtaining information?
   a. Obtaining verbal and nonverbal input from the child
   b. Observing the relationship between parents and child
   c. Using broad, open-ended questions
   d. Avoiding the use of guiding statements to direct the focus of the interview

6. The receptionist at the clinic where you are employed as a nurse has forwarded a call to you from Mrs. Garcia, mother of 4-year-old Maria. Mrs. Garcia tells you that Maria has had a fever all morning of around 37.8° C (100° F) and that she now has diarrhea and vomiting. As you provide triage by phone, which of the following actions is appropriate?
   a. Reassure Mrs. Garcia that Maria is not very sick and will be fine in a day or two.
   b. Confer with the practitioner at once.
   c. Wait to document in Maria's medical record until she comes in for a visit.
   d. Offer advice for home care and instruct Mrs. Garcia to call or come to the clinic if Maria's symptoms do not improve.

7. _____ is the capacity to understand what another person is feeling by experiencing the situation from that person's frame of reference.
   a. Sympathy
   b. Empathy
   c. Reassurance
   d. Encouragement

8. The nurse is conducting an interview with 8-year-old Jesus and his mother, Mrs. Lopez. Mrs. Lopez is worried because Jesus has been acting up at home and at school and disrupting everyone. An interpreter has been requested, because the mother speaks little English. When using an interpreter for communication with Mrs. Lopez, the nurse realizes that:
   a. the interpreter will have little to do because Jesus can interpret for his mother.
   b. when the interpreter and Mrs. Lopez speak for a long period, it will be necessary to interrupt to refocus the interview.
   c. the nurse needs to communicate directly with Mrs. Lopez and ignore the interpreter.
   d. the nurse needs to pose questions to elicit only one answer at a time from Mrs. Lopez.

9. Identify whether the following statements are true or false when planning how to communicate effectively with children.

   _____ Nonverbal components of the communication process do not convey significant messages.
   _____ Children are alert to their surroundings and attach meaning to gestures.
   _____ Actively attempting to make friends with children before they have had an opportunity to evaluate an unfamiliar person will increase their anxiety.
   _____ The nurse should assume a position that is at eye level with the child.
   _____ Communication through transition objects, such as dolls or stuffed animals, delays the child's response to verbal communication offered by the nurse.

10. To effectively provide anticipatory guidance to the family, the nurse should:
    a. provide information to deal with each problem as it develops.
    b. provide teaching and interventions based on needs identified by the professional.
    c. be suspicious of the parent's ability to deal effectively with the child's needs.
    d. assist the parents in building competence in their parenting abilities.

11. Communication with children must reflect their developmental thought process. Match each developmental stage with the communication guidelines important at that stage. (Stages may be used more than once.)

    a. Infancy
    b. Early childhood

    c. School-age years
    d. Adolescence

    _____ Focus communication on the child; experiences of others are of no interest to children in this stage.

    _____ Children in this stage primarily use and respond to nonverbal communication.

    _____ Children in this stage interpret words literally and are unable to separate fact from fantasy.

    _____ Children in this stage assign human attributes to inanimate objects.

    _____ Children in this stage require explanations and reasons why procedures are being done to them.

    _____ Children in this stage have a heightened concern about body integrity, being overly sensitive to any activity that constitutes a threat to it.

    _____ Children in this stage are often willing to discuss their concern with an adult outside the family and often welcome the opportunity to interact with a nurse.

12. Which of the following best describes the appropriate use of play as a communication technique with children?
    a. Small infants have little response to activities that focus on repetitive actions such as patting and stroking.
    b. Few clues about intellectual or social developmental progress are obtained from the observation of child's play behaviors.
    c. Therapeutic play has little value in reduction of trauma from illness or hospitalization.
    d. Play sessions serve as assessment tools for determining children's awareness and perception of illness.

13. Several creative communication techniques may be used with children. Identify which technique is being used in each of the following examples.

    a. _____ The nurse shows Tina a picture of a child having an intravenous infusion started and asks Tina to describe the scene.

    b. _____ The nurse says to Tina, "I am concerned about how the medicine treatments are going because I want you to feel better."

    c. _____ The nurse reads Tina a story from a book and asks her to retell the story.

    d. _____ The nurse provides Tina with crayons and paper and asks her to draw a picture of her family.

    e. _____ The nurse gives Tina a doll and a stethoscope and allows her to listen to the doll's heart.

14. A complete pediatric health history includes 10 expected components. List these components.

15. In eliciting the chief complaint, which of the following techniques is not appropriate?
    a. Limiting the chief complaint to a brief statement restricted to one or two symptoms
    b. Using labeling-type questions such as "How are you sick?" to facilitate information exchange
    c. Recording the chief complaint in the child's or parent's own words
    d. Using open-ended neutral questions to elicit information

16. Read the following entry from a pediatric health history: "Nausea and vomiting for 3 days. Started with abdominal cramping after eating hamburger at home. No pain or cramping at present. Unable to keep any food down but able to drink clear liquids without vomiting. No temperature elevation, no diarrhea." Which component of the health history does this entry represent?
    a. Chief complaint
    b. Past history
    c. Present illness
    d. Review of systems

17. Which of the following is not part of the past history to be included in a pediatric health history?
    a. Symptom analysis
    b. Allergies
    c. Birth history
    d. Current medications

18. What are the most important previous growth patterns to record when completing a child's history of growth and development?

19. What are the most important developmental milestones to record when completing the child's health history?

20. The nurse knows that the best description of the sexual history for a pediatric health history:
    a. includes a discussion of the patient's plans for future children.
    b. allows the patient to introduce sexual activity history.
    c. includes discussion of contraception methods only when the patient discloses current sexual activity.
    d. alerts the nurse to the need for sexually transmitted infection screening.

21. List five categories to include in an assessment of pain.

22. Indications for the nurse to conduct a comprehensive family assessment include which of the following?
    i. Children with developmental delays
    ii. Children with history of repeated accidental injuries
    iii. Children with behavioral problems
    iv. Children receiving comprehensive well-child care

    a. i, ii, iii, and iv
    b. ii, iii, and iv
    c. i, ii, and iii
    d. ii and iii

23. Assessment of family structure is best conducted:
    a. after the first meeting with the patient.
    b. only when a problem is suspected within the family.
    c. toward the end of the interview when rapport has been established.
    d. by interviewing the patient about other family members' roles within the family.

24. Assessment of family interactions and roles, decision making and problem solving, communication, and expression of feelings and individuality is known as assessment of:
    a. family structure.
    b. family function.
    c. family composition.
    d. home and community environment.

25. Describe four principal areas of concern the nurse should focus on when assessing family structure.

26. The dietary history of a pediatric patient includes:
    a. a 12-hour dietary intake recall.
    b. a more specific, detailed history for the older child.
    c. financial and cultural factors that influence food selection.
    d. criticism of parents' allowance of nonessential foods.

27. In pediatric examinations, the normal sequence of head-to-toe direction is often altered to accommodate the patient's developmental needs. Which of the following goals is least likely to guide the examination process?
    a. Minimizing the stress and anxiety associated with the assessment of body parts
    b. Recording the findings according to the normal sequence
    c. Fostering a trusting nurse-child relationship
    d. Preserving the essential security of the parent-child relationship

28. Mr. Alls brings his 12-month-old son Keith in for his regular well-infant examination. The nurse knows that the best approach to the physical examination for this patient will be to:
    a. have the infant sit in the parent's lap to complete as much of the examination as possible.
    b. place the infant on the examination table with parent out of view.
    c. perform examination in head-to-toe direction.
    d. completely undress Keith and leave him undressed during the examination.

29. Behavior that signals the child's readiness to cooperate during the physical examination does not include:
    a. talking to the nurse.
    b. making eye contact with the nurse.
    c. allowing physical touching.
    d. sitting on parent's lap or playing with a doll.

30. The National Center for Health Statistics has growth charts available for pediatric patients. These growth charts have been revised to include _____, _____, and _____.

31. The assessment method that the nurse expects to provide the best information about the physical growth pattern of a preschool-age child is:
    a. recording height and weight measurements of the child and comparing growth measurements over time.
    b. keeping a flow sheet for height, weight, and head circumference increases.
    c. obtaining a history of sibling growth patterns.
    d. measuring the height, weight, and head circumference of the child.

32. Describe how to measure recumbent length in a 14-month-old child.

33. Identify the following statements regarding the growth or development patterns of pediatric patients as true or false.

_____ Normal growth patterns may vary among children of the same age-group.

_____ A sudden weight increase in a 10-year-old whose weight has been steady before is not an area for concern.

_____ Growth is a continuous but uneven process, and the most reliable evaluation is based on comparison of growth measurements over a prolonged time.

_____ Growth measurements during the physical examination should be age-specific and include length, height, weight, skinfold thickness, and arm and head circumference.

_____ One convenient measurement of body fat is arm circumference.

34. Which of the following findings for growth is cause for potential concern and should be followed closely?
    a. Height and weight fall above the 5th percentile on the growth chart.
    b. Height and weight fall below the 5th percentile on the growth chart.
    c. Height and weight fall below the 95th percentile on the growth chart.
    d. Height and weight fall within the 50th percentile on the growth chart.

35. Head circumference is:
    a. measured in all children up to the age of 24 months.
    b. equal to chest circumferences at about 1 to 2 years of age.
    c. about 8 to 9 cm smaller than chest circumference during childhood.
    d. measured slightly below the eyebrows and pinna of the ears.

36. In infants and young children, the _____ pulse should be taken because it is the most

reliable. This pulse should be counted for _____ because of the possibility of irregularities

in rhythm. When counting respirations in infants, observe the _____ movements and

count for _____ because their movements are irregular.

37. Which of the following statements about temperature measurement in children is true?
    a. Rectal site is preferred in children under 1 month of age.
    b. The axillary site is recommended by the American Academy of Pediatrics as a screening test for fever in infants 1 month of age.
    c. Ear (tympanic) temperature is a precise measurement of core body measurement.
    d. Oral temperature is a better indicator for rapid changes in core body temperature and accuracy and is the preferred method when the patient is under 5 years of age.

38. The nurse should obtain the vital signs of an infant in what order?
    a. Measure temperature, then count the pulse, and then count respirations.
    b. Count the pulse, then count respirations, and then measure the temperature.
    c. Count respirations, then count the pulse, and then measure the temperature.
    d. Measure the temperature, then count respirations, and then count the pulse.

39. Which of the following findings should the nurse recognize as normal when measuring the vital signs of a 5-year-old child?
    a. Femoral pulses graded at +1
    b. Oral temperature of 100.9° F
    c. Blood pressure of 101/61
    d. Respiratory rate of 28 breaths/min

40. Which of the following observations should be eliminated when recording the general appearance of the child?
    a. Impression of child's nutritional status
    b. Behavior, interactions with parents
    c. Hygiene, cleanliness
    d. Vital signs

41. Match each term with its description or associated assessment findings. (Terms may be used more than once.)

    a. Cyanosis
    b. Pallor
    c. Erythema
    d. Ecchymosis
    e. Petechiae
    f. Jaundice
    g. Craniosynostosis
    h. Tissue turgor

    i. Barrel chest
    j. Pigeon chest
    k. Capillary refill time
    l. Wryneck, or torticollis
    m. Opisthotonos
    n. Genu valgum
    o. Genu varum
    p. Gynecomastia

    q. Wheezes
    r. Crackles
    s. Innocent murmur
    t. Functional murmur
    u. Organic murmur
    v. Polydactyly
    w. Syndactyly

    _____ Appears in dark-skinned patients as ashen-gray lips and tongue

    _____ Appears in light-skinned patients as purplish to yellow-green areas

    _____ May be a sign of anemia, chronic disease, edema, or shock

    _____ Fusion of digits

    _____ Redness of the skin that may be the result of infection, local inflammation, or increased temperature due to climatic conditions

    _____ Large, diffuse areas, usually blue or black and the result of injury

    _____ Small, distinct pinpoint hemorrhages

    _____ Yellow staining of the skin usually caused by bile pigments

    _____ Time it takes for the blanched area to return to its original color; used to test for circulation and hydration

    _____ Extra digit

    _____ Injury to the sternocleidomastoid muscle with subsequent holding of the head to one side with the chin pointing toward the opposite side

    _____ Hyperextension of the neck and spine

    _____ Round chest

    _____ Sternum that protrudes outward

    _____ Premature closure of the sutures of the head

    _____ Amount of elasticity to the skin

    _____ Breast enlargement

    _____ Lateral bowing of the tibia

    _____ Stance in which knees are close together but feet are spread apart; "knock-knee"

    _____ Result of the passage of air through fluid or moisture in the lungs

    _____ Result of the passage of air through narrowed passageways in the lungs

    _____ No anatomic or physiologic abnormality exists

    _____ A cardiac defect with or without a physiologic abnormality exists

    _____ No anatomic cardiac defect exists, but a physiologic abnormality such as anemia is present

42. You are assessing skin turgor in 10-month-old Ryan. You grasp the skin on the abdomen between the thumb and index finger, pull it taut, and quickly release it. The tissue remains suspended, or tented, for a few seconds, then slowly falls back on the abdomen. Which of the following conclusions can you correctly assume?
    a. The tissue shows normal elasticity.
    b. The child is properly hydrated.
    c. The assessment was done incorrectly.
    d. The child has poor skin turgor.

43. You are assessing 7-year-old Mary's lymph nodes. Using the distal portions of your fingers, you press gently but firmly in a circular motion along the occipital and postauricular node areas. You record the findings as "tender, enlarged, warm lymph nodes." Which of the following is true?
    a. Your findings are within normal limits for Mary's age.
    b. Your assessment technique was incorrect and should be repeated.
    c. Your findings suggest infection or inflammation in the scalp area or external ear canal.
    d. Your recording of the information is complete because it includes temperature and tenderness.

44. Which of the following assessment findings of the head and neck does not require a referral?
    a. Head lag before 6 months of age
    b. Hyperextension of the head with pain on flexion
    c. Palpable thyroid gland, including isthmus and lobes
    d. Closure of the anterior fontanel at the age of 9 months

45. Normal findings on examination of the pupils may be recorded as PERRLA, which means:

46. Match each term with its description.

    a. Palpebral conjunctiva
    b. Testing eyes for reaction to light
    c. Testing eyes for accommodation
    d. Permanent eye color
    e. Strabismus

    f. Amblyopia
    g. Testing eyes for malalignment
    h. Testing light perception
    i. Testing peripheral vision
    j. Testing color vision

    _____ Usually established by age 6 to 12 months

    _____ Performed by using pseudoisochromatic cards

    _____ Corneal light reflex test and cover test

    _____ Performed by having the child look at a shiny object—first at a distance, then closer to the eyes; pupils should constrict as the object is brought near the eyes

    _____ One eye deviating from point of fixation

    _____ Performed by quickly shining a light source toward the eye and removing it; pupils constrict and then dilate

    _____ Type of blindness resulting from uncorrected "lazy" eye

    _____ Performed by having child fixate on a finger directly in front of the eyes, then moving it from the child's field of vision

    _____ Inside lining of the eyelids

    _____ Performed by shining light in the eyes and noting responses; used in newborns to test visual acuity

47. Which of the following is an expected finding in the child's eye examination?
    a. Opaque red reflex of the eye
    b. Ophthalmoscopic examination revealing that veins are darker and about one-fourth larger than the arteries
    c. Strabismus in the 12-month-old infant
    d. A 5-year-old child who reads the Snellen eye chart at the 20/40 level

48. Match each type of eye chart with the procedure used for that chart.

   a. Snellen chart
   b. Tumbling chart
   c. HOTV chart

   _____ To "pass" a line, child must correctly identify four out of six letters on the line; used for children who can read letters.

   _____ Child is asked to point in the direction the letter is facing.

   _____ Child is asked to point to the correct letter on a board held in the hands.

49. Which of the following children meet(s) referral criteria?
   a. Jason, age 14 years, who identified fewer than four out of six correct letters with his right eye and five out of six correct with his left eye during visual acuity testing
   b. Sandra, age 3 years, who demonstrated eye movement with the unilateral cover test
   c. Tommy, age 4 years, who demonstrated a two-line difference between eyes on his visual acuity testing
   d. All of the above

50. When assessing the ear of a 2-year-old child, the nurse should:
   a. expect cerumen in the external ear canal.
   b. use the smallest speculum to prevent trauma to the ear.
   c. pull the pinna up and back to visualize the canal better.
   d. pull the pinna down and back to visualize the canal better.

51. The nurse is performing an otoscopic examination on 14-month-old Justin. Which of the following is recognized as an abnormal finding?
   a. The umbo, tip of the malleus, appears as a round, opaque, concave spot near the center of the drum.
   b. Light reflex is pointing away from the face.
   c. Tympanic membrane is translucent, light pearly pink or gray.
   d. Tympanic membrane is dull, nontransparent.

52. The nurse is assessing the mouth and throat of 7-month-old Alex. Which of the following is recognized as a normal finding?
   a. Membranes are bright pink, smooth, and glistening.
   b. White curdy plaques are located on the tongue.
   c. Redness and puffiness are present along the gum line.
   d. Tip of the tongue extends to the gum line.

53. When assessing 4-year-old Gail's chest, the nurse should expect:
   a. movement of the chest wall to be symmetric bilaterally and coordinated with breathing.
   b. respiratory movements to be chiefly thoracic.
   c. anteroposterior diameter to be equal to the transverse diameter.
   d. retraction of the muscles between the ribs on respiratory movement.

54. On auscultation of 8-year-old Tammie's lung fields, the nurse hears inspiratory sounds that are louder, longer, and higher pitched than on expiration. These sounds are heard over the chest, except over the scapula and sternum. These sounds are:
   a. bronchovesicular breath sounds.
   b. vesicular breath sounds.
   c. bronchial breath sounds.
   d. adventitious breath sounds.

55. On palpation of 3-year-old Jennifer's apical impulse, where would the nurse expect to place the fingers?
   a. At the lower left midclavicular line and fifth intercostal space
   b. Lateral to the left midclavicular line and fourth intercostal space
   c. Over the pulmonic valve
   d. Over the aortic valve

56. When listening over the aortic area of the heart, where should the stethoscope be placed?
    a. Second right intercostal space, close to sternum
    b. Second left intercostal space, close to sternum
    c. Fifth left intercostal space, close to sternum
    d. Fifth right intercostal space, left midclavicular line

57. Examination of the abdomen is performed correctly by the nurse in what order?
    a. Inspection, palpation, and auscultation
    b. Inspection, auscultation, and palpation
    c. Palpation, auscultation, and inspection
    d. Auscultation, inspection, and palpation

58. When examining a child's genitalia, the nurse should:
    a. conduct this examination first so that the child will not be as apprehensive.
    b. ask the parent to leave the room so that the young child will not be as shy.
    c. wait until the end of the examination before discussing findings with the parent and child.
    d. understand that this examination may provoke anxiety in the child.

59. In performing an examination for scoliosis, the nurse understands that one of the following is an incorrect method.
    a. The child should be examined only in his or her underpants (and a bra if an older girl).
    b. The child should stand erect with the nurse observing from behind.
    c. The child should squat down with hands extended forward so that the nurse can observe for asymmetry of the shoulder blades.
    d. The child should bend forward with the back parallel to the floor so that the nurse can observe from the side.

60. Identify the following physical findings as normal or abnormal (needing additional evaluation).

    a. _____ Asymmetric bowlegs before the age of 2 years

    b. _____ Knock-knee accompanied by short stature in a 9-year-old child

    c. _____ Flat feet in an 18-month-old toddler

    d. _____ Broad-based gait in a 20-month-old toddler

    e. _____ Positive Babinski sign in a 9-month-old toddler

61. Name the six areas included in the neurologic examination.

62. Two-year-old Drew is brought to the clinic by his mom, who tells the nurse that Drew's eyes "look funny." What tests should the nurse use to determine ocular alignment? What findings in each test would indicate abnormal findings?

CRITICAL THINKING—CASE STUDIES

Mrs. Brown brings her 11-year-old son Kenny for a physical at the clinic where you work as a nurse. She is concerned because Kenny comes home from school "very tired and only wants to watch television." Kenny's bedtime has not changed, he performs well in school, and his mother denies stress or problems within the home. On physical examination, you discover Kenny is above the 90th percentile for weight by 11.3 kg (25 lb).

63. To effectively establish a setting for communication, you enter the room, introduce yourself to Mrs. Brown and Kenny, and explain your role and the purpose of the interview. You include Kenny in the interaction as you ask his name and age and what he is expecting at his visit today. You next inform Mrs. Brown and Kenny that he is 25 lb overweight and that his diet and exercise plan must be "terrible" for Kenny to be in "such bad shape." Which aspect of effective communication have you, as a nurse, forgotten that will most significantly affect the exchange of information during this interview?
    a. Assurance of privacy and confidentiality
    b. Preliminary acquaintance
    c. Directing the focus away from the complaint of fatigue to one of obesity
    d. Injecting your own attitudes and feelings into the interview

64. Based on the information provided in the case study, you can correctly record which of the following?
    a. Chief complaint
    b. Present illness
    c. Past medical history
    d. Symptom analysis

65. Mrs. Brown, Kenny, and you agree to the need to conduct a more intensive nutritional assessment. Which of the following ways to record Kenny's dietary intake would you suggest as most reliable in providing needed information to assess his dietary habits?
    a. 12-hour recall
    b. 24-hour recall
    c. Food diary for 3-day period
    d. Food frequency questionnaire

66. During the physical examination, which of the following physical findings could be consistent with excess carbohydrate nutrition?
    a. Caries
    b. Skin elastic and firm
    c. Hair stringy, friable, dull, and dry
    d. Enlarged thyroid

67. The physical examination has been completed and reflects that, other than his obesity, Kenny is in excellent physical health with normal blood counts. The completed nutritional assessment reflects that Mrs. Brown has little knowledge about proper nutrition and that Kenny has a large intake of "junk" foods high in fat and calories but low in nutrients. Based on the data collected, which of the following nursing diagnoses are most appropriate?
    i. Altered Family Process related to parent's knowledge deficit
    ii. Altered Family Coping related to family's inability to purchase needed foods
    iii. Altered Individual Coping related to fatigue from poor dietary habits
    iv. Altered Nutrition: More Than Body Requirements, related to eating practices
    v. Altered Nutrition: More Than Body Requirements, related to knowledge deficit of parent

    a. i, ii, and iv
    b. iii and iv
    c. ii, iv, and v
    d. iv and v

68. Once the problem is defined, you include Mrs. Brown in the problem-solving process. Why is it important to include the parent in the problem-solving process?

Mary, a 13-year-old, has come to the clinic with her mother. She is complaining of right-sided abdominal pain of 24 hours' duration. Mary tells you, the nurse, that she has had some nausea and vomiting but no diarrhea. Her appetite is depressed and she feels hot and feverish. She has taken acetaminophen for pain but with little relief. A complete blood count has been ordered and results are pending.

69. You are preparing Mary for a physical examination. You know that during the examination, Mary, as an adolescent, will likely:
    a. prefer her parents to be present during the entire examination.
    b. wish to undress in private and feel more comfortable when provided with a gown.
    c. prefer that traumatic procedures such as ear and mouth examinations be performed last.
    d. need to have heart and lungs auscultated first.

70. You complete the physical examination and determine that one of the following is an abnormal finding.
    a. Bowel sounds are stimulated by stroking the abdominal surface with the fingernail.
    b. Mary has no abdominal discomfort when she is supine with the legs flexed at the hips and knees.
    c. Mary's eyes are open during palpation of the abdomen.
    d. When the nurse presses firmly over the area distal to the right side of the abdomen and quickly releases this pressure, pain is intensified in the lower right side.

71. Which of the following organs is located in the lower right quadrant of the abdomen?
    a. Bladder
    b. Liver
    c. Ovaries
    d. Appendix

72. Mary's mother is apprehensive about her daughter's condition and asks you whether "it is serious." Which of the following is your best response?
    a. "Mary has appendicitis and will need to have surgery immediately."
    b. "You will have to ask the doctor about her condition."
    c. "Mary has some abdominal pain that is not normal. We are watching her very carefully and will be able to tell you more when the laboratory tests are completed."
    d. "Mary should be able to go home as soon as the doctor finishes with the examination and the laboratory tests are completed."

73. While inspecting the abdomen, which one of the following is a normal finding?
    a. Peristaltic waves
    b. Silvery, whitish lines when the skin is stretched out
    c. Bulging at the umbilicus
    d. Protruding abdomen with skin pulled tight

    Gerald, age 16, has been complaining to the school nurse of chest pain during physical education class at school. The nurse is performing an assessment of the heart.

74. _____ is the sound caused by the closure of the tricuspid and mitral valves. It is heard loudest at the _____ of the heart. _____ is the sound heard as a result of the closure of the pulmonic and aortic valves. It is heard loudest at the _____ of the heart.

75. During auscultation of S_2 a split is heard that does not change during inspiration. Based on this, the nurse should suspect:
    a. a normal finding referred to as *physiologic splitting*.
    b. mitral valve prolapse.
    c. that no anatomic cardiac defect exists, but that a physiologic abnormality such as anemia is likely to be present.
    d. fixed splitting, which can be a diagnostic sign of atrial septal defect.

7 Pain Assessment and Management in Children

1. Several research studies have suggested that the inconsistency of pain management in children is related to four practices. List them below.

2. In regard to pain management, nurses tend to:
   a. overtreat children's pain.
   b. undertreat children's pain.
   c. overestimate the existence of pain in children undergoing procedures.
   d. realize that children are more likely to become addicted with opiate analgesics.

3. Identify the following statements about pain in children as true or false.

   _____ Children's ability to describe pain changes as they grow older and as they cognitively and linguistically mature.

   _____ The young infant responding to pain demonstrates no association between approaching stimulus and subsequent pain.

   _____ Young infants responding to pain can demonstrate the same facial expression as when they are angry.

   _____ The young child becomes restless and irritable with continuing pain.

   _____ The older infant responds to pain without purposeful movement away from the stimulus and with only muscular rigidity, such as clenched fists, white knuckles, gritted teeth, contracted limb, and body stiffness.

   _____ Physiologic measures for pain are more useful than behavioral measures in assessing pain in infants and toddlers.

   _____ Children ages 4 and 5 years are able to use self-report pain measures.

   _____ A pain scale is an appropriate tool to use to assess pain in a 3-year-old child.

   _____ Crying that is more intense and sustained is associated with pain in the preverbal child.

   _____ Children between the ages of 4 and 7 years cannot tell you where they hurt.

   _____ The primary caregiver is an important source of information when assessing pain in children with developmental delays.

   _____ Cultural background may influence the validity and reliability of pain assessment tools developed in a single cultural context.

   _____ The most important aspect of pain assessment in the child with chronic illness is the relationship developed with the child and the family.

   _____ Oral dosages of opioids must be larger than parenteral dosages to achieve equianalgesia.

   _____ Respiratory depression is rare with opioid analgesia administered epidurally.

   _____ Infants and young children become addicted to opioids easily.

   _____ The guiding principle in pain management is that prevention of pain is always better than treatment.

   _____ Harmful effects do not occur from unrelieved pain in the child.

   _____ Long-term exposure to chronic pain may lead to more biologic and clinical problems in critically ill preterm infants than acute pain.

4. In regard to behavioral and physiologic responses to pain, children:
   a. remain consistent from age to age.
   b. vary widely in their responses.
   c. exhibit typical behaviors at each development stage.
   d. are unaffected by temperament.

5. Which of the following characteristics is most likely to be exhibited by an adolescent who is in pain?
   a. Decreased verbal expression and withdrawal
   b. Requests to terminate the procedure
   c. Verbal expression such as "You're hurting me!"
   d. Facial expression of pain and anger

6. Which of the following behavioral pain measures includes five categories of behavior and uses a scoring system to quantify pain behaviors, with 0 being no pain behaviors and 10 being the most possible pain behaviors?
   a. FLACC Pain Assessment Tool (*F*acial expression, *L*eg movement, *A*ctivity, *C*ry, and *C*onsolability)
   b. Children's Hospital of Eastern Ontario Pain Scale (CHEOPS)
   c. Toddler-Preschooler Postoperative Pain Scale (TPPS)
   d. Parent's Postoperative Pain Rating Scale (PPPRS)

7. Which of the following pain assessment scales uses blood pressure as a variable?
   a. Behavior Pain Score (BPS)
   b. Children's Hospital of Eastern Ontario Pain Scale (CHEOPS)
   c. Nurses Assessment of Pain Inventory (NAPI)
   d. Objective Pain Score (OPS)

8. The Wong-Baker FACES Pain Rating Scale:
   a. is easy to use but less reliable than other methods.
   b. is a rating of how children are feeling.
   c. has a coding system from 0.4 to 0.97.
   d. consists of six cartoon faces.

9. The Oucher Pain Scale:
   a. consists of six cartoon faces.
   b. consists of six culturally specific photographs of faces.
   c. uses descriptive words.
   d. uses a straight line.

10. The Poker Chip Tool:
    a. is recommended for children who understand the value of numbers.
    b. does not offer an option for "no pain."
    c. uses a picture of four different colored poker chips.
    d. is recommended for children under 3 years of age.

11. The Adolescent Pediatric Pain Tool:
    a. is used in children over 6 years of age.
    b. is grouped by sensory, affective, and evaluative qualities.
    c. uses a straight line.
    d. uses the scale of 0 to 10 to rate the degree of pain.

12. The Pediatric Pain Questionnaire:
    a. is useful in infants.
    b. is used to assess patient and parental pain perceptions.
    c. consists of a series of four questions related to pain assessment.
    d. is completed jointly by the physician, child, and family.

13. List the five indicators used in the CRIES pain assessment tool:

    C:

    R:

    I:

    E:

    S:

14. Which of the following statements is true in regard to nonpharmacologic pain management?
    a. When used properly, nonpharmacologic measures are a good substitute for analgesics.
    b. Nurses and physicians are generally well educated about nonpharmacologic approaches to pain management.
    c. Nonpharmacologic approaches to pain management are not effective with children.
    d. Whenever possible, nonpharmacologic and pharmacologic measures should be combined to manage pain.

15. Identify three specific nonpharmacologic strategies that can be used to manage pain.

16. Which of the following has been shown to have calming and pain-relieving effects when used with invasive procedures in neonates?
    a. Allowing parent to hold neonate during procedure
    b. Allowing neonate quiet time in the bassinet before the procedure
    c. Administering concentrated sucrose with or without nonnutritive sucking before procedure
    d. Using relaxation techniques during the procedure

17. Which of the following is an acute manifestation of pain in the neonate?
    a. Increased transcutaneous oxygen saturation
    b. Increased heart rate; rapid and shallow respirations
    c. Decreased muscle tone and increased vagal nerve tone
    d. Increased skin dryness, decreased blood pressure, hyperglycemia

18. In administering medications for pain relief, the nurse knows that _____ act primarily

    on the peripheral nervous system, whereas _____ work on the central nervous system.

19. Which of the following opioids is considered the gold standard for severe pain management?
    a. Hydromorphone
    b. Gentanyl
    c. Oxycodone
    d. Morphine

20. If oral codeine with acetaminophen is not controlling a child's pain, which action should occur first?
    a. Change to morphine.
    b. Increase the dose of acetaminophen before increasing the codeine dose.
    c. Increase the dose of codeine before increasing the dose of acetaminophen.
    d. Add diazepam (Valium) to the current medication.

21. Children older than 6 months of age:
    a. metabolize drugs more rapidly than do adults.
    b. metabolize drugs less rapidly than do adults.
    c. require smaller doses of opioids to achieve the same analgesic effect.
    d. have greater pain relief when the nonopioid dosage is past the ceiling effect.

22. Describe the three typical methods of drug administration used with patient-controlled analgesia.

23. When patient-controlled analgesia is used with children, the:
    a. drug of choice is meperidine.
    b. patient should control the dosing.
    c. nurse should control the dosing.
    d. drug of choice is morphine.

24. When using epidural analgesia to manage pain, the nurse knows that:
    a. analgesia results from the drug's effect on the brain.
    b. respiratory depression is fast to develop, usually 1 to 2 hours after administration.
    c. the epidural spaces at the lumbar and caudal level are used most often.
    d. securing the catheter with an occlusive dressing does little to prevent infection.

25. The transdermal patch Duragesic may be used:
    a. in infants for acute pain management.
    b. for patients who are opioid tolerant.
    c. as a safe and effective medication for children of all ages.
    d. to provide prolonged pain relief for more than 96 hours.

26. Which of the following methods of analgesic drug administration is a liquid gel that provides anesthesia to nonintact skin in about 15 minutes?
    a. Midazolam
    b. EMLA (eutectic mixture of local anesthetics)
    c. LAT (lidocaine-adrenaline-tetracaine)
    d. Numby Stuff

27. The anesthetic EMLA is used:
    a. before invasive procedures.
    b. as preoperative oral sedation.
    c. for chronic cancer pain.
    d. postoperatively.

28. To manage opioid-induced respiratory depression in patients receiving opioids by continuous infusion, the nurse should:
    a. increase the infusion by 25%.
    b. allow the patient long periods of uninterrupted sleep.
    c. administer naloxone and discontinue the infusion.
    d. administer naloxone by continuous intravenous infusion and titrate to reach an acceptable respiratory rate.

29. For postoperative or cancer pain control, analgesics should be administered:
    a. whenever needed.
    b. around the clock.
    c. before the pain escalates.
    d. after the pain peaks.

30. The most common side effect of opioid therapy is:
    a. respiratory depression.
    b. pruritus.
    c. nausea and vomiting.
    d. constipation.

31. Treatment of tolerance to opioid therapy includes:
    a. discontinuing the drug.
    b. decreasing the dose.
    c. increasing the dose.
    d. increasing the duration between doses.

32. Which of the following terms describes a physiologic state in which abrupt cessation of an opioid results in a withdrawal syndrome?
    a. Tolerance
    b. Physical dependence
    c. Addiction
    d. Pseudoaddiction

33. List at least three nursing interventions useful in evaluating pain response.

34. Which of the following describes moderate sedation (previously called "conscious sedation")?
    a. Patient is not easily aroused but responds to verbal commands.
    b. Patient is easily aroused and responds normally to verbal commands.
    c. Patient retains partial control of protective reflexes.
    d. Patient is not able to maintain a patent airway independently.

35. Preemptive analgesia administered for postoperative pain:
    a. is associated with higher analgesic requirements.
    b. is administered immediately after surgery.
    c. increases analgesic requirements.
    d. decreases hospital stay.

36. The biggest challenge in management of burn pain is:
    a. providing analgesia without interfering with the patient's awareness during and after procedures.
    b. providing analgesia that allows safe sedation during and after procedures.
    c. adding additional medications that decrease anxiety without adversely affecting respirations.
    d. using psychologic interventions effectively.

37. The two main nonpharmacologic approaches to management of headache are:

38. Recurrent abdominal pain in children:
    a. occurs at least once per week.
    b. does not interfere with the child's normal activities.
    c. requires individualized management.
    d. requires the nurse to understand that because there is no organic cause for the pain, the reported pain is not a true pain.

39. Which of the following can the nurse expect to be included in the care plan for controlling acute pain in sickle cell crisis?
    a. Administration of long-term oxygen
    b. Application of cold compresses
    c. Use of opioids started early in childhood and continued throughout adult life
    d. Relieving the pain completely as the goal of treatment of the acute episode

40. Identify the following statements about cancer pain in children as true or false.

    _____ Pain is the most prevalent symptom with cancer.

    _____ Cancer pain in children is rarely present before diagnosis.

    _____ The major sources of pain in children with cancer are treatment related.

    _____ Oral mucositis occurs most often in patients undergoing bone marrow transplant, chemotherapy, and radiation.

    _____ Antihistamines, local anesthetics, and opioids provide long-lasting pain relief for lesions associated with oral mucositis.

    _____ Morphine administered as a continuous infusion may be necessary for pain until mucositis is resolved.

    _____ Postdural puncture headaches should be treated by administering nonopioid analgesics and keeping the patient supine for 1 hour.

CRITICAL THINKING—CASE STUDIES

Beverly is a 10-year-old child who is coming to the health clinic because she has been having recurrent headaches for more than 6 months. She is an honor student who loves to play the violin. Beverly lives at home with both her parents and her 13-year-old sister, Sharon, who is also an honor student.

Beverly's mother is with her during the interview and physical examination. Beverly describes the headaches as increasing in frequency and always occurring in the morning during her first-period advanced math class. She has been taking acetaminophen almost daily with only moderate relief. A physical examination done by the health care provider was within normal limits.

41. Describe interventions that could be helpful in assessing Beverly's headaches.

42. After reviewing information collected and talking with Beverly, her parents, and her math teacher, the nurse believes that the headaches could be related to Beverly pushing herself in math class. She is doing well in math class, however, and does not want to stop the advanced class. What interventions could be helpful for Beverly and her parents at this point to control her headaches?

Brian is a 5-year-old boy being readmitted to the hospital because of his cancer. He has been doing fairly well at home; he is eating and sleeping well. Brian's weight has increased to 25 kg (56 lb), and he is now 1.2 m (4 ft) tall. His mother is with him at the hospital and is his primary caregiver at home.

43. Brian is being scheduled for magnetic resonance imaging to check on the status of his cancer. The nurse knows that Brian has had trouble keeping still during past procedures. The nurse notifies the health care provider so that Brian can be medicated for the test. What medication does the nurse expect the health care provider to order, and what would be the expected route and dose of the medication prescribed?

44. If Brian becomes neutropenic, which of the following medications for pain should be avoided?
    a. Acetaminophen
    b. Morphine
    c. All intramuscular medications
    d. Codeine

45. If Brian develops thrombocytopenia, which of the following medications for pain should be avoided?
    a. Acetaminophen
    b. Nonsteroidal antiinflammatory drugs
    c. Morphine
    d. Codeine

8 Health Promotion of the Newborn and Family

1. The three chemical factors in the blood that stimulate the initiation of the first respiration in the neonate are:

2. The primary thermal stimulus that helps initiate the first respiration is:

3. The nurse recognizes that tactile stimulation probably has some effect on initiation of respiration in the neonate. Which of the following is of no beneficial effect?
   a. Normal handling of the neonate
   b. Drying the skin of the neonate
   c. Slapping the neonate's heel or buttocks
   d. Placing the infant skin-to-skin with the mother

4. Which of these neonates will most likely need additional respiratory support at birth?
   a. The infant born by normal vaginal delivery
   b. The infant born by cesarean birth
   c. The infant born vaginally after 12 hours of labor
   d. The infant born with high levels of surfactant

5. During the transition from fetal to neonatal circulation, the newborn's cardiovascular system accomplishes which of the following anatomic and physiologic alterations?
   i. Closure of the ductus venosus
   ii. Closure of the foramen ovale
   iii. Closure of the ductus arteriosis
   iv. Increased systemic pressure and decreased pulmonary artery pressure

   a. i, ii, iii, and iv
   b. i, ii, and iii
   c. ii, iii, and iv
   d. i, iii, and iv

6. Identify the following statements about infant adjustments to extrauterine life as true or false.

   _____ Factors that predispose the neonate to excessive heat loss are large surface area, thin layer of subcutaneous fat, and the lack of shivering to produce heat.

   _____ Nonshivering thermogenesis is an effective method of heat production in the neonate, because it is able to produce heat with little use of oxygen.

   _____ Brown fat, or brown adipose tissue, has a greater capacity to produce heat than does ordinary adipose tissue.

   _____ The longer the infant is attached to the placenta, the less blood volume will be received by the neonate.

   _____ Deficient production of pancreatic amylase impairs utilization of complex carbohydrates.

   _____ Deficiency of pancreatic lipase assists the neonate in the digestion of cow's milk.

_____ Most salivary glands are functioning at birth even though most infants do not start drooling until teeth erupt.

_____ The stomach capacity for most newborn infants is about 90 ml.

_____ The newborn should be expected to void within the first 48 hours.

_____ The liver is the most mature of the gastrointestinal organs at birth.

_____ At birth the skeletal system contains larger amounts of ossified bone than cartilage.

_____ After birth, development of the nervous system proceeds in a cephalocaudal-proximodistal pattern.

7. What three factors make the infant more prone to problems of dehydration, acidosis, and overhydration?

8. Match each term with its description.

   a. Meconium
   b. Breast-fed infant stools
   c. Formula-fed infant stools

   _____ Pale yellow to golden; pasty consistency

   _____ First stool; dark green with pasty, sticky consistency

   _____ Pale yellow to light brown; firmer in consistency with more offensive odor

9. Newborns receive passive immunity in the form of immunoglobulin G from the _____ _____

   and _____ _____.

10. The nurse recognizes that all of the following effects of maternal sex hormones in the newborn are normal except:
    a. hypertrophied labia.
    b. secretion of "witch's milk" from the newborn breasts.
    c. pseudomenstruation.
    d. bleeding from the breast nipples.

11. Fill in the blanks in the following statements pertaining to sensory functions in the normal newborn.

    a. The newborn can fixate on a bright object that is within _____ _____ and in the midline of the visual field.

    b. Infants have visual preferences for the colors _____ _____ and _____ and for

       designs such as _____ _____ and _____

    c. The newborn's response to _____-frequency sounds is one of decreased motor activity and crying.

       Exposure to _____-frequency sound elicits an alerting reaction.

    d. Newborn visual acuity is reported to be between _____ and _____.

12. The nurse is performing the 5-minute Apgar on a newborn. Which of the following observations is included in the Apgar score?
    a. Blood pressure
    b. Temperature
    c. Muscle tone
    d. Weight

13. Match each period of reactivity with the observations the nurse is likely to make during that period.

    a. First period of reactivity
    b. Second stage of first period of reactivity
    c. Second period of reactivity

   _____ This is an excellent bonding period and the best time to start breast-feeding.

   _____ During this period, infant sleep lasts 2 to 4 hours; heart rate and respiratory rate decrease.

   _____ Gastric and respiratory secretions are increased; passage of meconium commonly occurs.

14. The nurse is using the Brazelton Neonatal Behavioral Assessment Scale to assess the newborn's behavioral responses. How should the nurse define *habituation?*
    a. Responsiveness of the newborn to auditory and visual stimuli
    b. Process whereby the newborn becomes accustomed to stimuli
    c. The ability of the infant to be easily aroused from sleep state
    d. A reactive Moro reflex by the infant, with good muscle tone and coordination

15. Which of the following is not correct about the relationship of newborn weight to gestational age?
    a. All infants below the weight of 2500 g (5 lb, 8 oz) are preterm by gestational age.
    b. Gestational age is more closely related to fetal maturity than is birth weight.
    c. Classification of infants by both weight and gestational age can be beneficial for predicting mortality risks.
    d. Hereditary influences are a normal part of assessment.

16. On assessment of a 24-hour-old newborn, the nurse makes the following observations. Which is normal?
    a. Cyanotic color centrally and peripherally
    b. Axillary temperature of 35.5° C (96° F)
    c. Flexion of the infant's head and extremities, which rest on the chest and abdomen
    d. Respirations of 68 breaths/min

17. Temporal artery thermometers:
    a. are less accurate than tympanic thermometers.
    b. are more sensitive in detecting rectal fever in infants.
    c. are reliable as a screening tool for infants under 3 months.
    d. are reliable as a screening tool for infants 3 to 24 months.

18. Match each term with its description.
    a. Milia
    b. Erythema toxicum
    c. Harlequin color change
    d. Nevus flammeus
    e. Acrocyanosis
    f. Cutis marmorata
    g. Mongolian spots
    h. Telangiectatic nevi
    i. Caput succedaneum
    j. Cephalhematoma
    k. Vernix caseosa
    l. Lanugo

   _____ Irregular areas of deep blue pigmentation, usually in sacral and gluteal regions, seen in the newborn

   _____ Distended sebaceous glands that appear as tiny white papules on the cheeks, chin, and nose in the newborn

   _____ Condition in which the lower half of the body becomes pink and upper half is pale when the newborn lies on side

   _____ Edema of the soft scalp tissue

   _____ Pink papular rash with vesicles superimposed on thorax, back, buttocks, and abdomen in the newborn

_____ Port-wine stain

_____ Hematoma between periosteum and skull bone

_____ Cyanosis of hands and feet

_____ "Stork bites"; flat, deep pink, localized areas usually seen at back of neck

_____ Transient mottling when infant is exposed to decreased temperature, stress, or overstimulation

_____ Fine downy hair present on the newborn's skin

_____ Cheeselike substance; mixture of sebum and desquamating cell covering the skin at birth

19. Newborns lose up to 10% of their birth weight by 3 or 4 days of age. The factor that does not contribute to this process is:
    a. limited fluid intake in breast-fed infants.
    b. incomplete digestion of complex carbohydrates.
    c. loss of excessive extracellular fluid.
    d. passage of meconium.

20. When assessing blood pressure (BP) in the newborn, which of the following is true?
    a. BP is affected by gestational age and birth weight.
    b. Routine BP measurements of full-term neonates are an excellent predictor of hypertension.
    c. A normal BP reading for a 3-day-old infant is approximately 90/60.
    d. BP should be measured routinely on all healthy newborns as recommended by the American Academy of Pediatrics.

21. Which of the following is an abnormal finding when assessing the head of a newborn?
    a. Molding found in an infant after vaginal birth
    b. Inability to palpate the sphenoidal and mastoid fontanels
    c. Head lag and hyperextension when the infant is pulled into a semi-Fowler position
    d. Posterior fontanel palpated at about 2 to 3 cm

22. Assessment of the newborn includes which of the following?
         i. Clinical gestational age assessment
        ii. General measurements
       iii. General appearance
        iv. Head-to-toe assessment
         v. Parent-infant attachment

    a. i, ii, iii, iv, and v
    b. i, ii, iii, and iv
    c. ii, iii, iv, and v
    d. ii, iii, and iv

23. Which of the following observations from the eye assessment of a newborn is recognized as normal?
    a. Purulent discharge at age 48 hours
    b. Absence of the red reflex at age 24 hours
    c. No pupillary reflex at age 3 weeks
    d. Presence of strabismus at age 48 hours

24. a. How should the nurse assess auditory ability in the newborn?

    b. How can the nurse assess for hearing loss in the newborn?

25. It is important to assess for nasal patency in the newborn, because newborns are usually_____

_____.

26. The nurse correctly identifies the need to notify the physician for which of the following neonates?
    a. The 24-hour-old neonate found to have Epstein pearls on the side of the hard palate
    b. The 2-day-old neonate with periodic breathing
    c. The 24-hour-old neonate who has nasal flaring
    d. The 2-hour-old neonate who has a bluish, white, moist, umbilical cord with one vein and two arteries visible

27. Match each term with its description.

    a. Anal patency
    b. Periodic breathing
    c. Rooting reflex
    d. Babinski reflex
    e. Moro reflex
    f. Apnea
    g. Grasp reflex
    h. Lingual frenulum

    _____ Restriction can interfere with adequate sucking
    _____ Response in which touching cheek along the side of the mouth causes infant to turn head toward that side and begin to suck
    _____ Fanning of the toes and dorsiflexion of the great toe; disappears after 1 year of age
    _____ Symmetric abduction and extension of the arms; fingers fan out; thumb and index finger form a C
    _____ Passage of meconium from rectum during first 48 hours of life
    _____ Flexion caused by touching soles of feet near bases of digits or palms of hands
    _____ Rapid nonlabored respirations followed by pauses of less than 20 seconds
    _____ Period of no respiration for 20 seconds

28. Fill in the blanks in the following statements.
    a. The loss of heat to cooler solid objects in the environment that are not in direct contact with an infant is called

    _____.

    b. Heat loss from the body through direct contact of the skin with a cooler solid object is termed _____.

    c. Placing an infant in the direct flow of air from a fan causes rapid heat loss through _____.

    d. Loss of heat through skin moisture is termed _____.

29. The nurse implements all of the following actions to maintain a patent airway in a newborn. Which will be least effective?
    a. Maintaining the infant in a supine position during sleep
    b. Performing oropharyngeal suctioning for 5 seconds with sufficient time between attempts to allow infant to reoxygenate
    c. In the delivery room, suctioning the infant's pharynx first, then the nasal passages
    d. Continuing oral feedings for the infant with nasal flaring and intercostal retractions

30. Identify the following medications to be given as preventive care.

    a. _____ Prophylactic eye treatment against ophthalmia neonatorum

    b. _____ Administered by injection to prevent hemorrhagic disease of the newborn

    c. _____ First dose given between birth and 2 days of age to decrease incidence of hepatitis B

31. In screening for phenylketonuria, the nurse knows:
    a. blood samples should be taken after 24 hours of age and again at 2 weeks of age.
    b. blood should be drawn using a venous blood sample.
    c. preparation includes instructing parents to keep the infant NPO for 2 hours before the test.
    d. to completely saturate the filter paper by applying blood to both sides of the paper.

32. The nurse should involve the parents in the care of their newborn. Teaching is least likely to include:
    a. the use of Ivory soap, oils, powder, and lotions with each bath.
    b. bathing the infant, using plain warm water, no more than two or three times per week during the first 2 to 4 weeks of age.
    c. care of the umbilical stump, including placing the diaper below the cord to avoid irritation and wetness of the site.
    d. care of the circumcision site, explaining that on the second day a yellowish white exudate forms normally as part of the granulation process.

33. Describe the current policy of the American Academy of Pediatrics on circumcision of newborn male infants.

34. Human milk is preferable to cow's milk because:

    a. human milk has a nonlaxative effect.
    b. human milk has more calories per ounce.
    c. human milk has greater mineral content.
    d. human milk offers greater immunologic benefits.

35. Cultural beliefs and practices are significant influences on infant feeding. Identify which of the following statements is true.
    a. Many cultures do not give colostrum to newborns but wait until the milk has "come in" to start breast-feeding.
    b. U.S.-born Hispanic women are more likely to initiate breast-feeding than those recently immigrated.
    c. Muslim women typically continue exclusive breast-feeding until late in infancy.
    d. Jewish cultures place little value on breast-feeding their infants.

36. The nurse is instructing new parents about proper feeding techniques for their newborn. Indicate whether the following statements are true or false.

    _____ Infants need at least 2 hours of sucking daily.

    _____ Galactosemia in the infant is a contraindication for breast-feeding.

    _____ Breast-fed infants tend to be hungry every 2 to 3 hours.

    _____ Using a microwave oven to defrost frozen human milk destroys the antiinfective factors and vitamin C content in the milk.

    _____ Supplemental water is not needed in breast-fed infants, even in hot climates.

    _____ Propping the bottle is discouraged because it facilitates the development of middle ear infections in the infant.

37. Mrs. Gonzalez is a first-time mother. She comes to the clinic because of painful nipples and is afraid she will have to terminate breast-feeding. The breast physical examination is normal. Which of the following actions does the nurse recognize as most likely causing the painful nipples?
    i. Using an electric pump to express milk for the infant to drink when Mrs. Gonzalez is away from home
    ii. Washing the nipples before and after each feeding with soap and applying aloe vera gel
    iii. Using plastic-backed nipple pads
    iv. Letting warm water flow directly over the breast in the shower

    v. Leaving breast milk on the areola after feedings and letting it dry

    vi. Letting the infant breast-feed every 2 hours

  a. i and v

  b. iv and v

  c. iii and vi

  d. ii and iii

38. Which of the following actions by the nurse will least likely promote the attachment process between the infant and parent?

  a. Recognizing individual differences present in the infant and explaining these normal characteristics to the parent

  b. Helping the mother assume the en face position when she is presented with her infant

  c. Explaining to the parents how to respond to their infant with the use of reciprocal interacting

  d. Explaining to the parents the need for infants to have an organized schedule of daily activities that allows them to remain in their crib during awake periods

39. The feeding scale developed by the National Child Assessment Satellite Training (NCAST) program:

  a. is administered by the nurse before the newborn is discharged.

  b. focuses on concrete guidelines to identify successful interactions between child and parent.

  c. encourages parents to talk about their own parents' childrearing practices.

  d. looks at each parent's behavior regarding response to child's distress and sensitivity to cues.

CRITICAL THINKING—CASE STUDY

Michael was born by normal vaginal delivery to Marilyn and Doug Madison. Assessment at birth reflects the following: heart rate of 120 beats/min; respiratory effort good with a strong cry; well-flexed muscle tone with active movement and reflex irritability; turns head away when nose is suctioned; and color assessment of body pink with feet and hands blue. Michael's weight is 2700 g (6 lb), and his length is 53 cm (21 inches). Mrs. Madison is allowed to hold Michael and put him to breast in the delivery room. The Madisons do not plan to have Michael circumcised.

40. What is the Apgar score for Michael?

  a. 8

  b. 10

  c. 9

  d. 7

41. The nurse is conducting a gestational age assessment of Michael based on the six neuromuscular signs. What are these signs, and what results would indicate a higher maturity rating?

42. Listed below are nursing actions that the nurse would perform during the transitional period. Arrange these actions in order of highest to lowest priority.

    i. Taking head and chest circumference measurements

    ii. Assessing for neonatal distress

    iii. Administering prophylactic medications

    iv. Scoring for gestational age

    v. Assessing vital signs

  a. ii, v, i, iii, iv

  b. i, ii, v, iii, iv

  c. ii, iii, i, v, iv

  d. ii, v, iv, i, iii

43. Identify, in order of highest to lowest priority, four nursing goals that are considered the basics for safe and effective care of the newborn.

44. You are assigned to care for 1-day-old Michael in the newborn nursery. List six daily assessments that should be conducted and documented.

45. Mrs. Madison and Michael are being discharged tomorrow. You are preparing to provide Mrs. Madison with the newborn discharge teaching plan. Michael is Mrs. Madison's first infant, and on assessment you find that she has several questions about her techniques of breast-feeding. You show her how to hold Michael for feeding, how to position him properly to facilitate sucking, and how to care for her breasts. You also provide her with a video to reinforce your instruction. When you return later, Mrs. Madison asks you about the use of supplemental feedings. Which of the following is your best response?
    a. "It is okay to give Michael supplements but only after he is put to the breast."
    b. "Why would you think about that now? We'll discuss it tomorrow when you are ready to go home."
    c. "There is no need to give Michael supplemental feedings. Supplemental feeding may decrease your milk production."
    d. "You will need to give Michael supplemental feedings sometimes because you may not have enough milk."

46. You correctly evaluate the teaching plan you provided in question 44 as effective when:
    a. Mrs. Madison is discharged to take Michael home.
    b. Mrs. Madison explains to the nurse how to successfully breast-feed Michael.
    c. Mrs. Madison is seen by the nurse successfully breast-feeding Michael. Additionally, Mrs. Madison discusses with the nurse the information that the nurse had previously shared with her on breast-feeding.
    d. Mrs. Madison verbalizes that she has no further questions about breast-feeding and is able to describe to the nurse the teaching that had been provided.

47. Mrs. Madison and Michael are being discharged just 24 hours after birth. What should the nurse include in the early discharge newborn home care instructions for each of the following areas?

    a. Wet diapers:

    b. Stools:

    c. Activity:

    d. Cord:

    e. Position for sleep:

    f. Safe transport of the newborn home from the hospital:

48. Mrs. Madison is concerned because she thinks Michael is getting a cold. She tells you that he is "sneezing a lot." Your best response would be:
    a. "It is because the nose has been flattened while going through the birth canal. It will go away in another day or two."
    b. "Michael cannot get a cold; he is breast-feeding and this gives him a natural immunity."
    c. "Sneezing is abnormal and you will need to watch Michael for fever development and decreased sucking."
    d. "Most newborns are obligatory nose breathers, and sneezing is very common."

49. You are a nurse assigned to the newborn nursery. While assessing a newborn, you see white patches on the inside of the mouth. How would you correctly determine whether this is a normal or abnormal finding?

50. A nursing assistant has been assigned to work with you. Summarize what you would tell him or her about each of the following issues.
    a. The most important way to prevent cross-infection:

    b. Preventing transmission of *Pseudomonas* organisms:

    c. Handling newborn infants before the first bath:

9 Health Problems of the Newborn

1. Match each term with its description or associated term.

   a. Cephalopelvic disproportion
   b. Crepitus
   c. Moniliasis
   d. Staphylococcus aureus
   e. Icterus
   f. Hemolytic
   g. Phototherapy
   h. Bronze-baby syndrome

   i. Heterozygous
   j. Homozygous
   k. Hemangioma
   l. Port-wine stain
   m. Inborn errors of metabolism
   n. Phenylketonuria
   o. Teratogen

   _____ Causes impetigo

   _____ Occurs as a result of accumulation of or absence of essential by-products

   _____ Exposing the infant's skin to an appropriate light source

   _____ Agent that produces congenital malformations

   _____ Results in fetal head not being able to pass through the maternal pelvis

   _____ Rare reaction to phototherapy in which the serum, urine, and skin turn grayish brown

   _____ Associated with glaucoma

   _____ Candidiasis

   _____ Having one gene with a normal effect

   _____ Coarse, crackling sensation that can be produced by rubbing together fractured bone fragments

   _____ Vascular tumor

   _____ Having defective genes from both parents

   _____ Related to destruction of red blood cells

   _____ Genetic disease inherited as an autosomal recessive trait

   _____ Jaundice

2. Birth injuries may occur during the delivery of the infant. Birth injuries are not usually the result of:
   a. forceful extraction.
   b. dystocia.
   c. excess amniotic fluid.
   d. breech presentations.

3. Which of the following birth injuries is most likely to need further evaluation?
   a. Subcutaneous fat necrosis
   b. Ecchymoses
   c. Petechiae
   d. Scleral hemorrhage

4. Nursing care for soft tissue injury is not usually directed toward:
   a. assessing the injury.
   b. preventing breakdown and infection.
   c. providing explanations and reassurance to the parents.
   d. explaining the need for careful follow-up of injury after the infant's discharge.

5. Match each type of extracranial hemorrhagic injury with its description.

   a. Caput succedaneum
   b. Subgaleal hemorrhage
   c. Cephalhematoma

   _____ Bleeding into the area between the periosteum and bone; does not cross the suture line

   _____ Bleeding into the potential space that contains loosely arranged connective tissue

   _____ Edematous tissue above the bone; extends across sutures

6. An infant suffers a fracture of the clavicle during birth. Which of the following would the nurse expect to observe on the physical examination of this infant?
   a. Crepitus felt over the affected area
   b. Symmetric Moro reflex
   c. Complete fracture with overriding fragments
   d. Positive scarf sign

7. Match each type of paralysis with its correct description. (Types may be used more than once.)

   a. Facial paralysis
   b. Brachial palsy
   c. Phrenic nerve paralysis

   _____ Arm hangs limp with the shoulder, and arm is adducted and internally rotated.

   _____ The eye cannot close completely on the affected side; the corner of the mouth droops, and an absence of forehead wrinkling occurs. This type of paralysis is caused by injury to cranial nerve VII.

   _____ This usually disappears spontaneously in a few days but may take several months.

   _____ This causes diaphragmatic paralysis, with respiratory distress as the most common sign of injury; injury is usually unilateral, with affected side of lung not expanding.

   _____ Nursing care includes maintaining proper positioning and preventing contractures.

   _____ Nursing care is aimed at aiding the infant in sucking and the mother with feeding techniques.

   _____ Nursing care is aimed at assisting the infant with respiratory complications.

   _____ Artificial tears are instilled to prevent drying.

8. Which of the following is not correct in describing erythema toxicum neonatorum?
   a. It is a benign, self-limiting rash that appears within the first 2 days of life.
   b. The rash is most obvious during crying episodes.
   c. The rash may be located on all areas of the body, including the soles of the feet and the palms of the hands.
   d. Lesions appear as 1- to 3-mm, white or pale yellow pustules with an erythematous base. Smears of the pustules show increased numbers of eosinophils and lowered numbers of neutrophils.

9. You are preparing to teach a class to new parents about candidiasis. Identify whether each of the following statements is true or false.

   _____ Candidiasis is a yeastlike fungus that can be transmitted by maternal vaginal infection during delivery, through person-to-person contact, and from contaminated articles.

   _____ In the neonate, candidiasis is usually found in the oral and diaper areas.

   _____ It is difficult to distinguish between oral candidiasis and coagulated milk in the infant's mouth because both are easily removed by simple wiping.

   _____ Thrush appears when the oral flora are altered as a result of antibiotic therapy or poor hand washing by the infant's caregiver.

   _____ Oral candidiasis can be treated with the administration of oral nystatin four times a day, after feedings and at night.

_____ Candidiasis appears most often in the newborn's first week of life.

_____ It is not necessary to boil bottles or nipples for infants with oral candidiasis, because the fungus is heat resistant.

_____ Oral nystatin should be placed in the far back of the throat to allow the infant to swallow it easily.

_____ Oral nystatin should be administered before feedings to help the medication provide better coverage of the gastrointestinal lesions.

10. Neonatal herpes:
    a. rarely has a rash that affects the fetal scalp-monitoring sites.
    b. does not manifest with a rash found in a cluster formation.
    c. does not always manifest with a rash.
    d. always manifests with some type of rash.

11. Which of the following statements concerning impetigo is not correct and should be omitted by the nurse from the teaching plan?
    a. Impetigo is treated with oral antibiotics and topical application of mupirocin (Bactroban).
    b. Impetigo is an eruption of vesicular lesions that occur on skin that has not been traumatized.
    c. Distribution of impetigo lesions usually occurs on the perineum, trunk, face, and buttocks.
    d. The infected child or infant must be isolated from others until all lesions have healed.

12. Identify the type of birthmark described by each of the following statements.

    a. _____ These lesions are pink, red, or purple and often thicken, darken, and pro-portionately enlarge as the child grows.
    b. _____ These are red, rubbery nodules with a rough surface that are recognized as tumors that involve only capillaries.
    c. _____ These are multiple flat, light brown marks that are often associated with the autosomal dominant hereditary disorder neurofibromatosis.

13. Treatment for port-wine stain includes laser therapy. Which of the following should be included in the teaching plan for treatment expectations?
    a. The lesion will have a bright pink appearance for 10 days after treatment.
    b. Expose the infant to sunlight for 15 minutes daily after treatments.
    c. Administer salicylates before each treatment for pain.
    d. After treatment, gently wash the area with water and dab it dry.

14. _____ is an excessive accumulation of bilirubin in the blood and is characterized by

    _____, a yellow discoloration of the skin.

15. In discussing the pathophysiology of bilirubin, the nurse knows that red blood cell destruction results in

    _____ and _____. _____

    _____ is an insoluble substance bound to albumin. In the liver this is changed to a

    soluble substance, _____ _____.

16. The term used to describe the yellow staining of the brain cells that can result in bilirubin encephalopathy is:
    a. jaundice.
    b. physiologic jaundice.
    c. kernicterus.
    d. icterus neonatorum.

17. Which of the following statements about bilirubin encephalopathy is true?
    a. Development may be enhanced by metabolic acidosis, lowered albumin levels, intracranial infections, and increases in the metabolic demands for oxygen or glucose.
    b. It produces no permanent neurologic damage.
    c. Serum bilirubin levels alone can predict the risk for brain injury.
    d. It produces permanent liver damage by deposits of conjugated bilirubin within the cell.

18. A newborn develops hyperbilirubinemia at 48 hours of age. The condition peaks at 72 hours and declines at about age 7 days. The most likely cause of this hyperbilirubinemia is:
    a. physiologic jaundice.
    b. pathologic jaundice.
    c. hemolytic disease of the newborn.
    d. breast milk jaundice.

19. Of the four infants described below, which should the nurse recognize as being least likely to develop jaundice?
    a. An infant with subgaleal hemorrhage that is now resolving
    b. An infant with cephalhematoma that is now resolving
    c. An infant who has feedings started early, which will stimulate peristalsis and rapid passage of meconium
    d. An infant who is of Native American descent

20. Which of the following therapies should the nurse expect to implement for jaundice associated with breast-feeding?
    a. Increased frequency of breast-feedings
    b. Permanent discontinuation of breast-feedings
    c. Discontinuation of breast-feedings for 24 hours with the use of home phototherapy
    d. Increased frequency of breast-feedings and addition of caloric supplements

21. Newborns are more prone to produce higher levels of bilirubin because they:
    i. have higher concentrations of circulating erythrocytes.
    ii. have red blood cells with a shorter life span.
    iii. have reduced albumin concentrations.
    iv. have anatomically underdeveloped livers.

    a. i, ii, iii, and iv
    b. i, ii, and iii
    c. ii, iii, and iv
    d. iii and iv

22. Which of the following is true regarding diagnostic evaluations for bilirubin?
    a. Newborn levels of unconjugated bilirubin must exceed 5 mg/dl before jaundice is observable.
    b. Hyperbilirubinemia is defined as a serum bilirubin value of above 8 mg/dl in full-term infants.
    c. When jaundice occurs before 24 hours of age, bilirubin level assessment is unnecessary.
    d. Transcutaneous bilirubinometry is an effective cutaneous measurement of bilirubin in full-term infants being treated with phototherapy.

23. List the risk factors that place the term infant at high risk for hyperbilirubinemia.

24. Which of the following statements about phototherapy is false?
    a. For phototherapy to be effective, the infant's skin must be fully exposed to an adequate amount of light or irradiance.
    b. The initiation of phototherapy should always be based on clinical judgment rather than serum bilirubin levels alone.
    c. For best results, the goal of phototherapy is to increase irradiance to the 430- to 490-nm band.
    d. The color of the infant's skin influences the efficacy of phototherapy, with darker-skinned infants needing double or intensive therapy.

25. Implementation of phototherapy for an infant with jaundice does not include:
    a. shielding the infant's eyes with an opaque mask.
    b. recognizing that once phototherapy has been started, visual assessment of jaundice increases in validity; therefore fewer serum bilirubin levels will be necessary.
    c. repositioning infant frequently to expose all body surfaces to the light.
    d. assessing the infant for side effects, including loose, greenish stools; skin rashes; hyperthermia; dehydration; and increased metabolic rates.

26. Complete the following:
    a. Erythroblastosis fetalis is caused by _____ _____.

    b. Problems of Rh incompatibility may arise when the mother is _____

    _____ and the infant is _____

    _____. The most common blood group incompatibility in the neonate occurs

    when the mother has type _____ blood and the infant has either type

    _____ or type _____ blood.

    c. The nurse is reviewing maternal laboratory results. The nurse knows that the _____

    _____ test monitors anti-Rh antibody titers. The test performed postnatally to detect

    antibodies attached to the circulating erythrocytes of affected infants is called the _____

    _____ test.

    d. To be effective in preventing maternal sensitization to the Rh factor, the nurse must administer $Rh_o(D)$

    immune globulin (RhoGam) to the Rh-negative mother within _____

    _____ after the first delivery or abortion and with each subsequent pregnancy. To fur-

    ther decrease the risk for Rh alloimmunization, RhoGam is administered at _____

    to _____ weeks of gestation. RhoGam is administered by the

    _____ route.

    e. Exposure to Rh antigen with significant antibody formation occurring and causing a sensitivity response is known

    as _____.

27. Explain how the nurse is expected to assist the practitioner with a blood exchange transfusion in the newborn.

28. Which of the following statements about hypoglycemia in the newborn is true?
    a. Hypoglycemia is present when the newborn's blood glucose is lower than the baby's requirement for cellular energy and metabolism.
    b. In the healthy term infant who is born without complications, blood glucose is routinely monitored within 24 hours of birth to detect hypoglycemia.
    c. A plasma glucose level less than 60 mg/dl requires intervention in the term newborn.
    d. Pregnancy-induced hypertension and terbutaline administration have not been found to alter infant metabolism or increase the hypoglycemia risk in the newborn.

29. What assessment finding is the nurse most likely to see in the infant as a result of hypoglycemia?
    a. Forceful, low-pitched cry
    b. Tachypnea
    c. Jitteriness, tremors, twitching
    d. Vomiting, refusal to eat

30. Which of the following nursing interventions are recognized as appropriate for the infant with hypoglycemia?
    i. Institute early bottle-feeding or breast-feeding.
    ii. Increase environmental stimulants.
    iii. Protect from cold stress and respiratory difficulty that predispose the infant to decreased blood glucose levels.
    iv. Force early oral glucose feedings, avoiding formula and breast milk until newborn is stable.

    a. i, ii, iii, and iv
    b. i and iii
    c. iii and iv
    d. i, ii, and iii

31. Full-term infants at risk for hypoglycemia shortly after birth include which of the following?
    i. Those born to diabetic mothers
    ii. Those who are small for gestational age
    iii. Those with perinatal hypoxia

    a. i, ii, and iii
    b. i and ii
    c. ii and iii
    d. i and iii

32. Ben, a full-term newborn, has symptomatic hypoglycemia and inability to tolerate oral feedings. An intravenous glucose infusion has been ordered. Which of the following does the nurse recognize as correct?
    a. The infusion is administered through the umbilical catheter.
    b. An initial bolus infusion of 10% dextrose will be given over a 10-minute interval, followed by continuous dextrose infusion for 24 hours.
    c. Extravasation of the fluid into the surrounding areas can cause tissue sloughing.
    d. Termination of the glucose solution should be rapid to prevent hyperinsulinism.

33. Hyperglycemia in the newborn is defined as a blood glucose concentration greater than _____ in the full-term infant and greater than _____ in the preterm infant.

34. Infants at risk for early-onset hypocalcemia include:
    a. postterm infants.
    b. infants who develop jaundice.
    c. infants born to hypertensive mothers.
    d. small-for-gestational-age infants who experience perinatal hypoxia.

35. The care plan for the infant who has hypocalcemia and is receiving intravenous calcium gluconate should include:
    a. the scalp veins are the preferred site for intravenous administration of calcium gluconate.
    b. signs of acute hypercalcemia include vomiting and bradycardia.
    c. rapid infusion administration is best tolerated by the infant.
    d. calcium gluconate is compatible with sodium bicarbonate.

36. The nurse is assessing Sarah, a neonate born at home, and observes slight blood oozing from the umbilicus. What is the most likely cause of Sarah's hemorrhagic disease?
    a. The neonate was born with an anatomically immature liver.
    b. Coagulation factors (II, VII, IX, X) are deactivated in the neonate.
    c. Vitamin K was administered to the neonate shortly after birth.
    d. The newborn was born with a sterile intestine and was unable to synthesize vitamin K until feedings began.

37. The goal is to prevent hemorrhagic disease in the newborn by prophylactic administration of vitamin K (AquaMEPHYTON). How does the nurse correctly administer this drug?

38. Lucy has been diagnosed with congenital hypothyroidism. The nurse is instructing the parents on how to care for Lucy. Which of the following is the nurse least likely to include in the plan?
    a. The drug of choice is synthetic levothyroxine sodium.
    b. The drug is tasteless and can be crushed and added to formula, water, or food.
    c. If a dose is missed, twice the dose should be given the next day.
    d. Signs of overdose of the drug include slow pulse rate, lethargy, cool skin, and excessive weight gain.

39. When teaching the parents of the newborn about testing for phenylketonuria, the nurse should include one of the following key points.
    a. The test is performed only on infants expected to have the disorder.
    b. The test is performed on cord blood.
    c. The test is not reliable if the blood sample is taken after the infant has ingested a source of protein.
    d. The test should be performed on all newborns before they leave the hospital, and a repeat blood specimen should be obtained by 2 weeks of age if the first test was taken within the first 24 hours of life.

40. Dietary instructions for the parents of a child with phenylketonuria include:
    i. maintain a low-phenylalanine diet through adulthood.
    ii. increase intake of high-protein foods such as meat and dairy products.
    iii. measure vegetables, fruits, juices, breads, and starches.
    iv. illness and growth spurts will increase the need for phenylalanine.
    v. introduce solid foods such as cereal, fruits, and vegetables during infancy as usual.
    vi. use soy formula during infancy.

    a. i, ii, iii, and iv
    b. i, iii, iv, v, and vi
    c. iii, iv, and v
    d. i, iii, iv, and v

41. In educating the parents of a newborn with galactosemia, the nurse includes one of the following in the plan.
    a. All food labels should be read carefully for the presence of lactose.
    b. Once the diagnosis is made and the diet is altered, little follow-up of these infants is necessary.
    c. Breast milk is acceptable for infants with galactosemia.
    d. Signs of visual impairment are unlikely in children with this disorder.

42. Diagnostic evaluation testing for congenital hypothyroidism in the newborn includes:
    i. a low level of T4.
    ii. a high level of thyroid-stimulating hormone.
    iii. mandatory testing of all newborns within the first 24 to 48 hours or before discharge.
    iv. venous blood samples taken on two separate occasions.

    a. i and iii
    b. i, ii, and iii
    c. i, ii, and iv
    d. ii and iv

43. Which of the following has a teratogenic effect on the fetus?
    a. Folic acid
    b. X-rays taken of the pelvis and abdomen 1 week after menstruation
    c. Amoxicillin
    d. Valproic acid

CRITICAL THINKING—CASE STUDY

Mrs. Becker had a normal pregnancy and delivery without complications at 39 weeks of gestation. She is breast-feeding her 2-day-old neonate, Ben, when she notices that Ben's skin looks yellow. Tests reveal that Ben's total serum bilirubin level is 13 mg/dl.

44. Mrs. Becker asks the nurse about Ben's condition and the seriousness of his illness. Which of the following is the best response?
    a. "Ben has pathologic jaundice, a serious condition."
    b. "Ben has breast milk jaundice, and you will need to stop breast-feeding."
    c. "Ben probably has physiologic jaundice, a normal finding at his age."
    d. "Infants with serum bilirubin levels of 13 mg/dl will develop bilirubin encephalopathy and severe brain damage."

45. The physician tells Mrs. Becker to increase her frequency of breast-feeding to every 2 hours and to avoid supplementation. The nurse is discussing the rationale for this management with Mrs. Becker. Which of the following is the basis for the ordered treatment?
    a. The jaundice is related to the process of breast-feeding, probably from decreased caloric and fluid intake by breast-fed infants.
    b. The jaundice is caused by a factor in the breast milk that breaks down bilirubin to a lipid-soluble form, which is reabsorbed in the gut.
    c. The jaundice is caused by the mother's hemolytic disease.
    d. The jaundice is increased because the infant was put to breast early, which increases the amount of time meconium is kept in the gut before excretion.

46. Ben's serum bilirubin level has not decreased as the physician hoped, and phototherapy has been ordered. Which of the following is the priority goal at this time?
    a. The family will be prepared for home phototherapy.
    b. The infant will receive adequate intravenous hydration.
    c. The infant will experience no complications from phototherapy.
    d. The infant will have hourly bilirubin level testing completed.

47. When caring for Ben, the nurse should take all of the following actions to prevent complications *except:*
    a. making certain that eyelids are closed before applying eye shields; checking eyes at least every 4 to 6 hour for discharge or irritation.
    b. monitoring axillary temperature closely to detect hyperthermia and/or hypothermia.
    c. maintaining an 18-inch distance between infant and light.
    d. applying oil daily to skin to avoid breakdown.

48. Which of the following is the best expected patient outcome for Ben while he is on phototherapy?
    a. Newborn begins feeding soon after birth.
    b. Family demonstrates an understanding of therapy and prognosis.
    c. Newborn displays no evidence of infection.
    d. Newborn displays no evidence of eye irritation, dehydration, temperature instability, or skin breakdown.

49. Accurate charting is an important nursing responsibility when caring for the newborn receiving phototherapy. What is included in the charting?

50. Once phototherapy is considered permanently completed, what should occur in relation to the bilirubin level?

51. Ben's condition has improved, and the physician has ordered him off phototherapy and released him for discharge. What home care instructions should the nurse provide?

10 The High-Risk Newborn and Family

1. Provide the correct term for each of the following descriptions.
   a. An infant whose birth weight is less than 2500 g (5.5 lb), regardless of gestational age: _____

   _____-_____ _____

   b. An infant whose birth weight is less than 1000 g (2.2 lb): _____ _____

   _____-_____ _____

   c. An infant whose birth weight falls below the 10th percentile on intrauterine growth curves: _____-

   _____-_____-_____ _____

   d. An infant whose birth weight falls above the 90th percentile on intrauterine growth curves: _____-

   _____-_____-_____ _____

   e. An infant born before completion of 37 weeks of gestation: _____ _____

   f. An infant born between the 38th week and completion of the 42nd week of gestation: _____

   _____ _____

   g. An infant born after 42 weeks of gestation: _____ _____

   h. Death of a fetus after 20 weeks of gestation: _____ _____

   i. Death that occurs in the first 27 days of life: _____ _____

   j. Describes the total number of fetal and early neonatal deaths per 1000 live births: _____

   _____

   k. An infant born between 34 $^6/_7$ and 36 $^6/_7$ weeks of gestation, regardless of birth weight: _____

   _____ _____

   l. The capacity to balance heat production and conservation and heat dissipation: _____

   _____

   m. An environment that permits the infant to maintain a normal core temperature with minimum oxygen

   consumption and caloric expenditure: _____ _____ _____

   n. Heat loss that occurs when infants are exposed to drafts or increased air flow: _____

   _____ _____

   o. Heat loss that can be effectively reduced by use of double-walled incubator in high-risk newborn:

   _____ _____ _____

   p. Heat loss that can be reduced by warming all items that come into direct contact with newborn:

   _____ _____ _____

2. Which of the following is not used as a category in the classification of high-risk newborns?
   a. Birth size
   b. Gestational age
   c. Mortality
   d. Birth age

3. Which of the following is a neonatal intensive care facility that provides care for extremely low–birth-weight infants and also offers extracorporeal membrane oxygenation and surgical repair of serious congenital cardiac malformations?
   a. Level I facility
   b. Level IIB facility
   c. Level IIIC facility
   d. Level IV facility

4. When a high-risk neonate needs transportation to a facility that can provide intensive care, the nurse recognizes that priority care for this neonate must include:
   a. transfer of both the mother and infant.
   b. immediate transport, often before stabilization of the neonate.
   c. complete life support system available during transport.
   d. prevention of transport delay by carrying the infant in the nurse's arms to the waiting transport vehicle.

5. A thorough systematic physical assessment is a must in the care of the high-risk neonate. Subtle changes

   in _____ _____, _____, _____, _____

   _____, or _____ _____ often indicate an underlying problem.

6. At birth the newborn is immediately assessed to determine any apparent problems and to identify those that demand immediate attention. The assessment not usually conducted at birth or immediately after birth is:
   a. assignment of a gestational age score.
   b. assignment of an Apgar score.
   c. evaluation for obvious congenital anomalies.
   d. evaluation for neonatal distress.

7. Identify whether the following statements about high-risk care of the neonate are true or false.

   _____ Neonates under intensive observation are placed in a controlled environment and monitored for heart rate, respiratory activity, and temperature.

   _____ Sophisticated monitoring and life-support systems can replace the observations of the infant by nursing personnel.

   _____ When hydrogel electrodes are used on the neonate's skin, they are easily removed by lifting the edge and wiping with alcohol.

   _____ Infants who are mechanically ventilated and have low Apgar scores can have lower blood pressures.

   _____ An accurate output measurement can be obtained in the neonate by using a urine collecting bag or by weighing the infant's diaper. Regardless of the method used, a 40-g weight of urine would be recorded as 40 ml of urine.

   _____ The nurse is preparing the infant for a heel stick. This preparation is done to create adequate vasodilation and is accomplished by placing a heating pad on the infant's heel.

   _____ Nurses are allowed to turn off alarm systems for electronic monitoring devices when their sounds disturb the infant's parents.

8. Identify the two most critical goals in caring for the high-risk infant.

9. The major source of increased production of heat during cold stress in the high-risk neonate is _____

   _____.

10. Low-birth-weight infants are at a disadvantage for heat production when compared with full-term infants because they have:
    i. small muscle mass.
    ii. fewer deposits of brown fat.
    iii. less insulating subcutaneous fat.
    iv. poor reflex control of skin capillaries.

a. i, ii, iii, and iv
b. ii, iii, and iv
c. i, ii, and iii
d. i, iii, and iv

11. Identify three major consequences produced by cold stress that create additional hazards for the neonate.

12. Match each term with its description.
a. Thermal stability
b. Neutral thermal environment
c. Convective heat loss
d. Radiant heat loss
e. Conductive heat loss
f. Evaporative heat loss

_____ Capacity to balance heat production, heat conservation, and heat dissipation

_____ Allows one to maintain normal core temperature with minimal oxygen consumption and caloric use

_____ Occurs by transfer of body heat to a cooler solid object not in direct contact

_____ Occurs when infants are exposed to drafts or when surrounding air is cool

_____ Can be decreased by drying the neonate thoroughly with warm towels

_____ Loss of heat through direct contact with a cooler surface

13. Which of the following interventions is least likely to be effective for high-risk neonates?
a. Keeping the infant on servocontrol in an incubator or radiant warmer
b. Placing the heat-sensing probe on the infant's abdomen when the infant is in the prone position
c. Ensuring that the oxygen supplied to the infant via a hood around the head is warmed and humidified
d. Warming all items that come in direct contact with the infant, including the hands of caregivers

14. A primary objective in the care of high-risk infants is to maintain respiration. Describe how the nurse should complete the respiratory assessment.

15. The best way to prevent infection in the high-risk neonate begins with:
a. meticulous and frequent hand washing of all persons coming in contact with the infant.
b. observing continually for signs of infection.
c. requiring everyone working in the neonatal intensive care unit (NICU) to put on fresh scrub clothes before entering the unit.
d. performing epidemiologic studies at least monthly.

16. Baby girl Miller has been admitted to the NICU with low birth weight and possible infection. Parenteral fluids have been ordered for hydration and antibiotic administration.
a. What are the preferred sites for peripheral intravenous (IV) infusions for this infant?

b. In many neonatal centers a specially inserted catheter is used for IV hydration and medication administration because it is less expensive and decreases trauma to the neonate. What is this catheter called?

    c. The nurse starts a peripheral line and places the neonate on an infusion pump to regulate the rate of IV administration. Ten minutes later the nurse observes for signs of infiltration. The nurse should be looking for the following signs:

17. A complication that develops with the use of the umbilical catheter is thrombi. This complication is best recognized by the appearance of:
    a. blanching of the buttocks and genitalia.
    b. bluish discoloration seen in the toes, called "cath toes."
    c. bounding pedal pulses.
    d. hemorrhage from the umbilical catheter area.

18. Introduction of minimal enteral feedings in the metabolically stable preterm infant:
    a. increases incidence of necrotizing enterocolitis.
    b. increases mucosal atrophy incidence.
    c. stimulates the infant's gastrointestinal tract.
    d. maintains serum glucose homeostasis.

19. Identify whether the following statements are true or false.

    _____ Although infants demonstrate some sucking and swallowing activities before birth, coordination of these mechanisms does not occur until approximately 32 to 34 weeks of gestation, and they are not fully synchronized until 36 to 37 weeks.

    _____ Research has shown that infants receiving trophic feedings versus no feedings have an overall higher number of days to full feedings and a longer hospital stay.

    _____ Preterm infants receiving continuous feedings show better weight gain than those receiving intermittent bolus feedings.

    _____ Milk produced by mothers of preterm infants changes in content over the first 30 days postnatally, until its content is similar to that of full-term human milk.

    _____ Milk produced by mothers whose infants are born at term contains higher concentrations of protein, sodium chloride, and immunoglobulin A (IgA).

    _____ Low-birth-weight infants (<1500 g) who are fed only human milk demonstrate decreased growth rates and nutritional deficiencies.

    _____ Preterm infants who are fed fortified human milk have shorter hospital stays and less infection than infants given preterm formulas.

    _____ Fortified human milk is mixed as close to feeding time as possible and stored in the refrigerator.

    _____ IgA concentration is higher in the milk of mothers of term infants as compared with mothers of preterm infants.

    _____ Pasteurization of donor human milk serves little purpose, because all donors are carefully screened.

    _____ Preterm infants have the same capacity to digest and absorb protein, carbohydrates, and fats as full-term infants.

    _____ The amount of calories required for optimal growth in sick and very low-birth-weight infants is higher than for healthy infants.

    _____ Enfamil Human Milk Fortifier comes in a powder form and is mixed with human milk. It is not used as a separate formula.

20. The amount to be fed to the infant by nipple is:
    a. determined by the infant's tolerance to previous feedings.
    b. increased when the infant requires 25 minutes or more for feeding completion.
    c. increased when the infant reaches the postnatal age of 34 weeks.
    d. increased when prodding techniques are used to increase sucking and decrease aspiration.

21. Feeding facilitation techniques for preterm infants include:
    a. using a pliable nipple with faster flow.
    b. using a slightly firm nipple with slow flow.
    c. manipulating the nipple frequently by twisting and turning when the infants stops sucking.
    d. positioning the infant on the back with the head supported.

22. What is the best measurement of feeding success in the infant?
    a. Soft abdomen
    b. No aspirated gastric residual
    c. Ability to suck on pacifier
    d. Coordinated sucking and swallowing ability

23. An infant who weighs 1400 g appears to be ready for enteral feedings. Which of the following should the nurse include in the implementation of gavage feedings?
    a. Insert the tube into the unobstructed nares.
    b. Perform the procedure with the infant in a supine position with the head elevated 45 degrees.
    c. Aspirate the contents of the stomach, measure these contents, and replace the residual as part of the feeding.
    d. Allow the feeding to flow by gravity; then push a small amount of the feeding into the stomach; then allow the remainder of the feeding to flow by gravity.

24. _____ _____ decreases hospital stay, enhances transition from tube to bottle-feeding, and results in better bottle-feeding performance in preterm infants.

25. In caring for a preterm infant's skin, the nurse knows to:
    a. use scissors to remove dressings or tape from the infant's extremities.
    b. use solvents to remove tape from the neonate's skin.
    c. use alkaline-based soaps in removal of stool.
    d. use zinc oxide–based tape to secure monitoring equipment or intravenous infusions.

26. Which of the following is a correct nursing intervention to prevent skin damage in the neonate?
    a. Instruct parents before discharge on regular use of sunscreen for all infants under 6 months of age.
    b. Apply adhesive tape to protect arms, elbow, and knees from friction rubs.
    c. Use powders on diaper dermatitis areas as a moisture barrier.
    d. Use gel mattresses to decrease skin breakdown.

27. _____ _____, a common preservative in bacteriostatic water and saline, has been shown to be toxic to newborns and is not used to flush intravenous catheters or reconstitute medications.

    Oral or parental medications should be sufficiently diluted if they are _____ solutions to prevent necrotizing enterocolitis.

28. Identify the following as true or false.

    _____ Each infant is different; therefore supportive developmental care requires ongoing data collection by the nurse.

    _____ Developmentally supportive care uses both physiologic and behavioral information to evaluate the needs of the infant in an NICU setting.

    _____ Developmental maturation for the young preterm infant is seen by a decrease in quiet sleep.

    _____ Nursing care for the neonate should include modification of care to provide longer episodes of undisturbed sleep.

    _____ Prolonged "clustering" of care for the ill infant promotes physiologic stability.

    _____ The best time for care of an infant is when the infant is awake.

    _____ Containment or facilitated tucking positioning of the infant during procedures has been shown to increase physiologic and behavioral stressors.

    _____ Stroking a preterm infant who is not physiologically stable can result in distress, including oxygen desaturation.

_____ Preterm infants are less responsive to visual stimulation and have less acuity and accommodation than full-term infants.

_____ Therapeutic positioning for preterm and high-risk infants should provide support to maintain flexed and midline postures.

_____ Using earmuffs in the NICU is an important intervention to prevent later speech and language difficulties.

_____ Strong visual stimulation such as high-contrast black and white patterns can evoke an obligatory staring response by the immature infant who is unable to break away from it.

29. The _____ sleeping position is recommended by the American Academy of Pediatrics for healthy infants in the first year of life as a preventive measure for sudden infant death syndrome.

30. Which of the following is the best way for the nurse to promote a healthy parent-infant relationship for the family with a high-risk neonate?
    a. Reinforce parents during their caregiving activities and interactions with their infant.
    b. Help parents understand that the preterm infant offers no behavioral rewards.
    c. Reassure parents that the infant is doing well.
    d. Encourage the mother to stay by the infant's bedside to promote bonding.

31. The term _____ _____ _____ is applied to physically healthy children who are perceived by parents to be at high risk for medical or developmental problems.

32. Discharge instructions for the parents of the preterm infant should not include:
    a. warning parents that their infant may still be in danger and will need constant attention.
    b. providing information to the parents on how to contact personnel for later questions.
    c. instructions about car safety seats, including how these seats can be adapted for smaller infants with the placement of blanket rolls on each side of the infant to support the head and trunk.
    d. providing adequate information about immunization needs.

33. To help parents deal with neonatal death, the nurse should:
    a. discourage the parent from staying with the infant before death to prevent overattachment.
    b. explain to the parents that the infant would have had many developmental problems and it is better that the infant did not suffer.
    c. give the parents the opportunity to hold and talk with the infant before and after death.
    d. force the parents to see the infant after death because closure is necessary.

34. A physical characteristic usually observed in the preterm infant and not observed in the full-term infant is:
    a. proportionately equal head in relation to the body.
    b. skin that is translucent, smooth, and shiny with small blood vessels clearly visible underneath the epidermis.
    c. distinct creases extending across the entire palms of the hands and down the complete soles of the feet.
    d. absence of lanugo and little vernix caseosa.

35. Apnea in the preterm infant is defined as a lapse of spontaneous breathing lasting for:
    a. 5 seconds.
    b. 10 seconds.
    c. 15 seconds.
    d. 20 seconds.

36. Bryan, a 2-day-old preterm infant being cared for in the NICU, had some periods of apnea yesterday. Today when you arrive to work, you learn in report that the infant has had no further apneic episodes since yesterday. However, shortly after you begin your shift, Bryan's apnea monitor alarm sounds. What should you do first?
    a. Use tactile stimulation, rubbing on the infant's back to stop the apneic spell.
    b. Suction his nose and oropharynx.
    c. Assess the infant for color and for presence of respiration.
    d. Place the infant on his abdomen.

37. The preterm infant is having respirations with absence of diaphragmatic muscle function. This is causing a lack of respiratory effort because the central nervous system is not transmitting signals to the respiratory muscles. What is this type of apnea called?
    a. Obstructive apnea
    b. Central apnea
    c. Periodic apnea
    d. Mixed apnea

38. A late and serious sign of respiratory distress in the neonate is:
    a. central cyanosis.
    b. respiratory rate of 90 breaths/min.
    c. substernal retractions.
    d. nasal flaring.

39. Which of the following is a correct procedure to use when suctioning the nasopharyngeal passages, trachea, or endotracheal tube in a newborn?
    a. Pulse oximeter is observed before, during, and after suctioning to provide an ongoing assessment of oxygenation status.
    b. Continuous suction is applied as the catheter is withdrawn.
    c. The catheter is inserted gently and slowly, and suction is conducted to a point where the catheter meets resistance before the catheter is withdrawn.
    d. The time the airway is obstructed by the catheter is limited to no more than 10 seconds.

40. Discuss the importance of surfactant to the preterm infant's lungs.

41. Match each term with its description.
    a. Pulmonary interstitial emphysema
    b. Lung compliance
    c. Continuous positive airway pressure (CPAP)
    d. Intermittent mandatory ventilation (IMV)
    e. Positive end-expiratory pressure (PEEP)
    f. Nasal flaring
    g. Grunting
    h. Synchronized intermittent mandatory ventilation (SIMV)
    i. High-frequency ventilation (HFV) modalities
    j. Lecithin/sphingomyelin ratio

    _____ Method that infuses air or oxygen under a preset pressure by means of nasal prongs, a face mask, or an endotracheal tube

    _____ Perinatal diagnostic test for lung maturity

    _____ Method that allows infant to breathe spontaneously at his or her own rate but provides mechanical cycled respirations and pressure at regular preset intervals by means of an endotracheal tube and ventilator

    _____ Condition that develops in the preterm infant with respiratory distress syndrome and immature lungs as a result of overdistention of distal airways

    _____ Method that provides increased end-expiratory pressure during expiration and between mandatory breaths, preventing alveolar collapse

    _____ Lung distensibility

    _____ Abnormal sounds made on respiration as a result of increased effort required to fill the lungs; associated with atelectasis

    _____ Widening of the nostril during inspiration; signals respiratory distress

    _____ Infant-triggered ventilator with signal detector and assist/control mode

    _____ Method that delivers gas at very rapid rates to provide adequate minute volumes using lower proximal airway pressures

42. The administration of exogenous surfactant to preterm neonates with respiratory distress syndrome:
    a. shows no difference in improvement when synthetic surfactant is used versus natural surfactant.
    b. is done by intravenous infusion.
    c. requires adjustment of ventilator settings.
    d. requires suctioning the infant during administration.

43. Suctioning of the infant with respiratory distress syndrome:
    a. is performed by applying intermittent suction as the catheter is withdrawn.
    b. is performed routinely every 30 minutes to keep the airway open.
    c. is performed by slowly and gently inserting the catheter.
    d. is performed by advancing the catheter until resistance is met and then withdrawing.

44. Susie, a neonate born 20 minutes ago, was observed at birth to have meconium staining. If Susie has meconium in the lungs, this most likely will:
    a. prevent air from entering the lungs.
    b. trap inspired air in the lungs.
    c. cause no problems with breathing.
    d. lead to respiratory alkalosis.

45. An important nursing function is close observation of neonates at risk for developing air leaks. These infants include:
    a. those with respiratory distress syndrome.
    b. those with meconium-stained amniotic fluid.
    c. those receiving continuous positive airway pressure (CPAP) or positive-pressure ventilation.
    d. all of the above.

46. Infants diagnosed with bronchopulmonary dysplasia have special care needs. These needs include:
    a. adequate rest.
    b. avoiding diuretics.
    c. decreasing caloric intake.
    d. rapid weaning from ventilators.

47. Why are diagnosis and treatment of sepsis sometimes delayed in the neonate?

48. The laboratory evaluation for the diagnosis of sepsis is least likely to include:
    a. blood cultures.
    b. spinal fluid culture.
    c. urine culture.
    d. gastric secretions culture.

49. Clinical signs seen in necrotizing enterocolitis are:
    i. increased abdominal girth.
    ii. increased gastric residual.
    iii. positive stool hematest.
    iv. hypertension.

    a. i, ii, and iv
    b. i and iii
    c. ii, iii, and iv
    d. i, ii, and iii

50. Clinical manifestations of patent ductus arteriosus (PDA) include:
    a. increased $Paco_2$, decreased Pao_2, and decreased Fio_2.
    b. narrow pulse pressure with increased diastolic blood pressure.
    c. systolic or continuous murmur heard as a "machinery-type" sound.
    d. bradycardia.

51. Therapy for preterm infants who develop PDA often includes the administration of:
    a. theophyllin.
    b. indomethacin.
    c. digoxin.
    d. heparin.

52. Which of the following is a correct statement about persistent pulmonary hypertension of the newborn (PPHN)?
    a. PPHN is primarily a condition of preterm infants.
    b. PPHN is rarely associated with meconium aspiration.
    c. A loud pulmonary component of the second heart sound and often a systolic ejection murmur are present with PPHN.
    d. Vasodilators, such as tolazoline, are used to decrease cardiac output.

53. Why does the nurse carefully monitor and record amounts of all blood drawn for tests in the preterm infant?
    a. Early prevention of anemia
    b. Prevention of infection
    c. Prevention of polycythemia
    d. Detection of factors that contribute to hypothermia

54. Define *polycythemia* and identify the infants who are most at risk for this condition.

55. The treatment of retinopathy of prematurity includes _____ and _____ _____ by a pediatric ophthalmologist.

56. Brenda is a 1-hour-old newborn who suffered asphyxia before birth, resulting in hypoxic-ischemic brain injury. What signs can the nurse expect to see indicating encephalopathy?

57. Which of the following interventions is contraindicated in the preterm infant with increased intracranial pressure?
    a. Avoiding interventions that produce crying
    b. Avoiding rapid volume expansion following hypotension
    c. Administering analgesics to reduce discomfort
    d. Turning the head to the right without body alignment

58. _____, the most common type of intracranial hemorrhage, occurs in both term and preterm infants. Small hemorrhages of venous origin with underlying contusion may occur.
    a. Subdural hemorrhage
    b. Intracerebellar hemorrhage
    c. Subarachnoid hemorrhage
    d. Hematoma

59. Which of the following statements about neonatal stroke is true?
    a. It is the number-one leading cause of seizures in term neonates.
    b. It is more common in females, where there is a tendency toward left-sided involvement.
    c. Known risk factors include maternal and/or fetal factor V Leiden, antiphospholipid, and prothrombin factors.
    d. Diagnosis is most accurate with head ultrasonography.

60. The nurse must be able to distinguish between seizures and jitteriness in the neonate. Which of the following is true about seizures?
    a. Seizures are not accompanied by ocular movement.
    b. Seizures have their dominant movement as tremor.
    c. In seizures the dominant movement cannot be stopped by flexion of the affected limb.
    d. Seizures are highly sensitive to light manual stimulation.

61. John is a newborn just delivered of a diabetic mother. The nurse will watch John for signs that he is rapidly developing:
    a. hyperglycemia.
    b. hypoglycemia.
    c. failure of the pancreas.
    d. dehydration.

62. Infants born to drug-dependent mothers may exhibit all of the following clinical manifestations except:
    a. tremors and restlessness.
    b. frequent sneezing.
    c. coordinated suck and swallow reflex.
    d. high-pitched, shrill cry.

63. Which of the following is true about the infant diagnosed with neonatal abstinence syndrome (NAS)?
    a. Methadone treatment by the mother will prevent withdrawal reaction in neonates.
    b. Meconium sampling for fetal drug exposure is less accurate than neonatal urine sampling because it does not take into account recent drug use by the mother.
    c. Mothers of NAS infants usually do not want the pregnancy or the infant.
    d. The most severe symptoms are observed in the infants of mothers who have taken large amounts of drugs over a long period.

64. Identify the following as true or false.

    _____ Methadone withdrawal in the fetus is less severe than heroine withdrawal.

    _____ The methadone-exposed fetus shows no signs of congenital anomalies.

    _____ The mother using methadone is not allowed to breast-feed her infant.

    _____ Infants exposed to methadone have a higher-than-normal incidence of sudden infant death syndrome.

    _____ Cocaine can affect fetal cardiac function and suppress fetal immune system.

    _____ Infants exposed to cocaine in utero demonstrate immediate untoward effects at birth.

    _____ A higher incidence of preterm delivery and placental abruption are associated with methamphetamine use during pregnancy.

    _____ Infants exposed to methamphetamine in utero have significantly smaller head circumferences and birth weights than those not exposed.

    _____ Marijuana is the most common illicit drug used by women of childbearing age in the United States.

    _____ Marijuana use during pregnancy can result in infants with larger head circumference and developmental delays.

    _____ Fetal alcohol syndrome is the leading cause of cognitive impairment.

    _____ Fetal abnormalities are not related to the amount of the mother's alcohol intake but to the amount of alcohol consumed in excess of the liver's ability to detoxify it.

    _____ It is necessary for the woman wanting to become pregnant to understand that she should stop drinking 3 months before she plans to conceive.

65. The nurse can expect the infant with fetal alcohol syndrome to exhibit:
    a. normal prenatal growth patterns.
    b. normal feeding patterns.
    c. thicker upper lip and longer palpebral fissures.
    d. irritability.

66. When mothers smoke:
    a. their infants will have normal birth weights as long as the number of cigarettes smoked does not exceed one pack per day.
    b. their level of nicotine is higher than that of their newborn.
    c. their breast milk will not be affected.
    d. their rate of preterm births is increased.

67. TORCHS complex is a group of microbial agents that cause similar manifestations in the neonate. Identify what each letter stands for.

    T:

    O:

    R:

    C:

    H:

    S:

68. How can human immunodeficiency virus (HIV) be transmitted from the mother to the infant?

CRITICAL THINKING—CASE STUDY

Baby Mark was born at 36 weeks of gestation and weighed 2300 g (5 lb) at birth. At 1 minute of age, his Apgar score was 5. Mark was suctioned, and oxygen administration was started. He responded with spontaneous respirations. You are the nurse who has been assigned to care for Mark in the special care nursery. His admission vital signs are heart rate 150 beats/min, respirations 56 breaths/min, and axillary temperature of 35.8° C (96.4° F). Mark is placed in a radiant warmer and oxygen administration is continued by oxygen hood.

69. You would classify Baby Mark as a:
    i. full-term infant.
    ii. preterm infant.
    iii. low-birth-weight infant.
    iv. small-for-gestational-age infant.

    a. i and iv
    b. ii and iv
    c. ii and iii
    d. i and iii

70. You identify Mark as being at risk for developing respiratory distress syndrome based on his:
    i. gestational age.
    ii. low Apgar score.
    iii. hypothermia.
    iv. respiratory rate of 56 breaths/min.

    a. i, ii, iii, and iv
    b. i, ii, and iii
    c. ii, iii, and iv
    d. ii and iii

71. The nurse's plan for oxygen administration includes:
    a. frequent suctioning.
    b. frequent assessment to include unobstructed nares.
    c. nipple feeding with respiratory rates of 70 breaths/min and below.
    d. turning off monitor alarms to allow the neonate to rest.

72. Baby Mark's parents are visiting him for the first time. How can the nurse assist the parents in feeling more comfortable in the NICU atmosphere?
    a. Discourage questions of a technical nature.
    b. Tell the parents that Mark is going to be fine.
    c. Explain what is happening with Mark and why he is receiving this type of care.
    d. Leave the parents alone with the infant.

73. The nurse will develop a care plan for Mark that recognizes which of the following as the best expected outcome?
    a. Oxygen is administered correctly, and arterial blood gases are within normal limits.
    b. Monitor for changes in thermal environment.
    c. Record oxygen delivery rates every 2 hours.
    d. Assess respiratory status every hour.

74. Mark has had an apneic episode. What should the nurse include in the documentation of this episode?

CRITICAL THINKING—CASE STUDY

As a nurse in the NICU, you are assigned to care for a 1815-g (4-lb) preterm infant named Maria. In report you learn that Maria is still on gavage feedings and that tomorrow she is scheduled to begin bottle-feeding. If Maria tolerates her bottle-feedings well, she is scheduled to go home in a few days.

75. You observe the infant closely for behaviors that indicate readiness for bottle-feedings. Name these behaviors.

76. Describe how the nurse in the special care nursery should position the preterm infant. When giving parents discharge instructions, how should the nurse instruct the parents to place the infant while sleeping?

11 Conditions Caused by Defects in Physical Development

1. Match each term with its description.

   a. Growth
   b. Hyperplasia
   c. Hypertrophy
   d. Differentiation

   e. Organogenesis
   f. Teratogenesis
   g. Sensitive or critical period

   _____ Prenatal growth process disturbed to produce a structural or functional defect

   _____ Period with which the major impact of environmental factors coincides

   _____ Beginning of all major organ systems

   _____ Process during which cells divide and synthesize new proteins

   _____ Increase in cell number

   _____ Increase in cell size

   _____ Modification and specialization of early cells to form the individual

2. The most typical parental response to the birth of an infant with a physical disability includes:
   a. hostility and bitterness.
   b. disbelief and denial.
   c. strengthening of the psychologic attachment the mother has formed during pregnancy with the unborn child.
   d. establishment of realistic goals.

3. Which of the following actions can the nurse independently implement in the preoperative neonate?
   a. Start a peripheral intravenous line.
   b. Begin administration of prophylactic antibiotics.
   c. Provide accurate information to the newborn's parents regarding what to expect postoperatively.
   d. Begin pain management control.

4. Primary roles of the nurse in the care of an infant born with a physical defect include:
   a. discouraging the parents from talking about the infant.
   b. showing the parents photographs of other infants with similar defects and assuring them the defect can be corrected.
   c. supplying information only as requested by the parents.
   d. supporting and encouraging the parents in their caregiving tasks.

5. Identify the following statements about postoperative care of the neonate as true or false.

   _____ The newborn's poor chest wall stability, along with smaller and more reactive airways, contributes to postoperative respiratory compromise.

   _____ Most postoperative neonates require mechanical ventilation.

   _____ Neonates are highly subject to acidosis and hypoxia and require continuous monitoring of acid-base balance and oxygen status.

   _____ The preterm infant is at high risk for developing respiratory complications from general anesthesia.

   _____ The neonate is particularly sensitive to vagal stimulation, which can be induced by postoperative nasogastric tubes, endotracheal tubes, and suctioning.

   _____ The neonate's risk for rapid fluid shifts can be intensified by stress and loss of fluid during surgical procedures.

   _____ The more preterm or physiologically immature the infant, the more difficult to measure pain response.

6. Critical guidelines for neonatal postoperative care include continuous monitoring of oxygen and acid-base status. What actions would the nurse expect to take to achieve this goal?
   a. Monitor neonatal weight postoperatively and keep accurate intake and output records.
   b. Monitor axillary temperature, blood pressure, and heart rate every 15 minutes × 4, every 30 minutes × 2, every 1 hour × 6, and then every 2 hours for 24 hours.
   c. Monitor surgical site and skin status for drainage, bleeding, and amount of output from tubes.
   d. Monitor pulse oximetry and arterial blood gases.

7. The nurse has completed the physical assessment of an infant and has noticed a cutaneous dimple with dark tufts of hair between L5 and S1. Which of the following medical conditions should the nurse suspect?
   a. Spina bifida occulta
   b. Spina bifida cystica
   c. Meningocele
   d. Cranioschisis

8. Research has shown that supplemental folic acid can reduce the recurrence rates of spina bifida, anencephaly, or encephalocele. How should this supplement be administered?
   a. Daily folic acid dose to 4 mg beginning 1 month before conception and during the first trimester
   b. Daily folic acid dose of 0.4 mg as soon as pregnancy is confirmed
   c. Daily folic acid dose of 4 mg given through the use of multivitamin preparations beginning 1 month before conception and throughout the first trimester
   d. Daily folic acid dose of 4 mg beginning with the confirmation of pregnancy and continuing throughout pregnancy

9. Match each medical condition with its description.

   a. Anencephaly
   b. Myelodysplasia
   c. Myelomeningocele
   d. Hydrocephalus
   e. Cranioschisis
   f. Exancephaly

   g. Encephalocele
   h. Meningocele
   i. Setting-sun sign
   j. Rachischisis or spina bifida
   k. Pierre Robin sequence

   _____ Hernial protrusion of a saclike cyst, containing meninges, spinal fluid, and nerves

   _____ Defect characterized by retroposition of the tongue and mandible

   _____ Condition that results from disturbances in the dynamics of cerebrospinal fluid absorption and flow

   _____ Congenital malformation in which both cerebral hemispheres are absent

   _____ Any malformation of the spinal canal and cord

   _____ Marked by eyes rotated downward with sclera visible above the iris

   _____ Herniation of brain and meninges through a defect in the skull, resulting in a fluid-filled sac

   _____ Total exposure of the brain through a skull defect

   _____ Fissure in the spinal column that leaves the meninges and spinal cord exposed

   _____ Hernial protrusion of saclike cyst of meninges filled with spinal fluid

   _____ Skull defect with tissues protruding

10. The major anomaly associated with myelomeningocele is _____.

11. a. Name two methods by which prenatal neural tube defects can be diagnosed.

   b. When is the best time to perform these diagnostic tests?

12. Therapeutic management that provides the most favorable morbidity and mortality outcomes for the child born with myelomeningocele is:
    a. early physical therapy.
    b. closure of the defect within first 24 hours.
    c. vigorous antibiotic therapy.
    d. splint application to lower extremities.

13. a. What is the management goal for genitourinary function in the infant with myelomeningocele?

    b. What is the goal for the older child with the same condition?

14. Management of the genitourinary function in the patient with myelomeningocele includes clean intermittent catheterization (CIC) and anticholinergic medication. Which of the following statements about their use is correct?
    i. CIC is used to prevent spontaneous voiding.
    ii. Parents are taught to catheterize the infant every 4 hours during the day and once each night.
    iii. Anticholinergic medications enhance sphincter competence.
    iv. Anticholinergic medications reduce detrusor muscle tone and reduce bladder pressure.

    a. i and iii
    b. i and iv
    c. ii and iii
    d. ii and iv

15. Myelomeningocele may be associated with hydrocephalus. What should the nurse assess to identify an infant with hydrocephalus?
    a. Upward eye slanting
    b. Strabismus
    c. Wide or bulging fontanels
    d. Decreased head circumference

16. On delivery of an infant with myelomeningocele, which of the following nursing actions may be contraindicated?
    a. Examination of the membranous cyst for intactness
    b. Diapering the infant
    c. Keeping moist, sterile normal saline dressings on the defect
    d. Keeping infant in the prone position

17. An infant born with spina bifida who needs intermittent urinary catheterization has developed sneezing, wheezing, and a rash over his lower pelvic and genital area. The nurse should suspect this infant has developed:
    a. asthma.
    b. emphysema.
    c. latex allergy.
    d. anaphylaxis.

18. The primary diagnostic tool for detecting hydrocephalus in older infants and children is:
    a. computed tomography or magnetic resonance imaging.
    b. measuring head circumference.
    c. echoencephalography.
    d. ultrasonography.

19. Surgical shunts are often required to provide drainage in the treatment of hydrocephalus. What is the preferred shunt for infants?
    a. Ventriculoperitoneal shunt
    b. Ventriculoatrial shunt
    c. Ventricular bypass
    d. Ventriculopleural shunt

20. The nurse recognizes that the postoperative care of a patient with a shunt should include:
    a. positioning the patient in a head-up position.
    b. continuous pumping of the shunt to assess function.
    c. monitoring for abdominal or peritoneal distention.
    d. positioning the child on the side of the operative site to facilitate drainage.

21. The major complications of ventriculoperitoneal shunts are _____ and

    _____.

22. Posterior fontanel is closed by age _____. Anterior fontanel is closed by age

    _____ to _____ _____.

    Sutures are unable to be separated by intracranial pressure by age _____ to

    _____ _____.

23. Identify the following statements about microcephaly as true or false.

    _____ Microcephaly is defined as a head circumference greater than 5 standard deviations below the mean.

    _____ Primary microcephaly can be caused by an autosomal recessive disorder or a chromosome abnormality.

    _____ Secondary microcephaly can be caused by maternal infection or chemical agents.

    _____ All children with microcephaly have cognitive delays.

    _____ There is no treatment for microcephaly.

    _____ Nursing care is supportive and directed toward helping parents adjust to the infant.

24. Therapeutic management for craniosynostosis is:
    a. placement of ventriculoperitoneal shunt.
    b. removal of neoplasm.
    c. release of fused sutures.
    d. supportive assistance for parents.

25. Nursing care after surgery for the infant with craniosynostosis includes:
    a. careful monitoring of hematocrit and hemoglobin because of expected large blood loss during surgery.
    b. applying ice compresses for 5 minutes every hour because eyelids are often swollen shut.
    c. avoiding sedation and pain medications because neurologic status may be falsely altered.
    d. avoiding supine positioning.

26. In preparing the nursing care plan for the infant born with craniofacial abnormalities, which of the following is true?
    a. Children with this deformity face erroneous assumptions of cognitive impairment.
    b. Abnormalities include deformities involving the skull and facial bones.
    c. A helmet is often required after surgery to protect the operative site and bone grafts for 6 months to 2 years.
    d. All of the above.

27. What positioning instructions should be given to parents of an infant with positional plagiocephaly?

28. In severe cases of positional plagiocephaly, helmet therapy is advised. Describe this.

29. Match each degree of developmental hip dysplasia with its description.

    a. Acetabular dysplasia
    b. Subluxation
    c. Dislocation

    _____ Femoral head remains in contact with the acetabulum, but the head of the femur is partially displaced.

    _____ Femoral head remains in the acetabulum (mildest form).

    _____ Femoral head loses contact with the acetabulum.

30. The nurse observes which of the following signs in the infant with developmental hip dysplasia?
    a. Negative Ortolani test
    b. Asymmetric folds in skin of legs
    c. Lengthening of the limb on the affected side
    d. Limitation in adduction of the leg

31. Match each age-group with the expected therapeutic management for developmental hip dysplasia at that age.

    a. Newborn to 6 months
    b. 6 to 18 months
    c. Older child

    _____ More complex management, including operative reduction and innominate osteotomy procedures designed to construct an acetabular roof

    _____ Use of abduction devices such as Pavlik harness; can also include skin traction, hip spica cast

    _____ Gradual reduction by traction and individualized home traction program followed by attempted closed reduction of the hip

32. Why is the practice of double or triple diapering an infant with developmental dysplasia of the hip no longer recommended?

33. Which of the following is *correct* information to give when instructing parents on how to prevent skin breakdown for an infant in a Pavlik harness?
    a. Avoid massage of skin under the straps.
    b. Place the diaper above the straps.
    c. Put a piece of clothing between the strap and the skin.
    d. Adjust the harness daily as the child grows.

34. Match each skeletal congenital defect with its description or common name.

    a. Achondroplasia
    b. Osteogenesis imperfecta
    c. Pes planus
    d. Pes valgus
    e. Pes varus
    f. Metatarsus valgus

    g. Polydactyly
    h. Genu varum
    i. Genu recurvatum
    j. Klippel-Feil syndrome
    k. Arachnodactyly (Marfan syndrome)

_____ Commonly called "flatfoot"

_____ Inversion of entire foot, with sole resting on the ground

_____ Inherited defect of ossification at the epiphyseal plate, resulting in short limbs, large head, and lordosis

_____ Eversion of entire foot, with sole resting on the ground

_____ Eversion of forefoot, with heel remaining straight

_____ Inherited condition characterized by fragile, brittle bones

_____ Inherited abnormal length of extremities, fingers, toes; hypermobility of joints; defects of chest (pigeon breast) and spine

_____ Commonly called "back knee"

_____ Commonly called "bowleg"

_____ Excessive number of fingers, toes, or both

_____ Characterized by the absence of one or more cervical vertebrae and the fusion of two or more cervical vertebrae

35. Match each congenital clubfoot condition with its description.

a. Talipes varus
b. Talipes valgus
c. Talipes equinus
d. Talipes calcaneus

_____ Eversion, or bending outward

_____ Inversion, or bending inward

_____ Plantar flexion, in which the toes are lower than the heel

_____ Dorsiflexion, in which the toes are higher than the heel

36. Treatment of clubfoot includes:
    a. allowing the child to walk 2 weeks after surgical correction.
    b. surgical intervention at 3 months of age.
    c. casting extremity or extremities until 1 year of age.
    d. serial casting beginning immediately after birth.

37. Match each term with its description.

a. Metatarsus varus
b. Amelia
c. Meromelia
d. Phocomelia
e. Atresia

_____ Deficiency of long bones, with development of hands and feet attached at or near the shoulders; sometimes called "seal limbs"

_____ Absence of complete extremity

_____ Medial adduction of the toes and forefoot

_____ Partial absence of extremity

_____ Absence of a normal opening

38. An important assessment for the nurse to perform in identifying cleft palate is to:
    a. assess sucking ability of infant.
    b. assess color of lips.
    c. palpate the palate with the gloved finger.
    d. do all of the above.

39. Describe long-term problems often experienced by children with cleft lip or cleft palate.

40. Which feeding practices should be used for the infant with a cleft lip or palate?
    a. Use a large, hard nipple with a large hole.
    b. Use a normal nipple and position it sideways in the mouth.
    c. Use a special nipple, positioned so it is compressed by the infant's tongue and existing palate.
    d. Withhold breast-feeding until after surgical correction of the defect.

41. Which of the following is acceptable in providing postoperative care for the infant with a cleft lip or palate?
    a. Use of tongue depressor in the mouth to assess surgical site
    b. Continuous elbow restraints to prevent injury
    c. Placement of infant in the prone position after cleft lip repair
    d. Placement of infant in the prone position after cleft palate repair

42. In preparing the parents of a child with cleft palate, the nurse includes which of the following in the long-term family teaching plan?
    a. Explanation that tooth development will be delayed
    b. Guidelines to use for speech development
    c. Use of decongestants and acetaminophen to care for frequent upper respiratory tract symptoms
    d. All of the above

43. The priority nursing goal in the immediate care of a postoperative infant after repair of a cleft lip is to:
    a. keep the infant well hydrated.
    b. prevent vomiting.
    c. prevent trauma to operative site.
    d. administer medications to prevent drooling.

44. The nurse observes frothy saliva in the mouth and nose of the neonate, as well as frequent drooling. When fed, the infant swallows normally, but suddenly the fluid returns through the infant's nose and mouth. The nurse should suspect what medical condition?
    a. Esophageal atresia
    b. Cleft palate
    c. Anorectal malformation
    d. Biliary atresia

45. Discuss the nurse's role in the assessment of anorectal malformation.

46. The best definition of biliary atresia is:
    a. jaundice persisting beyond 2 weeks of age with elevated direct bilirubin levels.
    b. progressive inflammatory process causing intrahepatic and extrahepatic bile duct fibrosis.
    c. absence of bile pigment.
    d. hepatomegaly and palpable liver.

47. A hernia that is constricted and cannot be reduced manually is referred to as _____.

48. Identify the following statements about umbilical hernia as true or false.

_____ The disorder affects African-Americans more often than it does Caucasians.

_____ It affects preterm infants more than full-term infants.

_____ It may be present in association with Down syndrome.

_____ It is most prominent when the infant is crying.

_____ It usually resolves spontaneously by 3 to 5 years of age.

49. Which of the following is contraindicated as part of the therapeutic management for the neonate with congenital diaphragmatic hernia?
a. Endotracheal intubation
b. Gastrointestinal decompression
c. Positioning the infant with the head and chest elevated above the abdomen
d. Bag and mask ventilation

50. Match each condition with its description.

a. Gastroschisis
b. Omphalocele
c. Phimosis
d. Inguinal hernia
e. Femoral hernia
f. Cryptorchidism

g. Hypospadias
h. Epispadias
i. Hydrocele
j. Bladder extrophy
k. Hydronephrosis
l. Paraphimosis

_____ Prevents retraction of the foreskin

_____ Herniation of the abdominal contents through the umbilical ring

_____ Characterized by herniation lateral to the umbilical ring

_____ Externalization of the bladder

_____ Painless inguinal swelling

_____ Swelling in the groin area associated with severe pain (more common in females)

_____ Characterized by an inability to replace retracted foreskin in its normal position

_____ Fluid in the processus vaginalis

_____ Failure of one or both testes to descend

_____ Condition in which the urethral opening is located below the glans penis or along the ventral surface of the penile shaft

_____ Defect of urinary system characterized by failure of urethral canalization

_____ Distention of the renal pelvis and calyces

51. Identify the primary criteria used to assign gender to an infant born with ambiguous genitalia.

CRITICAL THINKING—CASE STUDY

Jane is a newborn diagnosed with myelomeningocele. She has been admitted to the neonatal intensive care unit (NICU).

52. Which of the following is the primary nursing goal for the care of Jane before surgical correction of the myelomeningocele?
    a. Observing for increasing paralysis
    b. Starting range-of-motion exercises to prevent muscle contractures
    c. Preventing skin breakdown
    d. Limiting environmental stimulus

53. Thirty-six hours after birth, the nurse notes that Jane is irritable and lethargic and has developed an elevated temperature. What should the nurse suspect?
    a. Hydrocephalus
    b. Infection
    c. Latex allergy
    d. Urinary retention

54. Which of the following nursing diagnoses is most relevant to Jane's care?
    a. Altered Bowel Elimination related to neurologic deficits
    b. High Risk for Infection related to the presence of infectious organisms
    c. Altered Nutrition related to immobility
    d. Altered Self-Concept related to physical disability

55. Develop goals related to Jane's care in the NICU.

56. Which of the following is the best way to meet Jane's tactile stimulation needs before repair of the myelomeningocele?
    a. Cuddling Jane frequently and encouraging parents to hold her in their arms
    b. Placing black and white drawings within Jane's view
    c. Caressing and stroking Jane frequently while she is placed on a pillow across her parent's lap
    d. Changing her diaper and dressing frequently

57. Jane has had corrective surgery and is now 6 hours postoperative. The nurse must observe her abdomen closely for

    the development of _____ _____.

58. After closure of the myelomeningocele, Jane's nursing care should include:
    a. measuring the head circumference daily.
    b. keeping external stimulus at a minimum.
    c. keeping strict limitation of leg movement.
    d. withholding breast- or bottle-feedings.

12 Health Promotion of the Infant and Family

1. Match each biologic development term with its description or example.

a. Binocularity	k. Amylase	u. Thermoregulation
b. Depth perception	l. Lipase	v. Thermogenesis
c. Visual preference	m. Trypsin	w. Total body fluid
d. Respiratory rate	n. Suckling	x. Renal structures
e. Heart rate	o. Sucking	y. Endocrine system
f. Sinus arrhythmia	p. Swallowing	z. Righting reflexes
g. Hematopoietic changes	q. Infantile swallow reflex	aa. Crawl position
h. Physiologic anemia	r. Mature swallow reflex	bb. Creeping
i. Digestive process	s. Santmyer swallow	
j. Ptyalin	t. Immunologic system	

_____ Immature at birth; human milk compensates for the first several months

_____ Stereopsis; begins to develop by age 7 to 9 months

_____ Receives a significant amount of maternal protection until infant is about 3 months of age

_____ Begins to slow in infants and is relatively stable

_____ Heart rate that increases with inspiration and decreases with expiration

_____ The fixation of two ocular images into one cerebral picture (fusion); begins to develop by 6 weeks of age and should be well established by age 4 months

_____ The presence of fetal hemoglobin for the first 5 months

_____ For infants, looking at the human face

_____ Caused by high levels of fetal hemoglobin, which is thought to depress the production of erythropoietin

_____ During infancy, this rate slows down, with sinus arrhythmia commonly seen

_____ Amylase; present in small amounts in the newborn but usually has little effect

_____ Deglutition; the ability to collect the food and propel it into the esophagus

_____ The term often used to denote breast-feeding

_____ Propelling forward on hands and knees with belly off floor; usually occurs at around 9 months

_____ Enzyme needed to achieve adult levels of fat absorption

_____ Pancreatic enzyme needed for digestion of complex carbohydrates

_____ Secreted in sufficient quantities to catabolize protein into polypeptides and some amino acids in infants

_____ Appears in utero as early as 15 to 18 weeks of gestation with maturation synchronized with swallowing and breathing patterns by 36 to 38 weeks

_____ Somatic reflex in which the tongue remains behind the central incisors and the mandible no longer thrusts forward; tongue pressure and movement against the hard palate push the food back into the pharynx

_____ Elicit postural responses of flexion or extension that are responsible for motor activities such as rolling over, assuming the crawl position, and maintaining normal head-trunk-limb alignment during activities

_____ Visceral reflex in which food lies in a shallow groove on the top of the tongue and the fluid flows by gravity down the tongue and along the sides of the mouth; efficient for fluids but not for solids

_____ Complete maturity of this system occurs during the latter half of the second year; predisposes the infant to dehydration

_____ Shivering

_____ A special reflex exhibited by infants when a puff of air is directed at the face

_____ Comprises 78% of the body weight at birth

_____ The symmetric tonic neck reflex, which is evoked by flexing or extending the neck, helps the infant assume this position

_____ More efficient during infancy than in the newborn stage

_____ Adequately developed at birth but functions are immature

2. Match each psychosocial development term with its description.

a. Acquiring a sense of trust, overcoming a sense of mistrust
b. Primary narcissism
c. Grasping
d. Biting
e. Cognition
f. Sensorimotor phase
g. Separation

h. Object permanence
i. Symbols
j. Use of reflexes
k. Primary circular reactions
l. Secondary circular reactions
m. Imitation
n. Play
o. Affect
p. Secondary schemas

q. Reactive attachment disorder (RAD)
r. Solitary play
s. Revised Infant Temperament Questionnaire (ITQ)
t. Spoiled child syndrome
u. Weaning
v. Graduated extinction

_____ A stage of the sensorimotor period; lasts until 8 months of age; primary circular reactions are repeated and prolonged for the response that results; phase in which grasping and holding become shaking, banging, and pulling

_____ The phase with which the infant is concerned, according to Erikson

_____ Process of giving up one method of feeding for another; usually refers to relinquishing the breast or bottle for a cup

_____ Reaching out to others; initially reflexive; has powerful social meaning for the parents

_____ Total concern for oneself; at its height in the newborn

_____ The ability to know; most commonly explained by Piaget's theory of development

_____ Mental representations; a major intellectual achievement of the sensorimotor period

_____ Occurs in the second stage of infancy; infants learn they can hold onto what is their own and more fully control their environment; also brings internal relief from teething discomfort and a sense of power or control

_____ A crucial event in the sensorimotor phase, in which infants learn to detach themselves from other objects in the environment

_____ The term used by Piaget to describe the period from birth to 24 months

_____ Marks the beginning of the replacement of reflexive behavior with voluntary acts in the sensorimotor period; occurs from 1 to 4 months; sucking and grasping become deliberate acts to elicit certain responses

_____ The realization that objects which exit the visual field still exist; a major accomplishment for the infant in the sensorimotor phase

_____ Identifies the first stage of the sensorimotor period; the experience of perceiving patterns or ordering; provides a foundation of the subsequent stages

_____ Occurs during the fourth sensorimotor stage of Piaget; characterized by infants using previous behavior achievements as the foundation for adding new skills

_____ Human behavior that requires the differentiation of selected acts from several events; developed by infants in the second half of the first year

_____ The type of play that infants engage in; denotes one-sided play

_____ Activity in which infants take pleasure in performing acts after they have mastered them; consumes most of the infant's waking hours

_____ Excessive self-centered and immature behavior resulting from the failure of parents to enforce consistent age-appropriate limits

_____ Outward manifestation of emotion and feeling; seen as infants begin to develop a sense of permanency

_____ A psychologic and developmental problem that stems from maladaptive or absent attachment between the infant and parent (or caregiver)

_____ Approach to dealing with night crying; to let the child cry for progressively longer times between brief parental interventions that consist only of reassurance

_____ A screening tool that focuses on nine temperament variables

3. Match each child care term with its description.

a. In-home child care
b. Family daycare home
c. Center-based child care
d. Work-based group child care
e. Sick-child care

_____ Available for times when the youngster is ill; often located in community hospitals or in work settings

_____ Usually refers to a licensed daycare facility that provides care for six or more children, for 6 or more hours a day

_____ May consist of a full-time babysitter who lives in the home or comes to the home

_____ An option that is becoming increasingly popular to provide high-quality and convenient child care to employees

_____ Typically provides child care and protection for up to six children for part of a day without informal arrangements such as exchange baby-sitting.

4. Match each immunization term with its description.

a. Attenuate
b. Whole-cell pertussis vaccine
c. Acellular pertussis vaccine
d. Vaccine-associated polio paralysis (VAPP)
e. Vaccination
f. Comvax
g. Vaccine
h. Toxoid

_____ Contains one or more immunogens derived from the *Bordetella pertussis* organism; the highly purified acellular vaccine

_____ Often used interchangeably with the term *immunization,* but these terms are not synonymous

_____ To reduce the virulence of a pathogenic microorganism by treating it or cultivating it on a certain medium

_____ A rare complication of the oral polio vaccine (OPV); prompted the change from the exclusive use of OPV to the exclusive use of inactivated polio vaccine (IPV)

_____ A combination vaccine for *Haemophilus influenzae* that decreases the number of injections the infant receives

_____ A modified bacterial toxin that has been made nontoxic but retains the ability to stimulate the formation of antitoxin

_____ A suspension of live (usually attenuated) or inactivated microorganisms (e.g., bacteria, viruses, rickettsiae) or fractions of the microorganisms administered to induce immunity

_____ Prepared from inactivated cells of *Bordetella pertussis;* contains multiple antigens

5. Match each term with its description related to potential pediatric injury.

   a. Small objects; small food items
   b. Syringe cap
   c. Infant seats, stairs, walkers
   d. Cords

   e. Latex balloons
   f. Bed or crib safety hazards
   g. Plastic bag

   _____ Poses a suffocation danger because it is lightweight and can be easily become wrapped around the head of an active infant

   _____ The leading cause of pediatric choking deaths from children's products

   _____ Common causes of aspiration in infants because they are often small, cylindric, and/or pliable

   _____ A tamper-resistant safety device that can be aspirated and is difficult to locate because it is clear; a potential aspiration hazard when using a syringe to accurately measure and dispense oral liquid medication to young children

   _____ Items that present opportunities for the danger of falling

   _____ Should be less than 30 cm (12 inches) to decrease the risk for strangulation

   _____ Items that pose a number of hazards from suffocation to strangulation

6. If the infant weighs 8 kg at age 5 months, about how many kilograms was his or her probable birth weight?
   a. 7.0
   b. 6.0
   c. 4.0
   d. 15.0

7. If the infant's head circumference is 46 cm at 6 months, how many centimeters would you expect his or her head circumference to be at 8 months?
   a. 46.5
   b. 47
   c. 47.5
   d. 49

8. The infant's posterior fontanel usually closes by:
   a. 6 to 8 weeks.
   b. 3 to 6 months.
   c. 12 to 18 months.
   d. 9 to 12 months.

9. Match each neurologic reflex with its expected behavioral response and with the age of its appearance in infancy. (Each reflex will be used twice.)
   a. Labyrinth righting
   b. Neck righting
   c. Body righting
   d. Otolith righting
   e. Landau
   f. Parachute

Expected Behavioral Response

_____ When infant is suspended in a horizontal prone position and suddenly thrust downward, hand and fingers extend forward as if to protect against falling.

_____ When body of an erect infant is tilted, head is returned to upright erect position.

_____ This is a modification of the neck righting reflex in which turning hips and shoulders to one side causes all other body parts to follow.

_____ When infant is suspended in a horizontal prone position, the head is raised and legs and spine are extended.

_____ While infant is supine, head is turned to one side. Shoulder, trunk, and finally pelvis will turn toward that side.

_____ Infant in prone or supine position is able to raise head.

Age of Appearance

_____ 7 to 12 months; persists indefinitely

_____ 6 months; persists until 24 to 26 months

_____ 2 months; strongest at 10 months

_____ 6 to 8 months; persists until 12 to 24 months

_____ 7 to 9 months; persists indefinitely

_____ 3 months; persists until 24 to 36 months

10. Which of the following statements is true about the proportion of the chest at the end of the infant's first year?
    a. The contour of the chest is more like a neonate's than an adult's.
    b. The anteroposterior diameter is larger than the lateral diameter.
    c. The chest is small in relation to the size of the heart.
    d. The chest circumference is about equal to the head circumference.

11. Of the following characteristics of vision, the one that is developed at the earliest age is:
    a. binocularity.
    b. stereopsis.
    c. corneal reflex.
    d. convergence.

12. The characteristic of the respiratory system that predisposes the infant to middle ear infection is the:
    a. short, angled eustachian tube.
    b. short, straight eustachian tube.
    c. close proximity of the trachea to the bronchi.
    d. size of the lumen of the eustachian tube.

13. The nurse can expect that an infant will begin to respond discriminately to others, particularly the mother, and respond by crying, smiling, and vocalizing at about:
    a. 10 months of age.
    b. 8 months of age.
    c. 2 months of age.
    d. birth.

14. Of the following hematopoietic changes, the one that is considered abnormal in the first 5 months of life is:
    a. low iron levels.
    b. physiologic anemia.
    c. presence of fetal hemoglobin.
    d. low hemoglobin level.

15. All of the following digestive processes are deficient in an infant until about 3 months *except:*
    a. amylase.
    b. lipase.
    c. saliva.
    d. trypsin.

16. The _____ is the most immature of all the gastrointestinal organs throughout infancy.

17. The purpose of nonnutritive sucking is to:
    a. satisfy the basic sucking urge.
    b. take in food.
    c. collect food and propel it into the esophagus.
    d. provide an efficient way to process fluids.

18. Which of the following is a characteristic of the somatic swallow reflex?
    a. The mandible does not thrust forward.
    b. The tongue remains in front of the central incisors.
    c. The tongue is concave and inclined against the palate.
    d. It is efficient for fluids but not for solids.

19. After birth, maximum levels of immunoglobulin A, D, and E in humans are:
    a. reached during infancy.
    b. attained in early childhood.
    c. transferred from the mother.
    d. reached before 9 months of age.

20. During the first 6 months, the infant is gradually better insulated by:
    a. increased shivering.
    b. increased adipose tissue.
    c. dilation of the capillaries.
    d. constriction of the capillaries.

21. The infant is predisposed to a more rapid loss of total body fluid and dehydration because:
    a. of a high proportion of extracellular fluid.
    b. of a high proportion of intracellular fluid.
    c. total body water is at about 40%.
    d. extracellular fluid is 20% of the total.

22. Complete maturity of the kidney occurs:
    a. at birth.
    b. by 6 months.
    c. by 1 year.
    d. by 24 months.

23. Until the renal structures mature, the range of specific gravity for the infant ranges from _____ to

    _____.

24. The expected immaturity of the infant's functioning endocrine system will be demonstrated in the infant's:
    a. growth patterns.
    b. thyroid levels.
    c. homeostatic control.
    d. immunoglobulin levels.

25. Fine motor development is evaluated in the 10-month-old infant by observing the:
    a. ability to stack blocks.
    b. pincer grasp.
    c. righting reflexes.
    d. tonic neck reflex.

26. Of the following characteristics, the one that disappears by about 3 months of age and prevents the infant from rolling over is the:
    a. ability to stack blocks.
    b. pincer grasp.
    c. righting reflexes.
    d. tonic neck reflex.

27. Which of the following assessment findings would be considered most abnormal?
    a. Infant displays head lag at 3 months of age.
    b. The motor quotient is 65.
    c. Infant begins to sit unsupported at 9 months of age.
    d. The motor quotient is 86.

28. If parents are concerned about the fact that their 14-month-old infant is not walking, the nurse should evaluate the cephalocaudal gross motor skill patterns and particularly evaluate whether the infant:
    a. pulls up on the furniture.
    b. uses a pincer grasp.
    c. transfers objects.
    d. has developed object permanence.

29. The factor that best determines the quality of the infant's formulation of trust is the:
    a. quality of the interpersonal relationship.
    b. degree of mothering skill.
    c. quantity of the mother's breast milk.
    d. length of suckling time.

30. According to Piaget's theory of cognitive development, the three crucial events of the sensorimotor phase are:
    a. trust, readjustment, and the regulation of frustration.
    b. separation, object permanence, and mental representation.
    c. imitation, personality development, and temperament.
    d. ordering, comfort, and satisfaction with his or her body.

31. The development of gender identity is reported to begin:
    a. after the first year.
    b. during the phallic stage.
    c. in utero.
    d. at puberty.

32. Parenting:
    a. is an instinctual ability.
    b. is a learned, acquired process.
    c. begins shortly after birth.
    d. shapes the infant's environment positively.

33. Separation anxiety and stranger fear normally begin to appear by:
    a. 4 weeks.
    b. 6 months.
    c. 14 months.
    d. 4 years.

34. A maltreated child who manifests behaviors such as limited eye contact and poor impulse control may be suffering from:
    a. separation anxiety.
    b. stranger fear.
    c. reactive attachment disorder.
    d. spoiled child syndrome.

35. Which of the following play activities would be least appropriate to suggest to parents for their 3-month-old infant?
    a. Provide bright objects.
    b. Use rattles.
    c. Use an infant swing.
    d. Place infant on floor to crawl and roll.

36. Knowledge of the infant's temperament should not be used in helping parents to:
    a. see an organized view of the child's behavior.
    b. choose childrearing techniques.
    c. identify a difficult child.
    d. see their child from a better perspective.

37. If parents are concerned about "spoiling" their child, the nurse should encourage them to respond to the newborn's crying episodes with:
    a. a delayed response of holding the infant.
    b. a prompt response of holding the infant.
    c. letting the infant cry a little.
    d. maintaining a feeding schedule.

38. Which of the following examples provides the best evidence that the child is being spoiled by the parents?
    a. The child who has a difficult temperament and a short attention span
    b. The toddler who has a temper tantrum
    c. The infant who has colic
    d. The child who always exhibits intrusive manipulative behavior

39. Limit setting and discipline should begin in:
    a. middle childhood or adolescence.
    b. infancy, with voice tone and eye contact.
    c. early infancy, with voice tone and eye contact.
    d. infancy, with time-out in a chair for misbehavior.

40. In guiding parents who are choosing a daycare center, the nurse should stress that state licensure represents a program that maintains:
    a. optimal care.
    b. health features.
    c. minimum requirements.
    d. safety features.

41. To decrease dependence on nonnutritive sucking in young infants, the best strategy for the nurse to recommend would be to:
    a. provide a homemade pacifier.
    b. prolong the time the infant is fed.
    c. restrain the sucking fingers.
    d. prohibit the use of a pacifier.

42. A 12-month-old infant would be likely to have:
    a. 2 teeth.
    b. 4 teeth.
    c. 6 teeth.
    d. 12 teeth.

43. Which of the following techniques is recommended to assist in weaning an infant?
    a. Gradually replace one bottle-feeding or breast-feeding at a time.
    b. Always wean to a bottle first.
    c. Always wean directly to a cup.
    d. Eliminate the nighttime feeding first.

44. From birth to 6 months of age, the breast-feeding mother should supplement the breast milk with:
    a. formula.
    b. nothing.
    c. water.
    d. vitamin D.

45. The greatest threat to successful breast-feeding for the employed mother is:
    a. lack of feeding options.
    b. danger of bacterial contamination.
    c. fatigue.
    d. inefficient breast pumping.

46. Which of the following is not acceptable because of the risk for falls?
    a. Using a changing table
    b. Keeping necessary articles within easy reach
    c. Changing the infant's diaper on the floor
    d. Using an infant walker to strengthen walking muscles

47. The primary reason for introducing solid food to infants is to:
    a. increase their overall caloric intake.
    b. provide a substitute for the milk source.
    c. introduce a taste and chewing experience.
    d. increase their weight.

48. If sweetening of the infant's home-prepared foods is performed, the risk for botulism can be avoided by using:
    a. honey.
    b. corn syrup.
    c. refined sugar.
    d. none of the above.

49. Studies have shown that excessive fruit juice consumption increases the likelihood of:
    a. growth problems.
    b. scurvy.
    c. rickets.
    d. nursing caries.

50. When introducing new food, the parents should not:
    a. decrease the quantity of the infant's milk.
    b. mix food with formula to feed through a nipple.
    c. introduce new foods in small amounts.
    d. offer the new food by itself at first.

51. Which of the following techniques is recommended to provide atraumatic care for immunization administration to infants?
    a. Select a 25-mm needle to deposit vaccine deep into the muscle mass.
    b. Use an air bubble to clear the needle before injection.
    c. Use the deltoid muscle.
    d. Use the EMLA patch before administration.

52. Match each sleep disturbance with its management technique.

   a. Nighttime feeding
   b. Developmental night crying
   c. Trained night crying
   d. Refusal to go to sleep
   e. Nighttime fears

   _____ Check at progressively longer intervals each night.

   _____ Keep a night-light on.

   _____ Reassure parents that this is a temporary phase.

   _____ Establish a consistent prebedtime routine.

   _____ Put infant to bed awake.

53. To prevent aspiration in the infant, the nurse should avoid using:
   a. baby powder made from cornstarch.
   b. pacifiers made from padded nipples.
   c. syringes to dispense oral medication.
   d. pacifiers with one-piece construction.

54. Which of the following items is the children's product that is a leading cause of pediatric choking deaths?
   a. Plastic garment bags
   b. Ill-fitting crib slats
   c. Latex balloons
   d. Ill-fitting crib mattresses

55. Which of the following situations involving cords would be considered least hazardous?
   a. A bib that is not removed at bedtime
   b. A pacifier that is hung around the infant's neck with a 10-inch string
   c. A play telephone with a 10-inch cord
   d. A toy tied to the playpen with a 15-inch ribbon

56. The best place for the infant car restraint is in the:
   a. back seat of the car, facing back.
   b. back seat of the car, facing front.
   c. front passenger seat of the car, with an air bag, facing front.
   d. front passenger seat of the car without an air bag, facing back.

CRITICAL THINKING—CASE STUDY

Jennifer Klein, a 5-month-old infant, is admitted to the pediatric unit with bronchiolitis. Both of the parents work, and Jennifer attends daycare. Jennifer is the first child, and the parents seem anxious about the admission, as well as about her care at home and her normal development. It is clear that the parents need information about general health promotion for their infant.

57. Place a check next to each of the following areas that should be assessed to determine the status of the parents' current health promotion practices. (Check all that apply.)

   _____ Respiratory status (lung sounds)

   _____ Nutrition

   _____ Fever patterns

   _____ Sleep and activity

   _____ Number and condition of teeth

   _____ Fluid and hydration status

   _____ Condition of the mucous membranes of the mouth

   _____ Immunization status

   _____ Safety precautions used in the home

58. Which of the following nursing diagnoses would be used most often for health promotion related to development in an infant of Jennifer's age?
    a. Activity Intolerance
    b. Ineffective Thermoregulation
    c. High Risk for Injury
    d. Altered Parenting

59. Of the following strategies, the one used most often to help new parents like Jennifer's adjust to the parenting role is:
    a. parenting classes.
    b. anticipatory guidance.
    c. first aid courses.
    d. cardiopulmonary resuscitation courses.

60. By the time Jennifer is ready for discharge, the nurse concludes that her parents have achieved improved parenting skills. Which of the following would best confirm the plan's success?
    a. Jennifer is afebrile.
    b. Reports from the other staff are positive.
    c. Verbalizations from the parents indicate that they understand.
    d. A home visit demonstrates that positive changes have occurred.

13 Health Problems During Infancy

1. The following terms are related to nutritional disturbances and feeding difficulties. Match each term with its description.

   a. Atopy
   b. Lactase
   c. Congenital lactase deficiency
   d. Sensitization
   e. Lacto-ovo vegetarians
   f. Vegans
   g. Macrobiotics
   h. MyPyramid

   i. Dietary reference intakes (DRIs)
   j. Spitting up
   k. Late-onset lactase deficiency
   l. Diarrhea
   m. Regurgitation
   n. Food allergy
   o. Oral allergy syndrome
   p. Allergens

   _____ More restrictive than pure vegetarians in that cereals, especially brown rice, are the mainstay of the diet

   _____ Pure vegetarians who eliminate any food of animal origin, including milk and eggs

   _____ Allergy with a hereditary tendency

   _____ An interactive dietary guide that aims to simplify food choices designed to decrease fat and empty calorie intake and increase consumption of grains and vegetables

   _____ Those who exclude meat from their diet but eat milk and eggs and rarely fish

   _____ Quantitative estimates of nutrient requirements for planning and evaluating diets for healthy infants; involves four categories, including estimated average (EA) requirements for age and gender categories, tolerable upper-limit (TUL) nutrient intakes that are associated with a low risk of adverse effects, adequate intakes (AIs) of nutrients, and new standard recommended dietary allowances (RDAs)

   _____ A major factor in malnutrition in many developing and underdeveloped nations

   _____ Hypersensitivity; refers to those reactions to food that involve immunologic mechanisms, usually immunoglobulin E (IgE)

   _____ Lactose intolerance that occurs when the intestinal lumen is damaged, causing a decrease in or destruction of the enzyme lactase

   _____ Occurs when a food allergen (commonly fruits and vegetables) is ingested and subsequent edema and pruritus develop, involving the lips, tongue, palate, and throat; recovery from symptoms usually is rapid

   _____ An enzyme needed for the digestion of lactose in the small intestine

   _____ Return of undigested food from the stomach, usually accompanied by burping

   _____ Usually involve proteins capable of inducing IgE antibody formation

   _____ Dribbling of unswallowed formula from the infant's mouth immediately after a feeding

   _____ The initial exposure of an individual to an allergen, resulting in an immune response, after which subsequent exposure induces a much stronger response that is clinically apparent

   _____ A rare disorder that appears soon after the infant has consumed lactose-containing milk; an inborn error of metabolism that involves the complete absence or severely reduced presence of lactase

2. An instrument that could be used to assess failure to thrive and is designed to assess the feeding interaction of infants up to 12 months of age is the _____ _____ _____ _____

   _____ _____ _____ .

3. In the United States, vitamin D deficiency is most likely to occur in an infant who:
   a. belongs to a low socioeconomic group.
   b. consumes yogurt as the primary milk source.
   c. had measles in the neonatal period.
   d. has the diagnosis of rheumatoid arthritis.

4. When hypervitaminosis is suspected, of the following vitamins, which would be most likely to present problems for the infant or child?
   a. Folate
   b. Vitamin A
   c. Biotin
   d. Vitamin C

5. Vitamin A deficiency has been reported with increased morbidity and mortality in children:
   a. with sickle cell disease.
   b. exposed to environmental tobacco smoke.
   c. with measles.
   d. who are breast-fed.

6. The greatest concern with minerals is:
   a. deficiency.
   b. excess, causing toxicity.
   c. nervous system disturbances from excess.
   d. hemochromatosis.

7. Match each type of vegetarianism with its description.
   a. Lacto-ovo vegetarianism
   b. Lactovegetarianism
   c. Pure vegetarianism (veganism)
   d. Macrobiotics
   e. Semivegetarianism

   _____ This group eliminates any food of animal origin, including milk and eggs.
   _____ This group is the most restrictive of all. Only small amounts of fruits, vegetables, and legumes are consumed.
   _____ This group excludes meat from their diet but eats milk, eggs, and sometimes fish.
   _____ This group excludes meat and eggs but drinks milk.
   _____ This group consumes a lacto-ovo vegetarian diet with the addition of some fish and poultry.

8. Children on strict vegetarian and macrobiotic diets should be evaluated for _____ _____
   _____, _____ _____, and _____.

9. List the four categories of the dietary reference intakes (DRIs).

10. Adequate intakes (AIs), a category of the dietary reference intakes, are based on nutrient intake of:
    a. preterm breast-fed infants.
    b. preterm bottle-fed infants.
    c. full-term breast-fed infants.
    d. full-term bottle-fed infants.

11. To ensure the most complete protein, a strictly vegetarian family should combine:
    a. milk and chicken.
    b. sunflower seeds and rice.
    c. rice and red beans.
    d. eggs and cheese.

12. In the United States, protein and energy malnutrition (PEM) occurs where:
    a. the food supply is inadequate.
    b. the food supply may be adequate.
    c. the adults eat first, leaving insufficient food for children.
    d. the diet consists mainly of starch grains.

13. Kwashiorkor occurs in populations where:
    a. the food supply is inadequate.
    b. the food supply is adequate for protein.
    c. the adults eat first, leaving insufficient food for children.
    d. the diet consists mainly of starch grains.

14. Childhood nutritional marasmus usually results in populations where:
    a. the food supply is inadequate.
    b. the food supply is adequate for protein.
    c. the adults eat first, leaving insufficient food for children.
    d. the diet consists mainly of starch grains.

15. Kwashiorkor, PEM, and marasmus would be least likely to be managed by:
    a. providing a high-protein, high-carbohydrate diet.
    b. replacing fluids and electrolytes.
    c. providing a high-fiber, high-fat diet.
    d. providing for essential physiologic needs.

16. Which of the following foods would be considered the least allergenic?
    a. Orange juice
    b. Eggs
    c. Bread
    d. Rice

17. Sensitivity to cow's milk in an infant may be manifested clinically by:
    a. irritability.
    b. excessive crying.
    c. vomiting and diarrhea.
    d. all of the above.

18. Which of the following diagnostic strategies is the most definitive for identifying a milk allergy?
    a. Stool analysis for blood
    b. Serum IgE levels
    c. Challenge testing with milk
    d. Skin testing

19. The American Academy of Pediatrics recommends treating cow's milk allergy in infants by changing the formula to:
    a. soy formula.
    b. goat's milk.
    c. casein hydrolysate formula.
    d. milk pretreated with microbial-derived lactase.

20. Which of the following is a less expensive alternative to hydrolyzed formulas and may be recommended by health care providers for cow's milk allergy?
    a. Yogurt
    b. Soy formula
    c. Elecare formula
    d. Goat's milk

21. Congenital lactase deficiency is:
    a. a rare form of lactose intolerance.
    b. the form of lactose intolerance associated with giardiasis.
    c. an intolerance that is manifested later in life.
    d. a form of lactose intolerance caused by intestinal damage.

22. Late-onset lactase deficiency is also known as:
    a. congenital lactase deficiency.
    b. secondary lactase deficiency.
    c. primary lactase deficiency.
    d. congenital lactase intolerance.

23. One strategy for parents of infants with lactase deficiency would be to:
    a. substitute human milk for cow's milk.
    b. substitute soy-based formula for human milk.
    c. drink milk alone without other food or drink.
    d. substitute frozen yogurt for fresh yogurt.

24. If allergy to cow's milk is suspected as the cause of an infant's colic, the parents should:
    a. try substituting casein hydrolysate formula.
    b. try substituting soy formula.
    c. be reassured that the symptoms will disappear spontaneously at about 3 months of age.
    d. be assessed for areas of improper feeding techniques.

25. A positive association has been demonstrated between colic and:
    a. carbohydrate malabsorption.
    b. excessive air swallowing.
    c. colonic fermentation.
    d. infant temperament.

26. Which of the following phrases best defines *spitting up?*
    a. It is the return of undigested food from the stomach, usually accompanied by burping.
    b. It is abdominal pain or cramping that is manifested by loud crying and drawing the legs up to the abdomen.
    c. It is the dribbling of unswallowed formula from the infant's mouth immediately after a feeding.
    d. It is the same as vomiting.

27. Other terms for *failure to thrive* include:
    a. growth failure and pediatric undernutrition.
    b. growth failure and organic failure to thrive.
    c. pediatric undernutrition and nonorganic failure to thrive.
    d. organic failure to thrive and nonorganic failure to thrive.

28. List at least three etiologic factors associated with growth failure.

29. Which of the following categories of failure to thrive is based on pathophysiology rather than etiology?
    a. Growth failure related to inadequate caloric intake
    b. Growth failure related to inadequate absorption
    c. Growth failure related to increased metabolism
    d. All of the above

30. If failure to thrive has been a longstanding problem, the infant will show evidence of:
    a. both weight and height being depressed.
    b. weight depression only.
    c. height depression only.
    d. neither height nor weight depression.

31. One important strategy for feeding a child with failure to thrive would be to:
    a. avoid having the same nurse feed the child.
    b. distract the child during meals with television and toys.
    c. maintain a calm, even temperament during feedings.
    d. vary the feeding routines to make the feeding time more interesting.

32. To increase the caloric intake of an infant with failure to thrive, the nurse might recommend:
    a. using developmental stimulation by a specialist during feedings.
    b. avoiding solids until after the bottle is well accepted.
    c. being persistent through 10 to 15 minutes of food refusal.
    d. varying the schedule for routine activities on a daily basis.

33. The incidence of diaper dermatitis is generally reported as greater in bottle-fed infants than in breast-fed infants because in breast-fed infants there is a lower:
    a. ammonia content in the urine.
    b. pH content of the feces.
    c. microbial content of the feces.
    d. number of stools per day.

34. Parents of an infant with diaper dermatitis should be encouraged to:
    a. wash the skin frequently.
    b. mix zinc oxide thoroughly with antifungal cream.
    c. use a hand-held dryer on the open lesions.
    d. use diapers with super-absorbent gel.

35. Seborrheic dermatitis is usually not manifested as:
    a. eczema.
    b. cradle cap.
    c. blepharitis.
    d. otitis externa.

36. Which of the following recommendations for the care of atopic dermatitis is controversial?
    a. Apply emollient within the first few minutes after bathing.
    b. Apply cool wet compresses to sooth the skin.
    c. Limit the infant's exposure to allergens.
    d. Administer antihistamines to control pruritus.

37. Identify the following statements as true or false.

    _____ The incidence of sudden infant death syndrome (SIDS) is associated with diphtheria, tetanus, and pertussis vaccines.

    _____ Maternal smoking during and after pregnancy has been implicated as a contributor to SIDS.

    _____ Parents should be advised to position their infants on their abdomen to prevent SIDS.

    _____ The nurse should encourage the parents to sleep in the same bed as the infant who is being monitored for apnea of infancy in order to detect subtle clinical changes.

    _____ To prevent SIDS, parents should avoid using soft, moldable mattresses and pillows in the bed.

CRITICAL THINKING—CASE STUDY

Six-month-old Jason has come to the office today for his routine immunizations. His mother says she thinks everything is just fine, except that Jason seems to have a lot of food intolerances. The nurse continues the assessment and finds that Jason is eating many of the food items the rest of the family eats, including milk products in very small amounts. There is no particular pattern to the way the new foods are being introduced. Jason exhibits a variety of symptoms related to skin irritations. He is developing rashes around his mouth and rectum and elsewhere on his body when he eats certain foods.

38. Based on the prevalence of the common health problems of infancy, what areas should the nurse include in an initial assessment of a 6-month-old?
    a. Nutrition
    b. Temperament
    c. Sleep patterns
    d. All of the above

39. Based on the data from the assessment interview, which of the following goals is best for the nurse to establish?
    a. To prevent outbreaks of food allergy
    b. To prevent death from anaphylaxis
    c. To prevent genetic transmission
    d. All of the above

40. Which of the following recommendations would be most appropriate for Jason's mother?
    a. Reconsider breast-feeding.
    b. Eliminate cow's milk.
    c. Add only one new food at each 5-day interval.
    d. Eliminate solids until 9 months of age.

41. At an earlier visit, the nurse had determined that there was altered parenting related to lack of knowledge in Jason's family. Which of the following outcome criteria would help the nurse evaluate the mother's ability to provide a constructive environment for Jason?
    a. Jason's mother is able to identify eating patterns that contribute to symptoms.
    b. Jason's mother is able to share her feelings regarding her parenting skills.
    c. Jason's mother is able to practice appropriate precautions to prevent infection.
    d. Jason's mother is able to identify the rationale for prevention of the skin rashes.

14 Health Promotion of the Toddler and Family

1. Match each term with its description.

a. Terrible twos
b. Weight
c. Height
d. Head circumference
e. Chest circumference
f. Autonomy versus doubt and shame
g. Negativism
h. Ritualism
i. Ego
j. Id
k. Superego
l. Tertiary circular reactions
m. New means through mental combinations
n. Domestic mimicry
o. Egocentrism

p. Preoperational phase
q. Egocentric speech
r. Collective monologue
s. Socialized speech
t. Preoperational thinking
u. Operations
v. Punishment and obedience orientation
w. Separation
x. Individuation
y. Parallel play
z. Toddler Behavior Assessment Questionnaire
aa. Sibling rivalry
bb. Regression
cc. Fears

_____ Imitation of household activity

_____ The average at 2 years of age is 86.6 cm (34 inches)

_____ Refers to the toddler years; period from 12 to 36 months of age

_____ Increases in size during the toddler years; also changes shape

_____ The persistent negative response to requests; characteristic of the toddler's behavior

_____ The average at 2 years of age is 12 kg (26.5 lb)

_____ The developmental task of the toddler years

_____ The toddler's need to maintain sameness and reliability; provides a sense of comfort

_____ The impulsive part of the psyche

_____ The fifth stage of the sensorimotor phase of development, when the child uses active experimentation to achieve previously unattainable goals

_____ May be thought of as reason or common sense during the toddler phase of psychosocial development

_____ The conscience

_____ Growth slows somewhat at the end of infancy; total increase during the second year is 2.5 cm (1 inch).

_____ The final sensorimotor stage that occurs during ages 19 to 24 months

_____ The inability to envision situations from perspectives other than one's own

_____ Consists of repeating words and sounds for the pleasure of hearing oneself and is not intended to communicate

_____ The ability to manipulate objects in relation to each other in a logical fashion

_____ Spans ages 2 to 7 years; characterized by egocentrism, transductive reasoning, magical thinking, and inability to conserve

_____ Those achievements that mark children's assumption of their individual characteristics in the environment

_____ The child's emergence from a symbiotic fusion with the mother

_____ Playing alongside, not with, other children

_____ Egocentric speech that reflects the child's lingering self-centeredness

_____ The natural jealousy and resentment of children to a new child in the family

_____ Common during the toddler stage; includes problems with sleep, animals, engines, strangers, and separation

_____ Implies that children think primarily based on their own perception of an event; phase in which problem solving is based on what children see or hear directly, rather than on what they recall about objects and events

_____ A retreat from a present pattern of functioning to past levels of behavior; usually occurs in instances of stress, when the child attempts to cope by reverting to patterns of behavior that were successful in earlier stages of development; common in toddlers

_____ One of the two types of speech used by children in the toddler years; used for communication; egocentric in that children communicate about themselves to others

_____ Tool that assists in identifying temperamental characteristics; reliable instrument used to assess toddler temperament and behaviors

_____ The most basic level of moral judgment, in which an action is judged as good or bad depending on whether it results in reward or punishment

2. Match each term with its description.

a. Booster
b. Plaque
c. Dental caries
d. Periodontal disease
e. Scrub method
f. Padded shield

g. Swish-and-swallow method
h. Fluorosis
i. Nursing caries
j. Convertible restraint
k. Five-point harness

_____ Device that depends on the vehicle belts to hold the child in place

_____ Baby bottle caries; early childhood caries; occurs when the child is placed in the crib or bed with a bottle of milk, juice, soda pop, or sweetened water at nap or bedtime or uses the bottle as a pacifier while awake

_____ A harness system that consists of a strap over each shoulder, one on each side of the pelvis, and one between the legs

_____ May be used to clean teeth when brushing is impractical

_____ A car seat that is suitable for infants in the rearward-facing position and for toddlers in the forward-facing position

_____ A condition characterized by an increase in the degree and extent of the enamel's porosity as a result of excessive fluoride ingestion by young children

_____ A brushing technique in which the tips of the bristles are placed firmly at a 45-degree angle against the teeth and gums and are moved back and forth in a vibratory motion; suitable for cleaning primary teeth

_____ A harness system that uses shoulder straps attached to a shield held in place by a crotch strap

_____ Tooth decay

_____ Gum disease

_____ Soft bacterial deposits that adhere to the teeth and cause decay

3. If the chest circumference of a toddler at age 1 to 2 years is 50 cm, what would you expect the head circumference to be?
   a. 25 cm
   b. 35 cm
   c. 50 cm
   d. 60 cm

4. Which of the following characteristics most predispose toddlers to frequent infections?
   a. Short, straight internal ear canal and large lymph tissue
   b. Slower pulse and respiratory rate and higher blood pressure
   c. Abdominal respirations
   d. Less efficient defense mechanisms

5. One of the most important digestive system changes completed during the toddler period is the:
   a. increased acidity of the gastric contents.
   b. voluntary control of the sphincters.
   c. protective function of the gastric contents.
   d. increased capacity of the stomach.

6. Which of the following statements is most characteristic of a 24-month-old child in regard to motor development?
   a. Motor skills are fully developed but occur in isolation from the environment.
   b. The toddler walks alone, but falls easily.
   c. The toddler's activities begin to produce purposeful results.
   d. The toddler is able to grasp small objects, but cannot release them at will.

7. Using Erikson's theory as a foundation, the primary developmental task of the toddler period is to:
   a. satisfy the need for basic trust.
   b. achieve a sense of accomplishment.
   c. learn to give up dependence for independence.
   d. acquire language or mental symbolism.

8. Piaget's theory of cognitive development depicts the toddler as a child who:
   a. repeatedly explores the same object each time it appears in a new place.
   b. is able to transfer information from one situation to another.
   c. has a persistent negative response to any request.
   d. has the rudimentary beginning of a superego.

9. The principal characteristics of Piaget's preoperational phase are:
   i. dependence on perception in problem solving.
   ii. egocentric use of language.
   iii. the ability to manipulate objects in relation to one another in a logical way.
   iv. the ability to solve problems based on what is recalled about objects and events.

   a. i, ii, and iii
   b. i and ii
   c. ii and iii
   d. ii, iii, and iv

10. Match each characteristic of preoperational thought with its description.

   a. Egocentrism   e. Animism
   b. Transductive reasoning   f. Irreversibility
   c. Global organization   g. Magical thinking
   d. Centration   h. Inability to conserve

   _____ Focusing on one aspect rather than considering all possible alternatives

   _____ Inability to envision situations from perspectives other than one's own

   _____ Inability to undo the actions initiated physically

   _____ Attributing lifelike qualities to inanimate objects

   _____ Thinking from the particular to the particular

   _____ Lack of understanding that a mass can be changed in size, shape, volume, or length without losing or adding to the original mass

   _____ Belief that thoughts are all-powerful and can cause events

   _____ Belief that changing any one part of the whole changes the entire whole

11. According to Kohlberg, the best way to discipline children is to:
    a. use a punishment and obedience orientation.
    b. withhold privileges.
    c. use power to control behavior.
    d. give explanations and help the child to change.

12. By the age of 3, the toddler generally:
    a. has clear body boundaries.
    b. participates willingly in most procedures.
    c. has as sense of maleness and femaleness.
    d. is unable to learn correct terms for body parts.

13. Which of the following skills is not necessary for the toddler to acquire before separation and individuation can be achieved?
    a. Object permanence
    b. Lack of anxiety during separations from parents
    c. Delayed gratification
    d. Ability to tolerate a moderate amount of frustration

14. The usual number of words acquired by the age of 2 years is:
    a. 50.
    b. 100.
    c. 300.
    d. 500.

15. The 2-year-old child living in a bilingual environment can:
    a. have advanced speaking ability without adequate comprehension.
    b. have advanced speaking ability along with advanced comprehension.
    c. achieve early linguistic milestones in each language at the same time.
    d. have delayed speaking without adequate comprehension.

16. As the child moves through the toddler period, there is a decrease in the frequency of:
    a. solitary play.
    b. imitative play.
    c. tactile play.
    d. parallel play.

17. List at least five characteristics of an 18- to 24-month-old child that would indicate readiness for toilet training.

18. Of the following techniques, which is the best to use when toilet training a toddler?
    a. Limit sessions to 5 to 8 minutes of practice.
    b. Remove child from the bathroom to flush the toilet.
    c. Ensure the toddler's privacy during the sessions.
    d. Place the potty chair near a television to help distract the child during the sessions.

19. Which of the following statements is false in regard to toilet training?
    a. Bowel training is usually accomplished after bladder training.
    b. Nighttime bladder training is usually accomplished after bowel training.
    c. The toddler who is impatient with soiled diapers is demonstrating readiness for toilet training.
    d. Fewer wet diapers signals that the toddler is physically ready for toilet training.

20. Of the following strategies, which is most appropriate for parents to use to prepare a toddler for the birth of a sibling?
    a. Explain the upcoming birth as early in the pregnancy as possible.
    b. Move the toddler to his or her own new room.
    c. Provide a doll for the toddler to imitate parenting.
    d. Tell the toddler that a new playmate will come home soon.

21. The best approach to stop a toddler's attention-seeking behavior of a tantrum with violent head banging is to:
    a. ignore the behavior.
    b. provide time-out.
    c. offer a toy to calm the child.
    d. protect the child from injury.

22. Of the following techniques, which is the best one to deal with the negativism of the toddler?
    a. Quietly and calmly ask the child to comply.
    b. Provide few or no choices for the child.
    c. Provide choices.
    d. Remain serious and intent.

23. Which of the following statements about stress in toddlers is true?
    a. Toddlers are rarely exposed to stress or the results of stress.
    b. Any stress is destructive because toddlers have a limited ability to cope.
    c. Most children are exposed to a stress-free environment.
    d. Small amounts of stress help toddlers develop effective coping skills.

24. List three sources of increased stress in toddlers.

25. Regression in toddlers occurs when there is:
    a. stress.
    b. a threat to their autonomy.
    c. a need to revert to dependency.
    d. all the above.

26. Which of the following statements is true in regard to nutritional changes from the infant to the toddler years?
    a. Growth rate increases.
    b. Caloric requirements decrease.
    c. Protein requirements are low.
    d. Fluid requirements increase.

27. Fluid requirement in toddlers represent:
    a. an increase in intracellular fluid.
    b. an increase in relative total body water.
    c. a decrease in intracellular fluid.
    d. an increase in fluid needs.

28. Which nutritional requirement may be difficult to meet in the toddler years?
    a. Calories
    b. Proteins
    c. Minerals
    d. Fluids

29. Physiologic anorexia in toddlers is characterized by:
    a. strong taste preferences.
    b. extreme changes in appetite from day to day.
    c. heightened awareness of social aspects of meals.
    d. all of the above.

30. Healthy ways of serving food to toddlers include:
    a. establishing a pattern of sitting at a table for meals.
    b. permitting nutritious nibbling in lieu of meals.
    c. discouraging between-meal snacking.
    d. all of the above.

31. Developmentally, most children at 12 months:
    a. use a spoon adeptly.
    b. relinquish the bottle voluntarily.
    c. eat the same food as the rest of the family.
    d. reject all solid food in preference for the bottle.

32. The best approach to use for the toddler who prefers the bottle to all solid food is to:
    a. require the toddler to eat something.
    b. allow the toddler to give up the bottle when ready.
    c. withhold all food and water until the child takes solids.
    d. puree the solids and feed them through the bottle.

33. For a toddler with sleep problems, the nurse should suggest:
    a. using a transitional object.
    b. varying the bedtime ritual.
    c. eliminating all bedtime snacks.
    d. all of the above.

34. Which of the following would be an inappropriate method to help a toddler adjust to the initial dental checkup?
    a. Explain to the child that a checkup won't hurt.
    b. Have the child observe his or her sibling's examination.
    c. Have the child perform a checkup on a doll.
    d. Ask the dentist to reserve a thorough examination for another visit.

35. The most effective way to clean a toddler's teeth is:
    a. for the child to brush regularly with toothpaste of his or her choice.
    b. for the parent to stabilize the chin with one hand and brush with the other.
    c. for the parent to brush the mandibular occlusive surfaces, leaving the rest for the child.
    d. for the parent to brush all except the mandibular occlusive surfaces.

36. Flossing is necessary:
    a. to remove plaque from below the gum margin.
    b. to remove debris from between the teeth.
    c. to reach areas where brushing is ineffective.
    d. all of the above.

37. Adequate fluoride ingestion:
    a. prevents gingivitis.
    b. prevents fluorosis.
    c. helps retain enamel protein.
    d. reduces the amount of plaque.

38. To prevent fluorosis, parents of toddlers should use all of the following strategies except:
    a. supervise the use of toothpaste.
    b. use fluoride rinses.
    c. store fluoride products out of reach.
    d. administer fluoride on an empty stomach.

39. One example of a treat that may damage the teeth is:
    a. aged cheese.
    b. celery sticks.
    c. sugarless gum.
    d. a handful of raisins.

40. Nursing bottle caries can result from:
    a. using a pacifier.
    b. feeding the last bottle just before bedtime.
    c. long, frequent nocturnal breast-feeding.
    d. all of the above.

41. Match each example of developmental status in a young child with its associated safety precaution that could be used to prevent injury.

    a. Has unrefined depth perception
    b. Is able to open most containers
    c. Has a great curiosity

    d. Walks, runs, and moves quickly
    e. Puts things in mouth
    f. Pulls on objects

    _____ Do not allow child to play near curb or parked cars.

    _____ Choose large toys without sharp edges.

    _____ Supervise closely at all times, especially near water.

    _____ Turn pot handles toward back of stove.

    _____ Remove unsecured or scatter rugs.

    _____ Know the number of the poison control center.

42. _____ _____ injuries cause more accidental deaths in all pediatric age-groups.

43. Children should use convertible car restraints until they:
    a. weigh 40 lb.
    b. reach the age of 1 year.
    c. reach the age of 8 years.
    d. weigh 60 lb.

44. The car restraint that consists of a standardized anchorage system uses a:
    a. five-point harness.
    b. convertible safety seat.
    c. universal child safety seat.
    d. belt-positioning model.

45. One of the best ways to prevent drowning in the toddler group is for parents to:
    a. learn cardiopulmonary resuscitation (CPR).
    b. supervise children whenever they are near any source of water.
    c. enroll the toddler in a swimming program.
    d. all of the above.

46. Prevention strategies have removed near-drowning as one of the leading causes of a vegetative state in children.
    a. True
    b. False

47. Burn injuries in the toddler age-group are most often the result of:
    a. flame burns from playing with matches.
    b. scald burn from hot liquids.
    c. hot object burns from cigarettes or irons.
    d. electric burns from electrical outlets.

48. The most fatal type of burn in the toddler age-group is:
    a. flame burn from playing with matches.
    b. scald burn from hot liquids.
    c. hot object burn from cigarettes or irons.
    d. electric burn from electrical outlets.

49. Poisonings in toddlers can be best prevented by:
    a. consistently using safety caps.
    b. storing poisonous substances in a locked cabinet.
    c. keeping ipecac syrup in the home.
    d. storing poisonous substances out of reach.

50. The parents should consider moving the toddler from the crib to a bed after the toddler:
    a. reaches the age of 2 years.
    b. will stay in the bed all night.
    c. reaches a height of 35 inches.
    d. is able to sleep through the night.

51. For each of the following potentially hazardous categories, give an example of an item that could cause aspiration or suffocation in the toddler (e.g., foods: hard candy).

    Foods:

    Play objects:

    Common household objects:

    Electrical items:

CRITICAL THINKING—CASE STUDY

Tasha Jackson is a 12-month-old infant who is visiting the clinic for her well-baby checkup. Tasha's mother, Dora, is expecting her second child in 3 months. Dora works full time and will be home for 6 weeks with the new baby. Tasha has been in daycare since she was a baby. Dora's husband also works full time during the day.

52. List four areas that the nurse should assess to obtain the information necessary to adequately provide anticipatory guidance for a toddler at Tasha's age.

53. The most appropriate initial nursing intervention would be to:
    a. allow Mrs. Jackson to express her feelings.
    b. give Mrs. Jackson advice about daycare.
    c. give Mrs. Jackson advice about sibling rivalry.
    d. all of the above.

54. Dora Jackson shares with the nurse that she is concerned about her daycare arrangements and is thinking about keeping Tasha at home for the 6 weeks after the baby is born. The highest priority intervention in this situation is to:
    a. stress the importance of preparing Tasha for the new sibling.
    b. recommend that Mrs. Jackson begin making plans to keep Tasha at home for the 6 weeks.
    c. recommend that any change in daycare should take place well before the new baby's arrival.
    d. explore Mrs. Jackson's concerns about her daycare arrangements.

55. The best way to evaluate and determine whether Mrs. Jackson's daycare concerns are warranted would be to:
    a. make a home visit after the baby is born.
    b. visit the daycare center.
    c. observe a return demonstration of baby care.
    d. solicit feedback from Mrs. Jackson that she is comfortable with her postpartum arrangements.

15 Health Promotion of the Preschooler and Family

1. Match each term with its description.

   a. Preschool period
   b. Placement stage
   c. Shape stage
   d. Design stage
   e. Combine
   f. Aggregate
   g. Pictorial stage
   h. Initiative
   i. Guilt

   j. Superego
   k. Oedipal stage
   l. Castration complex
   m. Oedipus/Electra complex
   n. Penis envy
   o. Preoperational phase
   p. Preconceptual phase
   q. Intuitive thought phase

   _____ Guilt that develops from a son's wish to marry his mother and kill his father or from a daughter's wish to marry her father and kill her mother

   _____ Occurs in the preschool years, resulting in conflict when children overstep the limits of their ability and inquiry

   _____ Time during which the child is 3 to 5 years of age

   _____ Phallic stage

   _____ The second stage of drawing development, in which the 3-year-old draws a single-line outline form, such as a rectangle, circle, oval, cross, or other odd shape

   _____ Period from ages 4 to 7 years, when the child begins to shift from totally egocentric thought to social awareness and the ability to consider other viewpoints

   _____ The conscience

   _____ The first stage of drawing development, in which a pattern of placing scribbles on paper appears by age 2 years; once developed, it is never lost

   _____ To create two united diagrams in a drawing

   _____ A girl's desire to have a penis

   _____ To create three or more united diagrams in a drawing

   _____ Guilt that develops regarding a son's feelings toward his father, making him fear the punishment of mutilation

   _____ The fourth stage of drawing development, in which designs are recognizable as familiar objects

   _____ Period from ages 2 to 4 years; the first phase of Piaget's preoperational phase

   _____ The chief psychosocial task of the preschool period

   _____ Period from ages 2 to 7 years; the stage of Piaget's cognitive theory that involves the preschooler

   _____ The third stage of drawing development, in which simple forms are drawn together to make structured designs

2. Match each term with its description.

   a. Play
   b. Right and left concepts
   c. Causality
   d. Time concepts
   e. Magical thinking
   f. Punishment and obedience orientation
   g. Naive instrumental orientation

   h. Sex typing
   i. Individuation-separation process
   j. Telegraphic speech
   k. Associative play
   l. Imitative play
   m. Imaginary companions
   n. Behavioral Style Questionnaire

o. Sexuality
p. Masturbation
q. Gifted-talented
r. Aggression
s. Frustration
t. Modeling
u. Reinforcement
v. Quantity
w. Severity

x. Distribution
y. Onset
z. Duration
aa. Stuttering
bb. Animism
cc. Desensitization
dd. Dyslalia
ee. Mutual play
ff. Denver Articulation Screening Examination

_____ Play that occurs between the child and an adult (often the parent); fosters development and enriched opportunities

_____ The process by which an individual develops the behavior, personality, attitudes, and beliefs appropriate for his or her culture and sex

_____ Different manifestations of behaviors that are used to differentiate between "normal" and "problematic" behavior

_____ Group play in similar or identical activities but without rigid organization or rules

_____ Actions directed toward satisfying the child's own needs and less commonly toward the needs of others

_____ Resembles logical thought superficially; the ability of preschoolers to explain a concept as they have heard it described by others, but with limited understanding

_____ The preschooler's belief that his or her own thoughts are all-powerful

_____ The child's way of understanding, adjusting to, and working out life's experiences

_____ The way that children from ages 2 to 4 years judge whether an action is good or bad; based on whether the action results in reward or punishment

_____ Ideas that a preschooler does not have the ability to understand

_____ Complete by the preschool years; marked by preschoolers being able to relate to unfamiliar people easily and to tolerate brief separations from parents with little or no protest

_____ Imaginative play; dramatic play; self-expression

_____ Idea that is completely misunderstood by preschoolers, who interpret it according to their own frame of reference

_____ Behavior that attempts to hurt a person or destroy property

_____ Can shape aggressive behavior; closely associated with modeling of "masculine" behavior

_____ Usually occurs between the ages of 2½ and 3½ years; usually relinquished when child enters school

_____ The number of occurrences

_____ Used to identify temperamental characteristics in children in the age range of 3 to 7 years

_____ A strategy to use to overcome fear; the child is exposed to a feared object in a safe situation

_____ Self-stimulation of the genitalia

_____ When a behavior starts; sudden changes in behavior are most significant

_____ The degree to which behavior interferes with social or cognitive functioning

_____ Stammering; a normal speech pattern in the preschooler

_____ A broad concept; the act of two people uniting intimately because of the special relationship they have

_____ Formation of sentences of about three or four words; includes only the most essential words to convey meaning

_____ The continual thwarting of self-satisfaction by parental disapproval, humiliation, punishment, and insults

_____ The amount of time a behavior lasts, significant periods being greater than 4 weeks

_____ Ascribing lifelike qualities to inanimate objects

_____ Refers to specific academic aptitudes, advanced memory skills, creative thinking, ability in the visual or performing arts, and psychomotor ability, either individually or in combination

_____ Imitating behavior of significant others; a powerful influencing force in preschoolers

_____ A tool for assessing articulation skills in the child and for explaining to parents the expected progression of sounds

_____ Articulation problems

3. The approximate age range for the preschool period begins at age _____ years and ends

at age _____ years.

4. The average annual weight gain during the preschool years is _____ to

_____ kg.

5. Which of the following statements about the preschooler's physical proportions is true?
   a. Preschoolers have a squat and potbellied frame.
   b. Preschoolers have a slender but sturdy frame.
   c. The muscle and bones of the preschooler have matured.
   d. Sexual characteristics can be differentiated in the preschooler.

6. Uninhibited scribbling and drawing can help to develop:
   a. symbolic language.
   b. fine muscle skills.
   c. eye-hand coordination.
   d. all of the above.

7. As preschool children begin to develop their own sense of morality, they primarily rely on:
   a. their association with other children.
   b. whether they are accepted for their attitudes.
   c. parental principles.
   d. all of the above.

8. The resolution of the Oedipus/Electra complex occurs when the child:
   a. identifies with the same-sex parent.
   b. realizes that the same-sex parent is more powerful.
   c. wishes that the same-sex parent were dead.
   d. notices physical sexual differences.

9. Because of the preschooler's egocentric thought, the best approach for effective communication is through:
   a. speech.
   b. play.
   c. drawing.
   d. actions.

10. Magical thinking, according to Piaget, is the belief that:
    a. events have cause and effect.
    b. God is an imaginary friend.
    c. thoughts are all-powerful.
    d. if the skin is broken, the child's insides will come out.

11. The moral and spiritual development of the preschooler is characterized by:
    a. concern for why something is wrong.
    b. actions that are directed toward satisfying the needs of others.
    c. thoughts of loyalty and gratitude.
    d. a very concrete sense of justice.

12. The preschooler's body image has developed to include:
    a. a well-defined body boundary.
    b. knowledge about his or her internal anatomy.
    c. fear of intrusive experiences.
    d. anxiety and fear of separation.

13. Sex typing involves the process by which the preschooler develops:
    a. a strong attachment to the same-sex parent.
    b. an identification with the opposite-sex parent.
    c. behavior and beliefs for his or her culture and sex.
    d. all of the above.

14. Language during the preschool years:
    a. includes telegraphic speech.
    b. is simple and concrete.
    c. uses phrases, not sentences.
    d. includes the ability to follow complex commands.

15. Research has shown that when two languages are presented to children simultaneously in early childhood, bilingual children are most likely to experience:
    a. adverse effects in their receptive language development.
    b. adverse effects in performance in the majority language.
    c. language milestones at similar stages to monolinguals.
    d. adverse effects to areas in addition to language.

16. Which of the following statements about social development of the preschooler is false?
    a. Imaginary playmates are a normal part of the preschooler's play.
    b. Preschoolers have overcome much of their anxiety regarding strangers.
    c. Preschoolers use telegraphic speech between the ages of 3 and 4 years.
    d. Preschoolers particularly enjoy parallel play.

17. Television and videotapes:
    a. hinder the preschooler's development.
    b. are a significant source for modeling.
    c. are not an interactive activity.
    d. do not promote learning for the preschooler.

18. In regard to the development of temperament in the preschool years:
    a. temperamental characteristics change considerably during the preschool years.
    b. the effect of temperament on adjustment in a group becomes important during the preschool years.
    c. children need to be treated the same regardless of differences in temperament.
    d. there really is no tool that will adequately identify temperamental characteristics during the preschool years.

19. List at least two strategies parents may use to help their child prepare for the preschool or kindergarten experience.

20. To guide parents in their quest to find a school with comprehensive services, the nurse should advise the parent to:
    a. find a school that focuses primarily on skill acquisition.
    b. visit the schools to observe their services personally.
    c. select a licensed program to ensure the highest standard.
    d. all of the above.

21. The best way for parents to respond to a child's questions about sexuality is to give the child:
    a. an honest answer and find out what the child thinks.
    b. one or two sentences that answer the specific question only.
    c. an honest, short, and to-the-point answer.
    d. an honest answer but a little less information than the child expects.

22. Which of the following characteristics is not typically seen in a gifted-talented child?
    a. Asynchrony across developmental domains
    b. Insatiable curiosity
    c. Less need for attention than other children
    d. Intensity of feelings and emotions

23. Which of the following factors influences aggressive behavior?
    a. Frustration
    b. Modeling
    c. Gender
    d. All of the above

24. Which of the following dysfunctional speech patterns is a normal characteristic of the language development of a preschooler?
    a. Lisp
    b. Stammering
    c. Nystagmus
    d. Echolalia

25. Which of the following sources of stress is typical of a 3-year-old?
    a. Insecurity
    b. Masturbation
    c. Jealousy
    d. Sexuality

26. Which of the following approaches is recommended to help prevent stress in children?
    a. Allow time for rest.
    b. Prepare the child for changes.
    c. Monitor the amount of stress.
    d. All of the above.

27. Which of the following examples would best help a preschooler dispel his or her fear of the water when learning to swim?
    a. Fear of the water is a healthy fear. It should not be dispelled.
    b. Allow the child to sit by the water with other children, play with water toys, and get splashed lightly with the water.
    c. Reassure the child as he or she is brought slowly into the water with an adult who knows how to swim.
    d. Throw the child in the water and have an adult keep the child's head above water.

28. Identify the following statements as true or false.

    _____ Sleep terrors can be described as a partial arousal from a very deep nondreaming sleep.

    _____ Nightmares usually occur in the second half of the night.

    _____ With sleep terrors, crying and fright persist even after the child is awake.

    _____ With nightmares the child is not very aware of another's presence.

29. When educating the preschool child about injury prevention, the parents should:
    a. set a good example.
    b. help children establish good habits.
    c. be aware that pedestrian–motor vehicle injuries increase in this age-group.
    d. do all of the above.

CRITICAL THINKING—CASE STUDY

Sheila Roth arrives at the office for a routine preschool physical. Her son Jacob, who is not quite 3 years old, will attend the 3-year-old preschool program at a local private school this year. Since he was a baby, Jacob has attended a home day-care program, while his mother managed her own interior decorating business. The preschool is run by an older woman who treats the 12 children in her program as if they were family. The helper at the daycare also seems very loving. The program is highly structured in regard to schedule and usual routines. Ms. Roth tells the nurse that she is looking forward to Jacob's new environment. His teacher is very creative and approaches the classroom from the perspective of the child's development. There will be a lot of choices for activities during the day.

30. Based on the information provided, which of the following is the best analysis?
    a. Jacob needs some preparation for this new preschool experience.
    b. Jacob will have less trouble adjusting than a child who has never attended daycare.
    c. Jacob is too young for such a drastic change.
    d. Jacob needs the individual attention he is getting at the daycare.

31. Which of the following expected outcomes would be most reasonable to establish?
    a. The nurse will help Ms. Roth assess Jacob's readiness for preschool.
    b. Jacob will attend preschool without any behavioral indications of stress.
    c. Ms. Roth will verbalize at least five strategies that can be used to help prepare Jacob for his preschool experience.
    d. Jacob will demonstrate behavior that indicates that he is adjusting to his preschool experience.

32. Which of the following interventions would be inappropriate for the nurse to suggest?
    a. Introduce Jacob to the teacher.
    b. Leave quickly on the first day.
    c. Talk about the new school as exciting.
    d. Be confident on the first day.

33. Which of the following of Jacob's characteristics would indicate that he is ready for preschool?
    a. Social maturity
    b. Good attention span
    c. Academic readiness
    d. All of the above

16 Health Problems of Early Childhood

1. The parents of Ivy, age 7 years, are concerned because Ivy has been diagnosed with fifth disease. Which of the following does the nurse recognize as being appropriate information for the parents?
   a. Ivy needs to be kept away from pregnant women.
   b. Ivy received the infection from insect bites.
   c. Ivy will have a "slapped face" appearance followed by a rash that subsides but reappears if skin is irritated by heat and cold.
   d. Ivy may develop serious complications leading to death from the disease.

2. Janie, age 6 years, has been diagnosed with a communicable disease. The nurse, in preparing the care plan, recognizes four goals. List them.

3. Match each communicable disease with its description or characteristics.

   a. Varicella   f. Mumps
   b. Diphtheria   g. Pertussis
   c. Fifth disease   h. Rubella
   d. Roseola   i. Scarlet fever
   e. Rubeola   j. Poliomyelitis

   _____ Rash appears in three stages; stage I is erythema on face, chiefly on cheeks.

   _____ This condition has a rash that begins as macules, rapidly progressing to papules and then to vesicles, eventually breaking and forming crusts.

   _____ Tonsillar pharyngeal areas are covered with white or gray membrane; complications include myocarditis and neuritis.

   _____ Rash is rose-pink macules or maculopapules, appearing first on trunk, then spreading to neck, face, and extremities; rash is nonpruritic.

   _____ Cough occurs at night, and inspirations sound like crowing.

   _____ This condition results in earache that is aggravated by chewing.

   _____ Rash appears 3 to 4 days after onset and maculopapular eruption on face with gradual spread downward; Koplik spots are present before the rash.

   _____ Discrete pinkish-red maculopapular rash appears on face and then spreads downward to neck, arms, trunk, and legs; greatest danger is teratogenic effect on fetus.

   _____ Permanent paralysis may occur.

   _____ Tonsils are enlarged, edematous, reddened, and covered with patches of exudate; rash is absent on face; desquamation occurs.

4. Which of the following assessments is not helpful in identifying potentially communicable diseases?
   a. Recent travel to foreign country
   b. Immunization history
   c. Past medical history
   d. Family history

5. Primary prevention of communicable disease is best accomplished by:
   a. immunization.
   b. control of the disease spread.
   c. adequate water supply.
   d. implementing good hand washing among hospital personnel.

6. Certain groups of children are at risk for serious complications from communicable diseases. Which of the following groups is not at risk?
   a. Children with an immunodeficiency or immunologic disorder
   b. Children receiving steroid therapy
   c. Children with leukemia
   d. Children who have recently undergone a surgical procedure

7. What antiviral agent is used to treat varicella infections in children at increased risk for complications associated with varicella?
   a. Varicella-zoster immune globulin
   b. Acyclovir
   c. Salicylates
   d. Steroids

8. Name the two diseases caused by the varicella zoster virus.

9. _____   _____   _____

   _____ (_____) or _____

   _____ _____ (_____) may

   be given to high-risk children who have no previous history of varicella and who are likely to contract the disease and have complications as a result.

10. The nurse knows, regarding pertussis, that:
    a. the incidence has decreased in infants less than 6 months of age.
    b. a booster vaccine (Tdap) is now recommended for all children ages 11 to 18 years of age.
    c. treatment should begin as soon as exposure is confirmed and includes the antibiotic amoxicillin.
    d. the disease is not contagious, so close household members do not need treatment.

11. The American Academy of Pediatrics has recommended vitamin A supplements for certain pediatric patients with measles. Correct dosage of vitamin A and instructions to parents of these children include:
    i. single oral dose of 200,000 international units in children 1 year old.
    ii. single oral dose of 100,000 international units in children 6 to 12 months old.
    iii. dosage may be associated with vomiting and headache for a few hours.
    iv. safe storage of the drug to prevent accidental overdose.

    a. i, ii, iii, and iv
    b. i, ii, and iv
    c. i, iii, and iv
    d. ii and iv

12. The nurse is conducting an educational session for the parents of a child diagnosed with varicella. Which of the following is not an appropriate comfort measure to include in this session?
    a. Use Aveeno bath treatment or oatmeal in bath water for added skin comfort.
    b. Use Caladryl lotion on rash to decrease itching.
    c. Use hot bath water to promote skin rash healing.
    d. Keep nails short and smooth to decrease chances of infection from scratching.

13. Which of the following does the nurse recognize as contraindicated in providing comfort measures to children with communicable diseases?
    a. Use of acetaminophen for control of elevated temperature in child with varicella
    b. Use of diphenhydramine (Benadryl) or hydroxyzine (Atarax) for itching
    c. Use of aspirin to control elevated temperature and/or symptoms in child with varicella
    d. Use of lozenges and saline rinses in an 8-year-old child with sore throat

14. The nurse knows the child with chickenpox can return to school:
    a. 2 weeks after onset of rash.
    b. when all lesions have progressed to the vesicle stage.
    c. after administration of acyclovir.
    d. 5 days after onset of rash or when all lesions are crusted.

15. Clinical manifestations differentiate bacterial conjunctivitis from viral conjunctivitis. Which of the following is present with bacterial conjunctivitis but not usually found with viral conjunctivitis?
    a. Child awakens with crusting of eyelids.
    b. Child has increase in watery drainage from eyes.
    c. Child has inflamed conjunctiva.
    d. Child has swollen eyelids.

16. When instructing the parents caring for an infant with conjunctivitis, which of the following will the nurse include in the plan?
    a. Accumulated secretions are removed by wiping from outer canthus inward.
    b. Hydrogen peroxide placed on cotton swabs is helpful in removing crusts from eyelids.
    c. Compresses of warm tap water are kept in place on the eye to prevent crusting.
    d. Washcloth and towel used by the infant are kept separate and not used by others.

17. Identify the following statements about stomatitis as true or false.

    _____ Aphthous stomatitis may be associated with mild traumatic injury, allergy, and emotional stress.

    _____ Aphthous stomatitis is characterized by painful, small, whitish ulcerations that heal without complication in 4 to 12 days.

    _____ Herpetic gingivostomatitis is caused by herpes simplex virus, usually type 1.

    _____ Herpetic gingivostomatitis is commonly called "cold sores" or "fever blisters."

    _____ Treatment for stomatitis is aimed at relief of complications.

    _____ When examining herpetic lesions, the nurse uses her uncovered index finger to check for cracks in the skin surface.

    _____ Herpetic gingivostomatitis is associated with sexual transmission.

    _____ Treatment for children with severe cases of herpetic gingivostomatitis includes oral acyclovir.

    _____ Topical anesthetics like lidocaine (Xylocaine Viscous) can be prescribed for children who are old enough to keep the drug in the mouth for 2 to 3 minutes and then swallow the drug.

18. Anne, an 8-year-old, has been diagnosed with giardiasis. The nurse would expect Anne to have most likely been seen initially with which of the following signs and symptoms?
    a. Diarrhea with blood in the stools
    b. Nausea and vomiting with a mild fever
    c. Abdominal cramps with intermittent loose stools
    d. Weight loss of 5 lb in the past month

19. A drug used to treat children diagnosed with giardiasis is:
    a. metronidazole (Flagyl).
    b. mebendazole (Vermox).
    c. erythromycin.
    d. tetracycline.

20. The nurse is instructing parents on the test-tape diagnostic procedure for enterobiasis. Which of the following is included in the explanation?
    a. Use a flashlight to inspect the anal area while the child sleeps.
    b. Perform the test 2 days after the child receives the first dose of mebendazole.
    c. Test all members of the family at the same time using frosted tape.
    d. Collect the tape in the morning before the child has a bowel movement or bath.

21. Children with pinworm infections are seen with the principal symptom of:
    a. perianal itching.
    b. diarrhea with blood.
    c. evidence of small ricelike worms in their stool and urine.
    d. abdominal pain.

22. The nurse has an order to administer 100 mg of mebendazole (Vermox) to 5-year-old Megan for a positive pinworm test. Which of the following is an appropriate action when administering this medication?
    a. Mebendazole should be withheld in all children under 6 years of age.
    b. Treatment is limited to Megan until other family members have tested positive.
    c. Mebendazole will also effectively treat giardiasis.
    d. Treatment should be repeated in 2 weeks to prevent reinfection.

23. Reduction of poisonings in children and infants can be accomplished by:
    a. use of child-resistant containers.
    b. educating parents and grandparents to place products out of reach of small children.
    c. educating parents to relocate plants out of reach of infants, toddlers, and small children.
    d. all of the above.

24. Ingestion of injurious agents by children:
    a. occurs most frequently at grandparent's or friend's home.
    b. occurs because infants and toddlers explore their environment through oral experimentation.
    c. has increased despite the use of child-resistant containers.
    d. can be avoided by teaching preschoolers which substances are dangerous.

25. The first action parents should be taught to initiate in a poisoning is to:
    a. induce vomiting.
    b. take the child to the family physician's office or emergency center.
    c. call the poison control center.
    d. follow the instructions on the label of the product.

26. Gastric lavage for pediatric poison ingestions:
    a. can be associated with serious complications of gastrointestinal perforation, hypoxia, and aspiration.
    b. is recommended in the emergency department for all cases of ingestion.
    c. has been proven to decrease morbidity.
    d. is most useful when the child comes to the emergency department within 3 hours of ingestion of the toxin.

27. Identify the general guidelines for emergency treatment for poisoning.

28. Which of the following statements about ipecac use for poisonous substance use is true?
    a. Ipecac helps to absorb the toxin.
    b. Ipecac is no longer recommended for routine home treatment of poisoning.
    c. Ipecac is useful when a corrosive substance has been ingested.
    d. Ipecac is useful when an overdose of a calcium channel blocker has been ingested.

29. Which of the following actions taken by the nurse is least likely to prevent recurrence of poisonings?
    a. In the emergency department, begin a discussion of ways to injury-proof the home.
    b. Do a home visit to assess safety before the child is discharged.
    c. Administer questionnaire for poison prevention to the parents when the child is discharged.
    d. Advise parents to kneel down to the child's level when determining what products need to be placed out of reach.

30. The nurse expects to assist with administration of a specific antidote for poisoning in which one of the following pediatric patients?
    a. The 8-month-old child admitted to the emergency department after eating 8 or 10 holly berries
    b. The 13-year-old girl who ingested an overdose of diazepam (Valium)
    c. The 8-year-old child who ingested three of his mother's birth control pills
    d. The 6-year-old child who ingested an overdose of an unidentified corrosive substance

31. Activated charcoal:
    a. is odorless, tasteless, and delivered with fewer complications via gastric lavage.
    b. stimulates the gastric mucosa,
    c. is often mixed with diet soda and served through a straw from an opaque container.
    d. has a bitter taste.

32. Potential causes of heavy metal poisoning in children include _____

    _____, and _____.

33. On routine physical examination, 2-year-old Zach is found to have an elevated blood lead level. The most likely cause for this finding is:
    a. Zach is allowed to play in the local sandbox at the park.
    b. Zach lives in a house built after 1980.
    c. Zach is fed from pottery that the family brought in Mexico.
    d. Zach's father is an artist and works at home.

34. Identify the following statements as true or false.

    _____ The neurologic system is of most concern when young children are exposed to lead, because the developing brain is very vulnerable.

    _____ Young children will absorb more of the lead to which they are exposed than will adults.

    _____ Lead-based nonintact paint in structures built before 1978 remains a common source of lead poisoning in children.

    _____ Lead-containing pottery or leaded dishes do not contribute to lead poisoning because food does not absorb lead.

    _____ If the venous blood value is below 10 mcg/dl of lead, the child is considered to have a safe blood lead value.

    _____ The exposure risk for children living in leaded environments is lower if their diet is deficient in iron and calcium and high in fats, because the diet slows the absorption of lead.

    _____ The primary nursing goal in lead poisoning is to prevent the child's initial or further exposure to lead.

    _____ Universal screening guidelines for blood lead level testing include all children between 1 and 2 years of age.

    _____ Mercury thermometers can cause toxicity if they are broken and vapors are inhaled.

    _____ Chelation treatment works by the use of a chemical compound that removes lead from circulating blood. It does not counteract any effects of the lead.

    _____ A level of lead not harmful to the pregnant woman is also not harmful to the fetus.

    _____ High lead levels are of most concern when they occur in children who are ages 12 and under.

    _____ Children who are iron deficient absorb lead more readily than those with sufficient iron stores.

35. The nurse is to give an injection of the chelation drug calcium disodium edentate. Which of the following does the nurse recognize as most appropriate?
    a. Keeping the child NPO for 24 hours after administration of the drug
    b. Mixing the drug with procaine to lessen the pain associated with the injection
    c. Maintaining seizure precautions at the bedside
    d. Making certain the patient has no peanut allergy before injection

36. Diagnostic evaluations for lead poisoning include:
    a. blood levels for lead concentration, including screening by finger and heel sticks, with blood collected by venipuncture to confirm diagnosis.
    b. recommended universal screening for all children, with those ages 6 years or older given priority.
    c. identifying children at high risk for anemia, because these children will most likely have higher lead levels.
    d. understanding that a blood level for lead in the 10 to 14 mcg/dl range is normal and needs no follow-up.

37. Therapeutic interventions for lead poisoning do not include:
    a. removal of the source of lead.
    b. improving nutrition.
    c. using chelation therapy.
    d. intravenous administration of dimercaprol.

38. Discharge planning for children with lead poisoning includes:
    a. confirmation that the child will be discharged to a home without lead hazards.
    b. immediate referral for development and speech therapy.
    c. visiting nurse care for continuation of intravenous treatment at home.
    d. explanation that there is little need for follow-up because lead levels have returned to normal.

39. Match each term with its description.

    a. Child neglect   e. Physical abuse
    b. Physical neglect   f. Munchausen syndrome by proxy
    c. Emotional neglect   g. Shaken baby syndrome
    d. Emotional abuse

    _____ Deliberate attempt to destroy a child's self-esteem

    _____ Violent shaking of infant that can cause fatal intracranial trauma

    _____ Failure to meet the child's needs for affection

    _____ Deprivation of necessities such as food and clothing

    _____ Failure to provide for the child's basic needs and adequate level of care

    _____ Deliberate infliction of physical injury on a child

    _____ An illness that one person fabricates or induces in another person

40. Identified characteristics of parents who are at higher risk for abusing their children do not include:
    a. older parents who waited until their mid-30s before having their first child.
    b. isolated parents with few supportive relationships.
    c. parents who grew up with poor role models.
    d. single-parent families.

41. A child who unintentionally contributes to an abusive situation most likely:
    a. fits into the "easy-child pattern."
    b. has demands, both physical and emotional, that are incompatible with the parent's ability to meet these needs.
    c. has low self-esteem.
    d. comes from a low socioeconomic background.

42. Which of the following statements is false?
    a. Most reporting of abuse has been from the middle socioeconomic population.
    b. One child is usually the victim in an abusive family; removal of this child often places the other sibling at risk.
    c. The abusive family environment is one of chronic stress, including problems of divorce, poverty, unemployment, and poor housing.
    d. Child abuse is a problem of all social groups.

43. Match each term with its description.

    a. Incest
    b. Molestation
    c. Exhibitionism
    d. Pedophilia
    e. Sexual abuse

    _____ The use, persuasion, or coercion of any child to engage in sexually explicit conduct
    _____ Preference for a prepubertal child by an adult as a means of achieving sexual excitement
    _____ Any physical sexual activity between family members
    _____ "Indecent liberties" such as touching or fondling
    _____ Indecent exposure

44. Identify each of the following statements related to sexual abusers as true or false.

    _____ The typical abuser is a male who is unknown to the victim.
    _____ Boys are less likely to report both intrafamilial and extrafamilial abuse than are girls.
    _____ Many sexual offenders are active in the community and hold full-time jobs.
    _____ The incestuous relationship between stepfather and stepdaughter is generally shorter and more often reported than the incestuous relationship between biologic father and daughter.
    _____ Sexual abuse by relatives who have a strong emotional bond with the victim is the least devastating to the child.
    _____ The youngest daughter is typically the child in the incestuous relationship.
    _____ Children may not reveal the truth about the abuse because they fear their parents would not believe them.

45. The nurse is talking with 13-year-old Amy, who has revealed that she is being sexually abused. Which of the following is a correct guideline for the nurse to follow?
    a. Promise Amy not to tell what she tells you.
    b. Assure Amy that she will not need to report the abuse.
    c. Avoid using leading statements that can distort Amy's reporting of the problem.
    d. It is okay for the nurse to express anger and shock and to criticize Amy's family.

46. In identification of the abused child, the nurse knows:
    a. physical abuse can be readily identified during the physical examination.
    b. specific behavioral problems can be seen in the abused child.
    c. maltreated children easily admit to the abuse they received from their parents.
    d. incompatibility between the history and the injury is probably the most important criterion on which to base the decision to report suspected abuse.

47. In obtaining a history pertaining to an incident of abuse, the nurse should:
    a. expect the child to betray the parents by admitting to the abuse received.
    b. expect the child to defend the parents out of a sense of loyalty.
    c. recognize that the child will have a sense of relief after telling someone about the abuse.
    d. recognize that the child's thinking can be shaped by the types of interrogations conducted after the report of abuse.

48. Which of the following parental behavioral responses should alert the nurse to the possibility of maltreatment of the child?
    a. Parent displays extreme care for the child, not wanting to leave the child's side.
    b. Parent displays signs of guilt, not being able to eat or sleep.
    c. Parent displays abnormal interest in the incident, going over each detail repeatedly.
    d. Parent displays anger at the child for being injured.

49. Physical assessment for child physical abuse:
    a. should identify all injuries.
    b. should always begin with rapid assessment of airway, breathing, circulation, and neurologic systems.
    c. should recognize that all forms of physical abuse have obvious signs.
    d. should occur only after legal authorities have been notified.

50. Physical assessment for child sexual abuse:
    a. includes documentation of only abnormal genital findings.
    b. includes collecting forensic evidence obtained directly from a prepubertal victim's body as much as 3 days after the incident.
    c. includes examination of the anal area.
    d. includes documentation of the size of the hymeneal opening, because it is predictive of sexual abuse.

51. The nurse working with the abused child and family:
    i. should view the parent and child as victims.
    ii. should teach the parents through demonstration and example rather than lecture.
    iii. recognizes that parents need to correct abnormal behavior in the child—for example, "We told you not to go with strangers."
    iv. recognizes that the goal of the nurse-child relationship is to provide a role model for the parents in helping them to relate positively to their child.

    a. i, ii, iii, and iv
    b. ii, iii, and iv
    c. i and iii
    d. ii and iv

CRITICAL THINKING—CASE STUDY

Jimmy is a 4-year-old preschool student who is brought to the school nurse's office by his teacher. She is concerned because Jimmy has purulent discharge in the corner of both eyes, with inflamed conjunctiva. The nurse observes Jimmy wiping his eyes frequently with his hands.

52. Based on the information provided, the nurse suspects that Jimmy has:
    a. bacterial conjunctivitis.
    b. viral conjunctivitis.
    c. allergic conjunctivitis.
    d. conjunctivitis caused by a foreign body.

53. Based on knowledge of communicable diseases, the nurse identifies which of the following as the priority goal for Jimmy's plan of care?
    a. Patient will not become infected.
    b. Patient will not spread disease.
    c. Patient will experience minimal discomfort.
    d. Patient will maintain skin integrity.

54. The nurse calls Jimmy's parents to request that they come and pick Jimmy up from school. What is the best rationale for this action?
    a. Jimmy is tired and needs additional rest because of the infection.
    b. Jimmy is at high risk for spreading the disease because of his age and his inability to wash his hands after touching his eyes.
    c. Jimmy needs immediate medical attention to prevent complications.
    d. The nurse needs to discuss causes of this disease with Jimmy's mother so that its recurrence can be prevented.

55. What information is important to include in the teaching plan for Jimmy's parents?
    a. Jimmy needs to have his own face cloth and towel.
    b. Eye medication will need to be administered before the eyes are cleaned.
    c. Jimmy cannot return to school until all symptoms have stopped.
    d. Jimmy will need his own eating utensils.

56. The nurse can expect treatment for Jimmy's condition to include:
    a. use of continuous warm compresses held in place on each infected eye.
    b. application of fluoroquinolone ophthalmic agents.
    c. oral broad-spectrum antibiotics.
    d. all of the above.

57. Which of the following evaluations best demonstrates the effectiveness of nursing interventions for Jimmy's condition?
    a. There is no spread of the disease within the school and family.
    b. Parents are able to demonstrate appropriate eye care.
    c. Jimmy reports no eye discomfort.
    d. Child engages in normal activities.

58. Albert, age 7, has been diagnosed with pinworms, and mebendazole (Vermox) has been ordered. The nurse knows that this drug should probably also be administered to:
    a. only Albert's siblings.
    b. only family members who test positive.
    c. all family members who are not under 2 years of age.
    d. everyone who uses the same toilet facilities as Albert.

17 Health Promotion of the School-Age Child and Family

1. Middle childhood is also referred to as the middle years, the school years, or the school-age years. What ages does this period represent?
   a. Ages 5 to 13 years
   b. Ages 4 to 14 years
   c. Ages 6 to 12 years
   d. Ages 6 to 16 years

2. Identify when the middle childhood years physiologically begin and end.

3. Which finding should the nurse expect when assessing physical growth in the school-age child?
   a. Weight increase of 2 to 3 kg per year
   b. Height increase of 3 cm per year
   c. Little change in refined coordination
   d. Decrease in body fat and muscle tissue

4. Identify the following statements about the school-age child as true or false.

   _____ In middle childhood there are fewer stomach upsets, better maintenance of blood glucose levels, and an increased stomach capacity.

   _____ Caloric needs are higher in relation to stomach size when compared with the needs of preschool years.

   _____ The heart is smaller in relation to the rest of the body during the middle years.

   _____ During the middle years, the immune system develops little immunity to pathogenic microorganisms.

   _____ Backpacks, when worn correctly, are preferred to other book totes during middle years.

   _____ Physical maturity correlates well with emotional and social maturity during the middle years.

   _____ School-age children's muscles are still functionally immature compared with those of the adolescent and are more easily damaged by muscular injury and overuse.

   _____ Wider physical differences between children are seen at the beginning of middle childhood than at the end.

   _____ There is no universal age at which the child assumes the characteristics of preadolescence.

   _____ Early appearance of physical sexual characteristics in girls and late appearance in boys have been linked to participation in risk-taking behaviors.

5. What period begins toward the end of middle childhood and ends at age 13?
   a. Puberty
   b. Preadolescence
   c. Early maturation
   d. All of the above

6. According to Freud, middle childhood is described as which one of the following periods?
   a. Anal
   b. Latency
   c. Oral
   d. Oedipal

7. According to Erikson, what is the developmental goal of middle childhood?
   a. Autonomy
   b. Trust
   c. Initiative
   d. Industry

8. Which of the following descriptions of school-age children is most closely linked to Erikson's theory?
   a. During this time, children experience relationships with same-sex peers.
   b. During this time, there is an overlapping of developmental characteristics between childhood and adolescence.
   c. During this time, temperamental traits from infancy continue to influence behavior.
   d. During this time, interests expand and children, with a growing sense of independence, engage in tasks that can be carried through to completion.

9. According to Piaget, what is the stage of development for middle childhood?
   a. Concrete operational
   b. Preoperational
   c. Formal operational
   d. Sensorimotor

10. Early appearance of secondary sex characteristics of girls during preadolescence may be associated with:
    a. satisfaction with physical appearance and higher self-esteem.
    b. increase in self-confidence and a more outgoing personality.
    c. dissatisfaction with physical appearance and lower self-esteem.
    d. increased substance use and reckless vehicle use.

11. Generally, the earliest age at which puberty begins in girls is age _____ _____; in boys, age

    _____ _____.

12. Middle childhood is the time when children:
    i. learn the value of doing things with others.
    ii. learn the benefits derived from division of labor in accomplishing goals.
    iii. achieve a sense of industry and accomplishment.
    iv. expand interests and engage in tasks that can be carried to completion.

    a. i, ii, iii, and iv
    b. i, iii, and iv
    c. i and iv
    d. ii and iii

13. Dillon is a 6-year-old starting in a new neighborhood school. On the first day of school, he complains of a headache and tearfully tells his mother he does not want to go to school. Dillon's mother takes him to school, and the nurse is consulted. The nurse recognizes that Dillon is slow to warm up to others and suggests:
    a. putting Dillon in the classroom with the other children and leaving him alone.
    b. insisting that Dillon join and lead the class song.
    c. including Dillon in activities without assigning him tasks until he willingly participates in activities.
    d. sending Dillon home with his mom because he has a headache.

14. Which of the following accurately describes the expected cognitive development during the concrete-operational period of middle childhood?
    a. Children are able to follow directions but unable to verbalize the actions involved in the process.
    b. Children are able to use their thought processes to experience events and actions and make judgments based on what they reason.
    c. Children are able to see things from an egocentric outlook that is rigidly developed around the action to be completed.
    d. Children progress from conceptual thinking to perceptual thinking when making judgments.

15. Children who are identified as having an easily distracted temperament:
    a. rarely pose a problem.
    b. usually exhibit discomfort when introduced to new situations.
    c. benefit from practice sessions before an event.
    d. should not be told when to stop activities, because this can trigger a reaction event.

16. The following terms relate to the accomplishment of cognitive tasks of middle childhood. Match each term with its description.

    a. Conservation
    b. Identity
    c. Reversibility
    d. Reciprocity
    e. Classification skills

    f. Serialize
    g. Combinational skills
    h. Metalinguistic awareness
    i. Perceptual thinking
    j. Conceptual thinking

    _____ Arrange objects according to some ordinal scale

    _____ Ability to manipulate numbers and to learn the skills of addition, subtraction, multiplication, and division

    _____ Ability to group objects according to the attributes they share in common

    _____ Ability to think through an action sequence, anticipate the consequences, and return and rethink the action in a different direction

    _____ Ability to deal with two dimensions at one time and to comprehend that a change in one dimension compensates for a change in another

    _____ Ability to distinguish a shape change when nothing has been added or subtracted

    _____ Ability to comprehend that physical matter does not appear and disappear by magic

    _____ Ability to think about language and to comment on its properties

    _____ Ability to make decisions based on what one reasons

    _____ Ability to make decisions based on what one sees

17. Which best describes major difference in moral development between young school-age children and older school-age children?
    a. Younger children believe that standards of behavior come from within themselves.
    b. Children 6 to 7 years of age know the rules and understand the reasons behind the rules.
    c. Older school-age children are able to judge an act by the intentions that prompted it and not only by the consequences.
    d. Rewards and punishments guide older school-age children's behavior.

18. Which of the following best identifies the spiritual development of school-age children?
    a. They have little fear of "going to hell" for misbehavior.
    b. They begin to learn the difference between the natural and the supernatural.
    c. They petition to God for less tangible rewards.
    d. They view God as a deity with few human traits.

19. Which of the following would the nurse not expect to observe as characteristic of peer group relationships of 8-year-old Mark?
    a. Mark demonstrates loyalty to the group by adhering to the secret code rules.
    b. Mark demonstrates a greater individual egocentric outlook when compared with other peer group members.
    c. Mark is willing to conform to the group's rule of "not talking to girls."
    d. Mark has a best friend within the peer group with whom he shares his secrets.

20. During the school-age years, children learn valuable lessons from age-mates. How is this accomplished?
    a. The child learns to appreciate the varied points of view within the peer group.
    b. The child becomes sensitive to the social norms and pressures of the group.
    c. The child's interactions among peers lead to the formation of intimate friendships between same-sex peers.
    d. All of the above

21. Which of the following is most characteristic of the relationship between school-age children and their family?
    a. Children desire to spend equal time with family and peers.
    b. Children are prepared to reject parental controls.
    c. The group replaces the family as the primary influence in setting standards of behavior and rules.
    d. Children need and want restrictions placed on their behavior by the family.

22. Ms. Jones is a single mother caring for her 10-year-old son, James. At an office appointment for James, his mother asks the nurse how to prevent her son from becoming involved in gang violence. The best response is:
    a. "Try to be more of a pal to James so that he won't seek outside approval."
    b. "Relax restrictions on James. He needs to increase his independence, and this will show that you trust him."
    c. "Become aware of any gang-related activities in your community."
    d. "Don't allow James to join any 'boys only' groups."

23. Children's self-concepts are developed by:

24. The nurse plans to conduct a sex education class for 10-year-olds. Which of the following does the nurse recognize as most appropriate for this age-group?
    a. Present sex information as a normal part of growth and development.
    b. Discourage question-and-answer sessions.
    c. Because sexual information supplied by parents usually produces feelings of guilt and anxiety in children, avoid parental assistance in conducting the program.
    d. Segregate boys from girls and include information related only to the same sex in the discussion.

25. In relation to body image, school-age children:
    a. are not aware of physical disabilities in others.
    b. pay little attention to their own body capabilities.
    c. seldom express concerns about their bodies to their families.
    d. do not model themselves after their parents or compare themselves with images observed in the media.

26. List team membership characteristics that promote child development during the middle years.

27. School-age children:
    a. have little interest in complex board, card, or computer games.
    b. rarely collect items.
    c. tire of having stories read aloud.
    d. participate in hero worship.

28. Identify the following statements as true or false.

    _____ Successful adjustment to school entrance has little relationship to the child's physical and emotional maturity.
    _____ Children's attitudes toward school are influenced by the attitudes of their parents.
    _____ Television can increase the child's vocabulary, extend the child's horizon, and enrich the school experience.
    _____ Television can encourage children to believe that violence is an effective solution to conflict.
    _____ Children respond poorly to teachers who have attributes of caring parents.

_____ The teacher's primary goal is guiding the child's intellectual development.

_____ The reward and punishment administered by the teacher has little effect on the child's self-concept.

_____ Interaction between teacher and individual pupil affects the pupil's acceptance by the other children.

_____ Being responsible for school work helps children learn to keep promises, meet deadlines, and succeed at jobs as adults.

_____ Punitive interactions and corporal punishment are associated with decreasing disruptive behaviors in children.

_____ Exposure to violence affects children's ability to concentrate and function.

29. A factor that most influences the amount and manner of discipline and limit-setting imposed on school-age children is:
    a. the parent's age.
    b. the parent's education.
    c. the child's response to rewards and punishments.
    d. the parent's ability to communicate with the school system.

30. List the purposes of discipline.

31. Seven-year-old Andy was caught taking a playmate's toy. Which of the following is an important understanding of this behavior?
    a. At this age, Andy's sense of property rights is limited, and he took the item simply because he was attracted to it.
    b. If Andy is caught and punished and promises "not to do it again," he will keep his promise.
    c. This stealing act is an indication that something is seriously lacking in Andy's life.
    d. Andy will learn the importance of respecting other's property if the parents unexpectedly give away an item that belongs to Andy.

32. To assist school-age children in coping with stress in their lives, the nurse should:
    i. be able to recognize signs that indicate the child is undergoing stress.
    ii. teach the child how to recognize signs of stress in herself or himself.
    iii. help the child plan a means for dealing with any stress through problem solving.
    iv. reassure the child that the stress is only temporary.

    a. ii, iii, and iv
    b. i, ii, and iii
    c. ii and iv
    d. i and iii

33. Identify which of the following statements describing fears in the school-age child is true.
    a. School-age children are increasingly fearful of body safety.
    b. Most of the new fears that trouble school-age children are related to school and family.
    c. School-age children should be encouraged to hide their fears to prevent ridicule by their peers.
    d. School-age children with numerous fears need continuous protective behavior by parents to eliminate these fears.

34. The term *latchkey children* refers to whom?

35. By the end of middle childhood, children should be able to assume personal responsibility for self-care in the areas of _____, _____, _____, _____, _____, and _____.

36. What are the current dietary guidelines for healthy middle school children, as suggested by the U.S. Department of Agriculture?

37. Sleep problems in the school-age child are often demonstrated by:
    a. delaying tactics because the child does not wish to go to bed.
    b. night terrors that awaken the child during the night.
    c. the development of somatic illness that awakens the child during the night.
    d. the increasing need for larger amounts of sleep compared with preschool and adolescent children.

38. Which of the following best describes sleepwalking in childhood?
    a. During sleepwalking, the movements are clumsy and repetitive.
    b. Sleepwalking occurs in the first 1 to 2 hours of sleep.
    c. During sleepwalking, speech is comprehensible.
    d. The child remembers the episode in the morning.

39. The nurse is planning to advise a school-age child's parents about appropriate physical activity for their child. Which fact does the nurse include?
    a. School-age children have the same stamina and control as 15-year-old teens.
    b. School-age children are prepared for participation in strenuous competitive athletics.
    c. Activities that promote coordination in the school-age child include running and skipping rope.
    d. Most children need continued encouragement to engage in physical activity.

40. Identify the following as true or false.

    _____ In children 6 and 7 years old, the task of going to bed can be facilitated by encouraging quiet activity before bedtime.

    _____ Twelve-year-old children usually offer the most difficulty in regard to bedtime.

    _____ The best approach to sleepwalking is to awaken the child and put him or her back to bed.

    _____ Nightmares are a part of the normal developmental process and more common in children ages 6 to 12 than in younger children.

    _____ Sleepwalking is usually self-limiting and requires no treatment.

    _____ Eruption of permanent teeth begins with the first, or 6-year, molar.

    _____ Children under 10 years of age often need parental assistance to brush back teeth.

    _____ Toothbrushes for school-age children should be soft nylon brushes with an overall length of about 8 inches.

    _____ School systems have contributed to the sedentary habits of children by devoting fewer resources to physical education programs, playgrounds, and after-school programs.

    _____ During middle childhood, girls and boys have the same basic structure and can compete against one another in sports.

    _____ Parents who pressure their children to perform beyond their capabilities risk injury and lowered self-esteem in their child.

    _____ School-age children demonstrate little ability and interest in music.

_____ Children under the age of 12 should ride in the front passenger seat of vehicles equipped with air bags.

_____ Children ages 5 to 9 years restrained in adult-type seatbelts are at increased risk for head injury from impact with interior vehicle parts.

_____ All-terrain vehicles (ATVs) have been approved by the American Academy of Pediatrics for children as young as 14 years of age.

_____ Skateboard, roller skate, or in-line skate injuries among children mostly involve the wrist and forearm.

41. What recommendations should be included in parent and teacher education relating to television, videogames, and the Internet?

42. List six components that should be included in the content of school health services.

43. The nurse is planning an educational session for a group of 9-year-olds and their parents aimed at decreasing injuries and accidents among this group. The nurse would best accomplish this goal by reviewing:
    a. safety rules to prevent burns when dealing with fire.
    b. safety rules to prevent poisonings when dealing with toxic substances.
    c. pedestrian safety rules and skills training programs to prevent motor vehicle accidents.
    d. safety rules for the use of all-terrain vehicles, encouraging their use only with supervision.

CRITICAL THINKING—CASE STUDY

Allen Thomas, age 9, is taken to the clinic by his mother for a school physical examination. Allen's mother is concerned because Allen wants to join the school soccer team this year. On physical examination, the nurse discovers that Allen has grown 5 cm (2 inches) in height and gained 5.4 kg (12 lb) since last year. His health history is unchanged from the previous year. Allen tells the nurse that he rides his bike more now than last year because he has a new best friend with whom to ride.

44. Based on the information given, the nurse should expand assessment with Allen in:
    i. his diet.
    ii. his knowledge and use of safety precautions when riding his bike.
    iii. his hygiene habits.
    iv. his reasons for wanting to play soccer.

    a. i, ii, and iii
    b. ii and iv
    c. i and ii
    d. i and iv

45. Which of the following would be the nurse's best response to the mother's concern about Allen playing soccer?
    a. "Allen is healthy, and playing soccer will allow him to increase strength and develop motor skill performance."
    b. "Allen is overweight for his age and should be encouraged to ride his bike less. Soccer is a better activity for him because it will help decrease his weight."
    c. "Allen is still too young to participate in strenuous sports like soccer. He should be able to participate in another year."
    d. "Let Allen play what he wants to. You worry too much about his activities."

46. Based on the information provided, the nurse plans an educational session for Allen and his mother. Which knowledge deficit would the nurse most likely identify for this family?
    a. Modified nutrition because of improper dietary habits
    b. Improper nutrition related to less daily intake than the body needs
    c. Lack of proper physical activity related to bike riding
    d. Improper parenting skills related to overprotective mother

47. Mrs. Thomas asks the nurse how she can foster Allen's development. What would be the best response by the nurse?
    a. "Don't interfere with Allen as long as he is doing well in school."
    b. "Give Allen recognition and positive feedback for his accomplishments."
    c. "Always point out to Allen how he incorrectly performs tasks so that he can improve his accomplishments."
    d. "Try not to set rules for Allen. He needs to set his own limits during this period of development."

48. The nurse realizes that Allen's weight gain:
    a. is normal during this growth period.
    b. is probably related to a high-fat diet, rich in junk food intake.
    c. will be corrected by the increase in exercise of soccer and bike riding.
    d. is not influenced by the mass media.

49. The nurse is discussing bicycle safety with Allen's mother. Mrs. Thomas says that Allen will soon need a new bike and helmet. Describe what should be included in the conversation about selecting the bike and safety helmet.

18 Health Problems of Middle Childhood

1. Skin in the infant and small child, as compared with skin in older children and adults:
   a. is tightly bound to the dermis.
   b. is less likely to have blister formation from an inflammatory process.
   c. is more likely to react to a sensitizing allergen than to a primary irritant.
   d. is more susceptible to superficial bacterial infection.

2. List four factors that can result in lesions of the skin in children.

3. Match each term related to assessment of the skin with its description.

   a. Pruritus   d. Paresthesia
   b. Anesthesia   e. Hypesthesia
   c. Hyperesthesia

   _____ Excessive sensitiveness

   _____ Absence of sensation

   _____ Diminished sensation

   _____ Itching

   _____ Abnormal sensation

4. Match each wound-related term with its description.

   a. Acute   g. Incision
   b. Chronic   h. Penetrating
   c. Pressure ulcer   i. Puncture
   d. Abrasion   j. Regeneration
   e. Avulsion   k. Allodynia
   f. Laceration

   _____ Rapid replacement by similar cells

   _____ Accidental cut, with either torn or jagged edges

   _____ Disruption of the skin that extends into the underlying tissue or into a body cavity

   _____ Heals uneventfully within the usual time frame

   _____ Does not heal in the expected time frame and can be associated with complications

   _____ Removal of the superficial layers of skin by scraping

   _____ Localized area of cellular necrosis that often becomes a chronic skin injury

   _____ Forcible pulling out or extraction of tissue

   _____ Wound with an opening that is small compared with its depth

   _____ Division of the skin made with a sharp object

   _____ Sensation of pain from normally nonpainful stimuli

5. Cindy, age 8 years, is brought to the clinic with a sore on her arm. She tells the nurse that she scratched it on a piece of metal at the playground about 1 week ago. Which of the following signs would the nurse expect to find if the sore has become infected?
   a. Itching at the site of the sore
   b. Rough edges around the sore
   c. No pain at the site
   d. Increased temperature around the sore

6. Epithelial wound healing:
   a. begins 72 hours after the wound is incurred.
   b. occurs by migration and proliferation of epithelial cells from the wound center toward the wound margins.
   c. occurs more rapidly when the wound is covered with a transparent or other occlusive-type dressing.
   d. occurs more rapidly when the skin is allowed to dry and to form an eschar, or scab.

7. High-quality patient outcomes for skin disorders include all of the following except:
   a. early, accurate diagnosis of the skin lesion.
   b. obtaining accurate accounts of child's symptoms.
   c. effective treatment and symptom relief.
   d. prevention of spread.

8. During wound healing, immature connective tissue cells migrate to the healing site and begin to secrete collagen into the meshwork spaces. What is this phase called?
   a. Scar contracture
   b. Inflammation
   c. Fibroplasia
   d. Scar maturation

9. Mary, age 7 years, fell and sustained a deep laceration to her chin. She was taken to the emergency department, where the laceration was sutured with the edges well approximated. The nurse expects the repair healing to take place by:
   a. primary intention.
   b. secondary intention.
   c. tertiary intention.

10. Which of the following is not indicated for use in promoting wound healing?
    a. Nutrition with sufficient protein, calories, vitamin C, and zinc
    b. Irrigation of wounds with normal saline
    c. Application of povidone-iodine daily
    d. Application of an occlusive dressing

11. Jimmy, age 9 years, has fallen and scraped his knee at school. He is brought to the school nurse for treatment. After cleaning the area and applying an over-the-counter first aid ointment, the nurse applies a transparent adhesive dressing. This type of dressing is considered to be:
    a. occlusive.
    b. semiocclusive.
    c. nonocclusive.
    d. permeable.

12. Which of the following statements about use of topical therapy in the pediatric population is true?
    a. Use of silver impregnated in dressing as foam decreases the bacterial burden and bioburden of the wound and has little absorption effect in the pediatric population.
    b. Application of heat provides a soothing effect to reduce inflammatory processes.
    c. The use of immunomodulators is suggested as first-line treatment in children younger than 2 years of age.
    d. Topical immunomodulators have been linked to possible skin cancer and lymphoma.

13. Which of the following does the nurse include in the educational plan when instructing parents about the use of topical corticosteroids?
    a. Do not use this cream on a fungal infection.
    b. Apply a thick layer of the cream and rub into the skin well.
    c. Do not use for longer than 3 days in chronic conditions.
    d. All of the above.

14. Which of the following is true about topical therapy for acute treatment of dermatologic problems?
    a. Application of heat to the area will relieve itching.
    b. Children's broken or inflamed skin is more absorbent than their intact skin.
    c. Chemicals that are nonirritating to intact skin will be nonirritating to inflamed skin.
    d. Emollient action of soaks, baths, or lotions increases skin irritation.

15. Skin disorder assessment includes the objective data collected by inspection and palpation. Which of the following is not an example of objective data?
    a. The lesion has an increased erythematous margin edge.
    b. The rash appears as macules and papules.
    c. The lesion is painful and itches.
    d. The lesion is moist.

16. List the signs of wound infection.

17. Wound care instructions to parents should include:
    a. Use betadine, alcohol, and hydrogen peroxide to prevent infection.
    b. Use hydrocolloid dressing that just covers the wound with little overlap.
    c. Formation of yellow gel with a fruity odor under hydrocolloid dressings is a sign of infection.
    d. Remove the hydrocolloid dressings by raising one edge of the dressing and pulling parallel to the skin to loosen the adhesive.

18. The nurse is applying wet compresses of Burow solution to Johnny's wound. Which of the following does the nurse recognize as correct information about this type of topical therapy?
    a. After application of the compresses, the wound is washed with soap and water and rubbed dry.
    b. Compresses loosen and remove crusts and debris.
    c. Burow solution is applied directly onto the wound and then covered with dry, soft gauze.
    d. When evaporation begins to dry out the dressings, more solution is poured directly over the dressings.

19. Care of bacterial skin infections in children may include all of the following except:
    a. good hand washing.
    b. keeping the fingernails short.
    c. puncturing the surface of the pustule.
    d. application of topical antibiotics.

20. Lisa, age 7, has been diagnosed with impetigo. Which of the following does the nurse recognize as being a manifestation of this bacterial infection?
    a. Inflammation of skin and subcutaneous tissues with intense redness
    b. Honey-colored, crusty exudate
    c. Lymphangitis
    d. Systemic effects of malaise

21. Which of the following is a fungal infection that lives on the skin?
    a. Tinea corporis
    b. Herpes simplex type 1
    c. Scabies
    d. Warts

22. Steve, age 8, has been diagnosed with tinea capitis. Which of the following does the nurse include in the teaching plan for Steve and his parents?
    a. No animal-to-person transmission is associated with this infection.
    b. Steve can continue to share hair grooming articles with his younger brother.
    c. Griseofulvin should be administered with high-fat foods.
    d. Cleanliness is the best way to prevent this disease.

23. Johnny has been diagnosed with tinea capitis. His mother asks how he got this infection. The best response would be:
    a. "Transmission is from person-to-person or from animal-to-person contact."
    b. "Transmission is from person-to-person contact only."
    c. "Transmission is from animal-to-person contact only."
    d. "It is more important to talk about treatment than how Johnny got the disease."

24. Which of the following statements about scabies is incorrect?
    a. Clinical manifestations include intense pruritus, especially at night, and papules, burrows, or vesicles on interdigital surfaces.
    b. Treatment is the application of 5% Elimite for all family members.
    c. After treatment, all previously worn clothing is washed in very hot water and dried at the high setting in the dryer.
    d. The rash and itching will be eliminated immediately after treatment.

25. a. What would the nurse look for in assessing whether a child has pediculosis?

    b. What is the current American Academy of Pediatrics guidelines regarding the no-nit policy in school?

26. In helping parents cope with pediculosis, the nurse should emphasize that:
    a. anyone can get pediculosis.
    b. lice will fly and jump from one person to another.
    c. cutting the child's hair short will prevent reinfestation.
    d. the condition can be transmitted by pets.

27. The nurse is instructing Angie's parents about using a pyrethrin shampoo for pediculosis. Which of the following should be included in these instructions?
    a. Only one application is needed.
    b. The shampoo is avoided in children with contact allergy to ragweed or turpentine.
    c. The shampoo kills the lice and nits on contact.
    d. The shampoo will kill all the nits.

28. The treatment of choice for pediculosis capitis in a 2-year-old child is:
    a. 5% permethrin cream (Elimite).
    b. 1% lindane shampoo (Kwell).
    c. selenium sulfide shampoos.
    d. permethrin 1% cream rinse (Nix).

29. Children with Lyme disease are not initially seen with:
    a. a small erythematous papule that has a circumferential ring with a raised, edematous, doughnut-like border.
    b. multiple, small secondary annular lesions with indurated centers on the palms and soles.
    c. flulike symptoms of headache, malaise, and lymphadenopathy.
    d. musculoskeletal pains that involve the tendons, bursae, muscles, and synovia.

30. Susan, age 10 years, has been diagnosed with Lyme disease. She has no allergies to medications. The nurse can expect the treatment to be:
    a. erythromycin.
    b. cefuroxime.
    c. ciprofloxin.
    d. doxycycline.

31. Match each term with its description.

    a. Histoplasmosis
    b. Coccidioidomycosis
    c. Rocky Mountain spotted fever
    d. Epidemic typhus
    e. Endemic typhus
    f. Rickettsialpox

    _____ Transmitted by flea bite or by inhaling or ingesting flea excreta

    _____ Transmitted from human to human by the body louse; requires that patient be isolated until deloused

    _____ Marked by maculopapular rash following primary lesion and eschar at site of bite; transmitted from house mouse to humans by infected mite

    _____ Infection caused by organism cultured from soil, especially where contaminated with fowl droppings

    _____ Transmitted by tick; maculopapular or petechial rash on palms and soles

    _____ Primary lung disease; endemic in southwestern United States

32. Children with cat scratch disease usually are seen with:
    a. headache, diarrhea, and fever.
    b. regional lymphadenopathy.
    c. maculopapular rash over the entire body.
    d. painful, pruritic papules at the site of inoculation.

33. Which of the following statements about cat scratch disease is true?
    a. It is caused by the scratch or bite of an animal, usually a cat or kitten.
    b. The animal will have a history of illness before transmission of the disease.
    c. Antibiotics shorten the duration of the illness.
    d. Analgesics are avoided during the disease process.

34. Billy has come in contact with poison ivy on a school picnic. The best intervention for the nurse to implement at this time is to:
    a. wash the area with a strong soap and water solution.
    b. apply Calamine lotion to the area.
    c. prevent spread by instructing Billy not to scratch the lesions.
    d. flush the area immediately with cold water.

35. When advising parents about the use of sunscreen for school-age children, the nurse should tell them that:
    a. a waterproof sunscreen with a minimum 15 SPF is recommended for children.
    b. the lower the number of SPF, the higher the protection.
    c. sunscreens are not as effective as sunblockers.
    d. the sunscreen should be applied 1 hour before the child is allowed in the sun.

36. Which of the following information about sunscreen containing PABA is false?
    a. It may stain clothes.
    b. It can cause an allergic reaction.
    c. It provides little protection when the child is swimming or sweating.
    d. It is an effective sunscreen against ultraviolet B.

37. Match each term with its description.
    a. Chilblain
    b. Frostbite
    c. Sunscreen
    d. Sunblocker
    e. Ultraviolet A (UVA)
    f. Ultraviolet B (UVB)
    g. Hypothermia
    h. Contact dermatitis

    _____ Blocks out ultraviolet rays by reflecting sunlight

    _____ Partially absorbs ultraviolet light

    _____ An inflammatory reaction of the skin to a substance that evokes a hypersensitivity response or a direct irritation

_____ Shorter light waves, responsible for tanning, burning, and most of the harmful effects attributed to sunlight

_____ Longest light waves, causing only minimal burning but playing a significant role in photosensitive and photoallergic reactions

_____ Condition in which ice crystals form in tissues

_____ Redness and swelling of the skin from cold exposure

_____ Cooling of the body's core temperature below 35° C (95° F)

38. In caring for the child with frostbite, the nurse remembers that:
    a. slow thawing is associated with less tissue necrosis.
    b. the frostbitten part appears white or blanched, feels solid, and is without sensation.
    c. rewarming produces a small return of sensation with a small amount of pain.
    d. rewarming is accomplished by rubbing the injured tissue.

39. A period of _____ _____ is usually required for a child to develop sensitivity to a drug that has never been previously administered. With prior sensitivity, the reaction

    appears _____ _____.

40. Erythema multiforme exudativum (Stevens-Johnson syndrome):
    a. is rare and occurs most often in females.
    b. is a hypersensitivity reaction to certain drugs.
    c. begins with generalized rash over the entire body except for palms, soles, and extensor surfaces.
    d. is caused by a bite from a flea.

41. Neurofibromatosis is:
    a. an autosomal dominant genetic disorder.
    b. suspected when the 5-year-old child is seen with six or more café-au-lait spots larger than 5 mm in diameter.
    c. suspected when the infant develops axillary or inguinal freckling.
    d. all of the above.

42. Johnny's mother is calling the clinic because Johnny has developed a rash over his entire body. Two days ago he was prescribed amoxicillin for an ear infection, and now his mother tells the nurse she thinks Johnny may have gotten a small rash with this medication when he previously took it. Which of the following would be the best intervention by the nurse at this time?
    a. Question the mother about other symptoms that Johnny may have developed.
    b. Continue the medication and have Johnny come in tomorrow to see the practitioner.
    c. Stop the medication and inform the practitioner.
    d. Tell the mother to give only half the prescribed dose of the medication until Johnny can return to the clinic to see the practitioner.

43. Cindy is 12 years old and is brought to the clinic because of a bald spot developing on her head. Cindy wears her hair tightly braided with beads. Which of the following should the nurse suspect?
    a. Alopecia from trauma
    b. Tinea capitis
    c. Psoriasis
    d. Urticaria

44. Billy has been stung by a bee. A small reaction has occurred at the site. What is the most appropriate action at this time?
    a. Wait until Billy is at home to completely remove the stinger with forceps.
    b. Remove the stinger as soon as possible by scraping it off the skin.
    c. Wash the area with hot water and soap.
    d. Arrange for Billy to undergo skin testing.

45. The most effective method for tick removal in a child is to:
    a. use curved forceps and grasp close to the point of attachment, then pull straight up with a steady, even pressure.
    b. apply mineral oil to the back of the tick and wait for it to back out.
    c. use the fingers to pull the tick out with a straight, steady, even pressure.
    d. place a hot match on the back of the tick and pick it up with gloved hands when the tick falls off.

46. Dog bites in children occur most often:
    a. in girls over 5 years of age.
    b. in children under 5 years of age.
    c. from stray dogs.
    d. in school yards and neighborhood parks.

47. Nora has been brought to the emergency department by her father after having been bitten by the family dog. Examination reveals three puncture wounds of the hand. Expected therapeutic management for these wounds includes:
    a. suturing the wounds.
    b. administering prophylactic antibiotics.
    c. irrigating with hydrogen peroxide.
    d. administering a tetanus toxoid booster, because Nora's last booster was given 13 months ago.

48. On a field trip to a remote area with his Boy Scout troop, Peter is bitten by a snake. Which of the following actions would be contraindicated?
    a. Remove Peter from the area and have him rest.
    b. Feel for a pulse distal to the bite area.
    c. Place ice from the ice cooler on the bite area.
    d. Apply a loose tourniquet above the bite area.

49. Human bites:
    a. are treatable at home.
    b. do not require tetanus immunization.
    c. should not have ice applied to the area.
    d. should receive medical attention if greater than ¼ inch.

50. During middle childhood:
    a. children are less susceptible to development of dental caries.
    b. plasticized sealant, applied to deep fissures and grooves of healthy teeth, can prevent cavity formation.
    c. periodontal disease contributes to tooth loss.
    d. regular administration of fluoride is no longer recommended.

51. The most common cause of malocclusion is:
    a. thumb sucking.
    b. tongue thrusting.
    c. hereditary factors.
    d. abnormal growth patterns.

52. Emergency care for tooth evulsion includes:
    a. replanting the tooth after bleeding has stopped.
    b. storing the tooth in tap water until it and the child can be transported to the dentist.
    c. holding the tooth by the root.
    d. rinsing the dirty tooth gently under running water before replanting.

53. The major nursing consideration in assisting the family of a child with nocturnal enuresis is to prevent the child from developing alterations in:
    a. body image.
    b. self-esteem.
    c. autonomy.
    d. peer acceptance.

54. The nurse is assisting the family of a child with a history of encopresis. Which of the following should be included in the nurse's discussion with this family?
    a. Instructing the parents to sit the child on the toilet at two daily routine intervals
    b. Instructing the parents that the child will probably need to have daily enemas for the next year
    c. Suggesting the use of stimulant cathartics weekly
    d. Reassuring the family that most problems resolve successfully with some relapses during periods of stress

55. Barbara has been diagnosed with attention deficit hyperactivity disorder and placed on methylphenidate (Ritalin) by her physician. Which of the following statements, made by the nurse to Barbara's parents, is correct?
    a. "This drug will ultimately lead to stimulation of the inhibitory system of the central nervous system by increasing dopamine and norepinephrine levels in the body."
    b. "Dosage is usually unchanged until adolescence."
    c. "This medication takes 2 to 3 weeks to achieve an effect."
    d. "Barbara's appetite will be increased with this drug."

56. Identify the following statements as true or false.

    _____ Dyslexia is a learning disability characterized by reading letters in reverse.

    _____ Children with learning disabilities have below-average intelligence.

    _____ Children with learning disorders grow up to be adults with learning disabilities.

    _____ Learning disabilities include learning problems that result from visual, hearing, or motor disabilities.

57. Therapeutic management for a child with a tic disorder primarily consists of:
    a. behavioral modification to teach the child to suppress the tic disorder.
    b. administration of haloperidol to suppress the tic disorder.
    c. education and support for the child and family with reassurance about the prognosis.
    d. genetic counseling for the parents.

58. Which of the following statements about Tourette syndrome (TS) is true?
    a. Manifestations are stable in intensity and rarely change once developed.
    b. Children with TS have no associated obsessive-compulsive symptoms.
    c. Tics lead to physical deterioration and affect life expectancy.
    d. Behaviors are involuntary.

59. Identify the following statements as true or false.

    _____ Posttraumatic stress disorder typically involves life-threatening events.

    _____ School phobia is more common in boys than in girls.

    _____ Children with school phobia are correctly viewed as delinquent children.

    _____ A frequent source of fear in school phobia is separation anxiety based on a strong dependent relationship between the mother and the child.

    _____ The primary goal for the child with school phobia is to return the child to school.

    _____ Prevention of dependency problems in childhood is based on encouraging independence at appropriate times during infancy and early childhood.

    _____ Recurrent abdominal pain of childhood is defined as three or more separate episodes of abdominal pain during a 3-month period interfering with function.

    _____ Children at risk for recurrent abdominal pain tend to be high achievers with great personal goals or those whose parents have unusually high expectations.

    _____ Parents of children with conversion reaction seldom display problems in communication or depression.

    _____ Depressed children usually exhibit low self-esteem, think of themselves as hopeless, and explain negative events in terms of their personal shortcomings.

    _____ Three risk factors identified for childhood schizophrenia are genetic characteristics, gestational and birth complications, and winter birth.

CRITICAL THINKING—CASE STUDY

Carol, age 9, went on a picnic yesterday with her family. Today she returns to school and is showing her classmates several leaves that she collected yesterday. The teacher notices that three of the leaves are from a poison ivy plant. The teacher takes Carol to the school nurse because of a rash that has developed on her arms and legs. Carol tells the nurse that the rash is "very itchy."

60. The nurse completes a diagnostic assessment of the skin rash to include a complete history and physical examination. The nurse knows that this history should include:
    a. inspection of the rash, including size and shape of lesions.
    b. symptoms, past and recent exposure to causative agents, medications taken, and history of previous similar rashes.
    c. palpation of the rash for increased heat, edema, and tenderness.
    d. skin scrapings from the site for microscopic examination.

61. The primary action the school nurse should take at this time is to:
    a. call Carol's parents to pick her up at school. Isolate Carol from other classmates until her parents arrive.
    b. give the poison ivy leaves to the school janitor to be destroyed in the school incinerator.
    c. instruct the teacher to make certain all classmates who had contact with the poison ivy plant wash these areas with mild soap and water.
    d. reassure Carol that everything is going to be fine, apply Calamine lotion to her rash, and instruct Carol not to scratch the rash.

62. What is the best nursing diagnosis for Carol at this time?
    a. Impaired Skin Integrity related to environmental factors
    b. High Risk for Infection related to presence of infectious organisms
    c. Pain related to skin lesions
    d. Body Image Disturbance related to presence of rash

63. Goals for Carol should include:
    a. Carol will not experience secondary damage, such as infection, from scratching.
    b. Carol will demonstrate acceptable levels of comfort from itching.
    c. Carol will be able to recognize and avoid precipitating agent in the future.
    d. All of the above.

64. In educating Carol and her parents about caring for the rash, the nurse should tell them to:
    i. bathe in tepid or cool water.
    ii. bathe in hot water.
    iii. apply hydrogen peroxide to the rash daily.
    iv. apply calamine lotion to the rash.
    v. administer over-the-counter diphenhydramine orally to decrease itching.
    vi. keep Carol's fingernails short.
    vii. wear heavy clothing to prevent contamination.
    viii. understand that the rash is contagious and will weep.

    a. i, iii, iv, vi, and vii
    b. i, iv, v, and vi
    c. ii, v, vi, and vii
    d. iii, iv, v, and viii

19 Health Promotion of the Adolescent and Family

1. In the female adolescent who has reached puberty, the luteinizing hormone initiates which of the following actions?
   a. Production of estrogen
   b. Growth of ovarian follicles
   c. Production of gonadotropin-releasing hormone
   d. Ovulation

2. The hormone in the female that causes growth and development of the vagina, uterus, fallopian tubes, and breasts is:
   a. estrogen.
   b. progesterone.
   c. follicle-stimulating hormone (FSH).
   d. luteinizing hormone (LH).

3. Identify the following statements regarding adolescence as true or false.

   _____ The adolescent is considered potentially fertile from the first menstrual period or first ejaculation.

   _____ Development of secondary sexual characteristics occurs in a predictable sequence.

   _____ The Tanner developmental stages are based on maturity of secondary sexual characteristics and can be used when assessing adolescent growth.

   _____ The hypothalamic-pituitary-gonadal system is maintained in an active state throughout childhood because of the low secretion of gonadotropin-releasing hormone.

   _____ The development of a small bud of breast tissue is the earliest, most visible change of puberty.

   _____ The average age for beginning menstruation is 13 years.

   _____ In girls, physical maturation leads to greater satisfaction with their appearance.

   _____ Initial menstrual periods usually last 2 or 3 days and are regular by the second month.

   _____ During puberty, FSH acting with LH stimulates the production of sperm.

4. Match each term with its description.

   a. Thelarche   e. Gynecomastia
   b. Pubarche   f. Puberty
   c. Physiologic leukorrhea   g. Ovulation
   d. Menarche

   _____ Biologic changes of adolescence

   _____ Onset of menstrual periods

   _____ Development of breast tissue

   _____ Male breast enlargement and tenderness

   _____ Development of pubic hair

   _____ Normal vaginal discharge

   _____ Release of an ovum by a follicle

5. Julie, 12 years old, is brought to the nurse practitioner's office by her mother. Julie has started to develop breast tissue and some pubic hair. Both the mother and daughter are concerned because Julie has been having increased vaginal discharge. Julie tells the nurse, "I wash my private area every day, but I still have fluid that comes out." What is the nurse's best response?
   a. "It sounds like you have an infection. We'll have the nurse practitioner check you to see what is causing this discharge."
   b. "Have you been using soap when you wash?"
   c. "This sounds like a normal discharge that happens to all girls as they start to mature. It is a sign that your body is preparing for your periods to begin."
   d. "This is probably not related to hygiene. Are you concerned that this discharge might be causing an odor?"

6. Girls may be considered to have _____ _____ if breast development has not occurred by age 13 or if menarche has not occurred within 2 to 2½ years of the onset of breast development. Girls may be considered to have _____ _____ if breast development or pubic hair appears before age 7 years.

7. The first pubescent change in boys is:
   a. appearance of pubic hair.
   b. testicular enlargement with thinning, reddening, and increased looseness of the scrotum.
   c. penile enlargement.
   d. temporary breast enlargement and tenderness.

8. Tommy is brought in by his father for his yearly physical. On examination, the nurse notes that since last year Tommy has developed pubic hair, testicular enlargement, and related scrotal changes. In planning anticipatory guidance, which of the following subjects would best be discussed with Tommy as soon as possible?
   a. Nocturnal emission
   b. Sexually transmitted infection prevention
   c. Pregnancy prevention
   d. Hygiene needs

9. The _____ _____ _____ refers to the increased development of muscles, skeleton, and internal organs that reaches a peak at about 12 years of age in girls and about 14 years of age in boys. _____ _____ is the most important determinant of the onset, rate, and duration of pubertal growth.

10. During assessment, the nurse observes that Gail has sparse growth of downy hair extending along the labia. Which of the following Tanner stages would be suspected?
    a. Stage 1
    b. Stage 2
    c. Stage 4
    d. Stage 5

11. Ben has just turned 16 years of age and is in for his routine physical. The nurse notes that Ben has pubescent changes and determines that Ben is in Tanner stage 3. What findings would best describe this Tanner stage?
    a. Testes, scrotum, and penis are adult in size and shape.
    b. No pubic hair is present.
    c. There is initial enlargement of scrotum and testes; reddening and texture changes of the scrotal skin; long, straight, downy hair at base of penis.
    d. There is initial enlargement of penis in length; testes and scrotum are enlarged; hair is darker, coarser, and curly over entire pubis.

12. Which of the following statements about pattern of growth during adolescence is true?
    a. Knowing the correct sequence of the growth pattern is useful only when assessing abnormal growth patterns versus normal growth patterns.
    b. Girls usually begin puberty and reach maturity about 2 years earlier than boys.
    c. Girls and boys experience an increase of muscle mass that begins during early puberty and lasts throughout adolescence.
    d. Girls and boys experience an increase in linear growth that begins for both during midpuberty.

13. On the average, girls gain _____ to _____ inches in height and _____ to _____ lb during adolescence, whereas boys gain _____ to _____ inches and _____ to _____ lb.

14. Which of the following best describes the formal operational thinking that occurs between the ages of 11 and 14 years?
    a. Thought process includes thinking in concrete terms.
    b. Thought process includes information obtained from the environment and peers.
    c. Thought process includes thinking in abstract terms, possibilities, and hypotheses.
    d. Thought process is limited to what is observed.

15. Jimmy, a 13-year-old, is sent to the school nurse because he and some of his peers were caught chewing tobacco while playing baseball. The nurse knows that the best way to influence Jimmy's behavior for health promotion would be to:
    a. tell Jimmy that he will be suspended from school if he continues to chew the tobacco.
    b. show Jimmy pictures of oral cancer from chewing tobacco.
    c. tell Jimmy about the dangers of chewing tobacco and stress the fact that girls do not like boys who chew tobacco.
    d. arrange for a local baseball hero to talk with Jimmy and his friends, stressing that he does not use chewing tobacco, his friends do not chew tobacco, and chewing tobacco causes ugly teeth.

16. Adolescent egocentrism may lead to a pattern of personal fable. An example of a personal fable is:
    a. "Everyone is coming to the play just to see me."
    b. "Mary Sue got pregnant, but it won't happen to me."
    c. "I hate taking my clothes off for gym class because everyone stares at me."
    d. "Mary is very envious of how I dress."

17. Adolescents develop the social cognition change of mutual role-taking. Which of the following is the best description of this ability?
    a. Heightened sense of self-consciousness
    b. Understanding the perspectives of others and that actions can influence others
    c. Beliefs that are more abstract and rooted in ideologic principles
    d. Realization that others have thoughts and feelings

18. The development of a personal value system or value autonomy during adolescence usually occurs by age:
    a. 14 to 16 years
    b. 18 to 20 years
    c. 13 to 14 years
    d. 16 to 18 years

19. Elements of principled moral reasoning emerge during adolescence. Which of the following is the best description of this moral development?
    a. Moral guidelines are seen to emanate from authority figures.
    b. Moral standards are seen as objective and not to be questioned.
    c. Absolutes and rules are questioned and subject to disagreement.
    d. A personal value system is developed.

20. Spiritual development during adolescent years can best be described as:
    a. placing less emphasis on what a person believes.
    b. placing more emphasis on whether a person attends religious services.
    c. becoming more focused on spiritual and ideologic matters and less on observing religious customs.
    d. becoming more focused on observing religious customs and less on ideologic matters.

21. According to Erikson, a key to identity achievement in adolescence is:
    a. related to the adolescent's interactions with others and serves as a mirror reflecting information back to the adolescent.
    b. linked to the role the adolescent plays within the family.
    c. related to the adolescent's acceptance of parental guidelines.
    d. related to the adolescent's ability to complete his or her plans for future accomplishments.

22. Expected characteristics of emotional autonomy during early adolescence include:
    a. increased independence from friends.
    b. increased need for parental approval.
    c. belief that parents are all-knowing and all-powerful.
    d. less emotional dependence on parents.

23. The formation of sexual identity development during adolescence usually involves:
    i. forming close friendships with same-sex peers during early adolescence.
    ii. developing intimate relationships with members of the opposite sex during middle adolescence.
    iii. developing emotional and social identities separate from those of families.
    iv. incorporating sexuality successfully into intimate relationships.

    a. i, ii, and iii
    b. ii, iii, and iv
    c. ii and iii
    d. i, ii, iii, and iv

24. Nationally, what percentage of boys and girls have had sexual intercourse by the twelfth grade?
    a. 67% of boys and 76% of girls
    b. 70% of boys and 58% of girls
    c. 68% of girls and 62% of boys
    d. 84% of girls and 58% of boys

25. The development of sexual orientation includes seven developmental milestones during late childhood and throughout adolescence. These milestones do not always occur in the same order or in the same time frame. List these milestones.

26. Intimate relationships are not necessarily characterized by:
    a. concern for each other's well-being.
    b. sharing of sexual intimacy.
    c. a willingness to disclose private, sensitive topics.
    d. sharing of common interests and activities.

27. Changes in family structure accompanied by changes in parental employment, with a dramatic increase in the percentage of mothers working outside the home, have resulted in changes for adolescents, including:
    a. adolescents having more time unsupervised by adults.
    b. adolescents having more time for communication and intimacy with parents.
    c. adolescents having less time to spend with peers.
    d. adolescents requiring more supervision by outside family members.

28. Adolescents who feel close to their parents show:
    i. more positive psychosocial development.
    ii. greater behavioral competence.
    iii. less susceptibility to negative peer pressure.
    iv. less tendency to be involved in risk-taking behaviors.

    a. i, iii, and iv
    b. i and ii
    c. iii and iv
    d. i, ii, iii, and iv

29. Describe authoritative parenting and results related to this type of parenting.

30. Internet chatrooms and social networking:
    a. have allowed adolescents a more public arena for developing interpersonal skills.
    b. have decreased the amount of bullying in the school setting.
    c. have increased the development of multitasking and longer attention spans in the adolescent.
    d. have decreased adolescents' risk-taking behaviors.

31. How do advances in cognitive development change during adolescence?
    a. Beliefs become more concrete and less rooted in general ideologic principles.
    b. Adolescents show an increasing emotional understanding and acceptance of parents' beliefs as their own.
    c. Adolescents encounter few new opportunities for decisions based on their past experiences.
    d. Adolescents develop a personal value system distinct from that of significant adults in their lives.

32. Compared with childhood peer groups, adolescent peer groups are:
    a. more likely to include peers from the opposite sex.
    b. less autonomous.
    c. less likely to influence members' socialization roles.
    d. more likely to require parental supervision.

33. Which of the following statements about adolescents and school is true?
    a. Transition from elementary school to middle school has no negative effects on adolescents.
    b. Dropout rates are highest among Hispanic and American Indian adolescents.
    c. Dropout rates are highest among Hispanic and African-American adolescents.
    d. Students with above-average grades have been identified as more likely to engage in suicide attempts.

34. While Jenny, age 16, is in for her routine checkup, her mother tells the nurse that Jenny wants to get a job at a local fast-food restaurant, where she would work 30 hours a week to earn extra money for clothes. The mother wonders whether this is a good idea. What is the nurse's best response?
    a. "Jenny is healthy, and there is no reason she could not take the job."
    b. "All adolescents are preoccupied with clothes, so let her go ahead."
    c. "That sounds like a dead-end job. Why would Jenny want to work there?"
    d. "Working 30 hours a week may take time away from her studies and extracurricular activities and increase fatigue. Looking together at Jenny's future career goals may help identify alternatives."

35. List three primary causes of mortality accounting for 75% of all adolescent deaths.

36. To best promote adolescent health, the nursing plan should incorporate:
    a. the adolescent's definition of health.
    b. the adolescent's past health promotion activities.
    c. a complete assessment of the adolescent's past medical treatment.
    d. a complete physical examination.

37. Health concerns consistent with middle adolescence include:
    a. school performance.
    b. emotional health issues.
    c. physical appearance.
    d. future career or employment.

38. Adolescents are more likely to participate in health care services when:
    a. they understand the potentially negative consequences of their health behavior.
    b. they rank confidential care and respect higher than site cleanliness.
    c. they view their health problems as not organic in nature.
    d. they see the health care provider as caring and respectful.

39. Identify the following statements as true or false.

    _____ Routine exercise can reduce risk for depression and emotional distress in adolescents.

    _____ Teens are less likely to seek sexual health care services when parental consent is required.

    _____ Media campaigns are most likely to be beneficial when targeted to appeal to parents rather than adolescents.

    _____ Protective factors that characterize adolescents who cope successfully with adverse life situations include the ability to adapt to new persons and situations.

    _____ The nurse involved with adolescent health promotion should plan interventions that decrease exposure to stressful life events and increase sources of emotional support.

    _____ The most successful adolescent health promotion programs are aimed at single issues presented with a focused educational approach.

    _____ When interviewing adolescents, the nurse should establish the boundaries around confidentiality and privacy at the beginning of the interview.

    _____ There is evidence to support the effectiveness of engaging adolescents by use of communication technology regarding health promotion.

    _____ School-based clinics have not increased adolescents' access to preventive services.

    _____ All adolescents who participate in homosexual activity will become homosexual adults.

    _____ Gay, lesbian, and bisexual adolescents need specific sexuality education that is different from that provided to other adolescents.

    _____ Students with below-average grades are more likely to engage in health-compromising behaviors.

    _____ Students who are exposed to repeated teasing and harassment are more likely to skip school and to attempt suicide.

    _____ Students who are regularly harassed are more likely to bring weapons to school.

    _____ The typical teenager's job provides neither continuity to adult employment nor links to adults who could serve as vocational mentors.

    _____ Parental involvement has not been shown to increase effectiveness of high schools.

    _____ The most likely cause of death for African-American teenagers is homicide involving firearms.

    _____ Excessive intake of calories, sugar, fat, cholesterol, and sodium is common among adolescents and is found at all income levels, in all racial or ethnic groups, and in both genders.

    _____ Of high school students nationwide, 11% report rarely or never using safety belts when riding in a car driven by someone else.

_____ Identified factors that promote resiliency among minority adolescents from disadvantaged backgrounds include coming from families and communities that provide nurturing, supportive, and culturally rich environments.

_____ Nurses should encourage teens to disclose their sexual orientations to their families as soon as the teens are sure of their orientation.

_____ Rural adolescents have higher rates of delinquency but less access to health care compared with urban adolescents.

40. Effective health care services for adolescents must be _____ and
_____.

41. List three strategies that nurses can use in school and clinical settings to promote adolescent self-advocacy skills.

42. List three elements that are critical in establishing a trusting relationship with an adolescent during a health interview.

43. During the adolescent health screening interview, the nurse can best address injury prevention by focusing on:
    a. drownings.
    b. burns.
    c. motor vehicle crashes.
    d. drug use.

44. The most appropriate way to prevent firearm injury among adolescents is:
    a. teaching the adolescent proper use of the firearm.
    b. counseling the adolescent on nonviolent ways to resolve conflict.
    c. passing laws to prevent parents from having guns.
    d. telling parents to keep the gun and the ammunition in separate locations within the house.

45. Adolescent girls of low socioeconomic status are particularly at risk for dietary deficiencies of:
    i. calories.
    ii. sodium.
    iii. calcium.
    iv. folic acid.
    v. iron.

    a. i, ii, and iii
    b. ii, iii, iv, and v
    c. iii, iv, and v
    d. i, iii, and v

46. When is a screening hemoglobin or hematocrit recommended for adolescents?
    a. At the first health provider encounter with an adolescent
    b. At the end of pubertal development
    c. At the end of puberty
    d. All of the above

47. Routine nutrition screening for all adolescents should include:
    a. a complete laboratory evaluation.
    b. questions about meal patterns and consumption of foods.
    c. a complete physical examination.
    d. a complete family history.

48. Adolescents with a body mass index (BMI) equal to or greater than the 95th percentile for age and gender are

    considered _____. Adolescents with a BMI between the 85th and 94th percentiles are

    considered _____.

49. Susan, age 15 years, comes to the school-based clinic and complains to the nurse practitioner about a vaginal discharge. After the nurse has established a trusting and confidential relationship, Susan confides that she has been sexually active with three different partners within the past 6 months. She thinks they used condoms every time, but she is not sure. Susan's last period was 4 weeks ago, and she has never had a Pap test. What tests would the nurse assisting the nurse practitioner expect to prepare for?
    i. Pap test
    ii. Gonorrhea test
    iii. Chlamydial test
    iv. Human immunodeficiency virus test
    v. Pregnancy test
    vi. Syphilis test

    a. ii, iii, iv, v, and vi
    b. i, ii, iii, iv, v, and vi
    c. ii, iii, iv, and vi
    d. i and v

50. The troubled adolescent thinking about suicide should be immediately referred for acute intervention when

    _____

    _____.

51. Cindy, age 16 years, reports that she has been sexually abused by her uncle. The nurse knows that the adolescent who has been a victim of sexual abuse:
    a. should be informed about the steps in the reporting process before information is disclosed to local authorities.
    b. is more likely to become a runaway.
    c. is more likely to remain in school and form ties with less threatening families.
    d. will usually attempt suicide within 1 month of reporting the incident.

52. The adolescent with body art:
    a. seeks body art as an expression of personal identity and style and to mark significant life events.
    b. is at lower risk for scarring if the piercing was done on the ear or nose because of the poor blood supply.
    c. should be advised to have the professional use the piercing gun for all piercing.
    d. should be advised that complications of piercing include infection and bleeding but rarely keloid formation, which occurs most often with tattoos.

53. Sleep patterns among adolescents:
    a. should be at least 10 hours nightly.
    b. shows that 1 in 8 is regularly sleep deprived.
    c. shows sleep deprivation contributes to school problems.
    d. shows that 1 in 4 reports use of the Internet as the major reason for lack of sufficient sleep.

54. Which of the following guidelines, if provided to the adolescent about tanning, is correct?
    a. If using self-tanning cream, no further sun protection is required.
    b. Sunscreens should include a sun protective factor (SPF) higher than 15 and a alcoholic base with lanolin.
    c. Long-term effects can include premature aging of the skin, increased risk for skin cancer, and, in some adolescents, phototoxic reactions.
    d. Dermatologists recommend tanning machines if used no more often than two times monthly.

CRITICAL THINKING—CASE STUDY

Shawna, a 16-year-old, visits the nurse practitioner for a routine checkup. Shawna is an A and B student in school and a member of the girls' drill team. She matured early and started to menstruate at the age of 10. Her menses are now regular. She has a boyfriend and has been dating since the age of 13. Shawna tells the nurse she has no specific concerns.

55. Based on risk factors associated with teens of Shawna's age, which of the following is the most important to discuss with Shawna at this time?
    a. Shawna's perception and concerns about health
    b. Shawna's nutritional habits
    c. Shawna's sexual activity
    d. Shawna's relationship with her family

56. The nurse establishes a trusting relationship with Shawna, who admits to having been sexually active with five boys since she started dating. Besides educating her on the risks for sexually transmitted infections and pregnancy, which of the following is most important for the nurse to include in her care plan for Shawna at this time?
    a. Discuss with Shawna how she can tell her parents about her sexual activity.
    b. Explore with Shawna possible reasons for her behavior.
    c. Assess Shawna's immunization status for hepatitis B and human papillomavirus.
    d. Assess how Shawna feels about the possibility of getting pregnant.

57. Mrs. Smith complains to you that her 15-year-old son, Ben, has begun to drift away from the family and that he finds fault with everything she and her husband do. She is worried about the relationship between them and Ben and does not understand what she and her husband have done wrong. "Why does Ben seem to suddenly dislike us so much?" Based on your knowledge of adolescent behavior, which of the following would be the best explanation?
    a. "Ben's behavioral standards are set by his peer group, and he is acting this way because of fear of rejection by this group."
    b. "Ben is defining his moral values, and you and your husband will need to have the same moral values as Ben if you want to continue to be close to him."
    c. "Ben is developing the capacity for abstract thinking and increasing his concern about social issues. He will return to share your views shortly."
    d. "Ben is defining independence-dependence boundaries and beginning to disengage from parents."

58. Christy, age 14, comes to the clinic for a physical examination. It has been longer than 2 years since her last examination. On review of Christy's immunization record, the nurse notes that Christy had a diphtheria-tetanus–acellular pertussis (DTaP) booster at age 4 years and a measles-mumps-rubella (MMR) vaccine at age 15 months. Past medical history reveals that Christy had been diagnosed with hepatitis A when she was 4 years of age and varicella at age 2 years. Since then, she has been healthy. Which of the following immunizations would you expect Christy to receive today?
    a. Influenza, pneumococcal, and chickenpox vaccines
    b. MMR, hepatitis B, and hepatitis A vaccines
    c. MMR, Tdap (acellular pertussis, diphtheria toxoid, and tetanus toxoid), meningococcal (MCV4), HPV (human papillomavirus), and hepatitis B vaccines
    d. Mantoux tuberculin, hepatitis B, Tdap vaccines, Tdap, and HPV vaccines

59. Carl, age 16 years, has been brought to the clinic after taking some drugs given to him by friends at school. He is now alert and, after talking to the nurse, confides that he is gay. Carl's parents do not know he is gay. Which of the following most likely explains Carl's drug-taking behavior?
    a. Carl is suicidal.
    b. Carl is a chronic drug user.
    c. Carl used the drugs as an escape from anxieties and emotional distress related to keeping his gay sexuality secret.
    d. Carl took the drugs as an attempt to call attention to himself and his gay lifestyle.

20 Physical Health Problems of Adolescence

1. Which of the following current beliefs about acne formation is true?
   a. Cosmetics containing lanolin and lauryl alcohol are not known to contribute to acne formation.
   b. There is scientific research to support the theory that stress will cause an acne outbreak.
   c. Exposure to oils in cooking grease can be a precursor to acne in adolescents working over fast-food restaurant oils.
   d. Acne usually worsens with dietary intake of chocolates and other foods high in sugars.

2. Nancy, age 16 years, comes to see the nurse because of acne on her face, shoulders, and neck areas. After talking with Nancy, the nurse makes a nursing diagnosis of Knowledge Deficit related to proper skin care. Which of the following would the nurse include in the instruction plan for Nancy?
   a. Wash the areas vigorously with antibacterial soaps.
   b. Brush the hair down on the forehead to conceal the acne areas.
   c. Avoid the use of all cosmetics.
   d. Gently wash the areas with a mild soap once or twice daily.

3. The practitioner has prescribed tretinoin cream (Retin-A) for Nancy's acne, and Nancy returns for a follow-up visit after 2 weeks of treatment because she feels she is not improving. During the nursing assessment, Nancy tells the nurse that she has "done everything" that she was told to do and asks, "Why is my acne no better?" The nurse's best reply is:
   a. "Because the medication prevents the formation of new comedones, it will take at least 6 weeks for improvement to be obvious."
   b. "You must not be using the medication right. Show me how you apply it to your face."
   c. "Acne is caused by dirt or oil on the surface of the skin. You will need to increase the number of times you wash these areas each day."
   d. "You will probably need to ask the practitioner about changing your medicine as soon as possible."

4. The nurse is conducting an educational session with Cindy and her parents on medications used for acne. Which of the following is correct information?
   a. Tretinoin gel has a bleaching effect on bed coverings and towels.
   b. Topical clindamycin is applied only to the individual lesions.
   c. Oral contraceptive medications contain estrogen, which will increase acne formation and should be avoided.
   d. Tretinoin requires that Cindy protect herself from sun exposure.

5. When using systemic antibiotic therapy for moderate to severe acne in adolescents, the nurse knows that:
   a. oral antibiotics are intended for short-term therapy and are not considered safe for long-term treatment.
   b. minocycline is more expensive but less likely to cause gastrointestinal side effects and is effective against severe inflammatory acne.
   c. results are better if systemic antibiotics are combined with topical antibiotic creams.
   d. resistance to amoxicillin and tetracycline usually develops.

6. The proper use of isotretinoin 12-*cis*-retinoic acid (Accutane) for adolescents includes:
   i. reserving its use for severe, cystic acne that has not responded to other treatments.
   ii. limiting treatment to 20 weeks.
   iii. watching for side effects, including mood changes, depression, and suicidal ideation.
   iv. watching for detrimental effects on bone mineralization.
   v. recognizing that it is contraindicated in pregnancy and in sexually active females not using an effective contraceptive method.
   vi. monitoring for elevated cholesterol and triglyceride levels before and during treatment.

   a. i, ii, iv, and v
   b. i, iii, and v
   c. i, ii, iii, v, and vi
   d. i, ii, iii, iv, v, and vi

7. The most common solid tumor in males 15 to 34 years of age is:
   a. varicocele.
   b. testicular torsion.
   c. priapism.
   d. testicular cancer.

8. The adolescent with testicular cancer is most likely to be initially seen with:
   a. Tender, painful swelling of the testes
   b. A mass in the posterior aspect of the scrotum that can be transilluminated
   c. A heavy, hard, painless mass palpable on the anterior or lateral surface of the testicle
   d. An asymptomatic scrotal mass that aches, especially after exercise or penile erection

9. Which of the following instructions should be included when teaching the adolescent male how to perform testicular self-examination?
   a. Perform the procedure once a month after a warm shower.
   b. A raised swelling palpated on the superior aspect of the testicle indicates an abnormality.
   c. Use the second and third fingers on each hand, holding each testicle between the fingers while palpating it with the other fingers.
   d. The normal testicle will feel soft with a round, smooth contour.

10. Which of the following adolescent females should be scheduled for her first pelvic examination?
    i. The 16-year-old who has not become sexually active
    ii. The adolescent who has been menstruating for 2 years
    iii. The adolescent who requests the examination because she wants to start taking birth control pills
    iv. The 21-year-old who has not become sexually active
    v. The adolescent who has been complaining of abdominal pain

    a. i, iii, and v
    b. ii, iii, and iv
    c. iii and v
    d. iii, iv, and v

11. Match each term with its definition. (Terms may be used more than once.)

    a. Varicocele   e. Human papillomavirus types 16 and 18
    b. Epididymitis   f. Priapism
    c. Testicular torsion   g. Penile fracture
    d. Gynecomastia

    _____ Breast enlargement that occurs during puberty

    _____ Wormlike mass that is palpated above the testicle and becomes smaller when the adolescent lies down

    _____ Benign and temporary disease that occurs in about 50% of adolescent boys

    _____ Associated with penile carcinoma

    _____ Inflammation that is a result of infection, local trauma, or chemical irritant

    _____ Rupture of the corpus cavernosum as a result of trauma to the erect penis

    _____ Marked by the testis hanging free from its vascular structure; results in partial or complete venous occlusion

    _____ Characterized by unilateral scrotal pain, redness, and swelling; may include urethral discharge, dysuria, fever, and pyuria; treated with antibiotics

    _____ Prolonged penile erection

    _____ Manifested by scrotum that is swollen, painful, red, and warm; pain radiating to groin, accompanied by nausea, vomiting, and abdominal pain; generally, an absence of fever and urinary symptoms; immediate surgery required to treat

    _____ The most common treatable cause of male-related impaired fertility

12. _____ _____ is defined as an absence of menses by age 15.

    _____ _____ is defined as an absence of menses for 6 months in a previously menstruating female, when pregnancy has been excluded.

    _____ is defined as abnormally light or infrequent menstruation.

    _____ is defined as painful menstrual flow.

13. Linda, age 16, started her menses at age 13 years. She comes into the school-based clinic with a history of secondary amenorrhea. Linda is an honor student and a long-distance runner who runs an average of 50 miles per week. The physical examination is normal, and Linda has been asked to decrease her running distance and to improve her nutrition. She is scheduled for a follow-up visit and told that if her menses are not more regulated, oral birth control pills will be prescribed. Linda wants to know why she would have to take the pills, because she is not sexually active. How would you respond?

14. The treatment of choice for adolescents with dysmenorrhea is:
    a. acetaminophen.
    b. oral contraceptives.
    c. nonsteroidal antiinflammatory drugs.
    d. estrogen-suppression drugs.

15. Adverse effects of intensive physical exercise on an adolescent's reproductive cycle may include all of the following except:
    a. delayed menarche.
    b. anovulation associated with dysfunctional uterine bleeding.
    c. amenorrhea.
    d. dysmenorrhea.

16. Match the term with its description.

    a. *Lactobacillus acidophilus*
    b. Premenstrual syndrome
    c. Endometriosis
    d. Dysfunctional uterine bleeding
    e. Vulvovaginal candidiasis
    f. *Trichomonas* vaginitis
    g. Leukorrhea
    h. Bacterial vaginosis (BV)
    i. Pelvic inflammatory disease (PID)

    _____ Condition that has more than 200 associated physical, psychologic, and behavioral symptoms

    _____ Condition that may be caused by the presence of endometrial tissue outside the uterine cavity

    _____ Abnormal vaginal bleeding, usually associated with anovulation

    _____ Symptoms that include thin, malodorous vaginal discharge; diagnosis confirmed by clue cells on microscopic examination

    _____ Infection of the upper genital tract (endometrium, fallopian tubes, and ovaries), most commonly caused by sexually transmitted bacteria, such as *Neisseria gonorrhoeae, Chlamydia trachomatis,* and a variety of other anaerobic bacteria

    _____ Predominant composition of normal vaginal flora

    _____ Condition that may manifest with vaginal pruritus and dysuria and is not a sexually transmitted infection (STI); treated with over-the-counter topical antifungal creams; characterized by "cottage cheese–like" discharge

    _____ An STI caused by an anaerobic parasitic protozoa

    _____ Glutinous, gray-white vaginal discharge caused by physical, chemical, or infectious agents

17. A recommended treatment for premenstrual syndrome to reduce water retention, food craving, and pain is:
    a. vitamin B$_6$, vitamin E, and primrose oil.
    b. an oral contraceptive pill containing drospirenone.
    c. 1200 mg/day of calcium and vitamin D.
    d. serotonin reuptake inhibitors.

18. *Trichomonas vaginalis* infection:
    a. is the most prevalent STI in adolescents.
    b. in females is linked with higher risks for human immunodeficiency virus (HIV), herpes, and PID.
    c. decreases the shedding of HIV among both men and women with HIV infection.
    d. involves treatment that includes both sexual partners and abstaining from sexual intercourse for 2 weeks after treatment.

19. Gail has been diagnosed with vaginitis. The nurse is preparing to instruct her on prevention. Describe what information the nurse should include in her instructions.

20. Indicate whether the following statements are true or false.

    _____ Easy access to cars, unsupervised time at home, and changing family composition have contributed to the incidence of sexual experimentation among adolescents.

    _____ There is evidence that low self-esteem in females and males is associated with sexual intercourse at an earlier age.

    _____ Instruction in the skills needed to resist sexual intercourse has less influence on reducing sexual activity than does providing information on dangers associated with sexuality activity (STIs or pregnancy).

    _____ The less familiar an adolescent is with his or her partner, the more likely they are to use contraception during intercourse.

    _____ Contraception use increases among girls as the duration of the relationship increases.

    _____ Adolescents who have at least one supportive parent engage in less risky behavior.

    _____ The pregnancies of adolescents under 15 years old are less frequently complicated by obstetric problems.

    _____ Adolescent mothers are just as likely to attend college as are other adolescents.

    _____ During a second pregnancy for a teenager, obstetric risk and risk to the infant are lower.

    _____ Teens between 12 and 16 years are at high risk for prolonged labor related to fetopelvic incompatibility.

    _____ Pregnant adolescents often have diets deficient in iron, calcium, and folic acid.

    _____ Effective parent-child communication about sexuality can delay the onset of first sexual intercourse.

    _____ The teenage pregnancy rate continues to increase for all age-groups.

21. Lesley is a sexually active adolescent. She comes to the clinic with abdominal pain and vaginal bleeding. Which of the following must be ruled out immediately?
    a. Ectopic pregnancy
    b. Ovarian cyst
    c. STIs
    d. Endometriosis

22. Ana, age 16, has not had a period for the past 3 months and her pregnancy test is positive. Which of the following is not an appropriate action for the nurse to take at this time?
    a. Inform Ana privately that her test is positive.
    b. Review with Ana facts about the pregnancy, including the duration of pregnancy and anticipated due date.
    c. Understand that Ana's reaction may be one of ambivalence, shock, fear, or apathy.
    d. Arrange for Ana's parents to be present when Ana is given the news.

23. Infants of adolescents are at risk because:
    a. teenage mothers often neglect their infants, leaving them for long periods with grandparents.
    b. teenage mothers supply excessive amounts of cognitive stimulation to their infants.
    c. adolescents often lack knowledge about normal infant growth and development.
    d. adolescents are less likely to treat their infant as love objects or playthings.

24. The first goal in nursing care of the pregnant teenager is:
    a. to arrange for the pregnant teen to register for food supplement programs to ensure proper nutrition.
    b. to assist the pregnant teen in obtaining health care.
    c. to involve the boyfriend and parents in the pregnancy so that the pregnant teen will have support during her pregnancy.
    d. to educate the pregnant teen regarding child care.

25. Postpartum care of adolescents should be directed toward the following goal:

26. A drug approved for medical abortion is mifepristone. Which of the following statements about this drug is true?
    a. The drug can be used to provide nonsurgical abortion at 49 days or less of pregnancy.
    b. The drug promotes receptor binding of endogenous or exogenous progesterone.
    c. The abortion completion rate is 100% in pregnancies if used correctly.
    d. The drug is administered intramuscularly up to 49 days after the last menstrual period.

27. Emily is an unmarried 17-year-old who is 6 weeks pregnant and has decided to have an abortion. One nursing action used to assist Emily would be:
    a. explaining to Emily that it is wrong for her to have an abortion and arranging for her to visit an adoption center.
    b. referring Emily to an appropriate abortion agency when she is 4 months pregnant.
    c. providing Emily with relaxation strategies to use during the abortion procedure.
    d. calling Emily's parents so that they can be present for the abortion.

28. In discussing prevention of STIs, the nurse tells the adolescent that the most effective is:
    a. birth control pills.
    b. norplant.
    c. spermicides.
    d. condoms.

29. Nancy, age 17, is brought to the family planning clinic by her mother for birth control. Which of the following is most important to include in a plan for Nancy at this time?
    a. Discussion of the effectiveness rates of various methods and importance of compliance
    b. Including Nancy's partner in the discussions
    c. Discussion of Nancy's perception of the likelihood of getting pregnant and her desire to prevent pregnancy versus her desire for pregnancy
    d. Cost of the various methods of contraception

30. According to the Centers for Disease Control and Prevention, which of the following statements about nonoxynol-9 is currently correct?
    a. It can be used in spermicides.
    b. It cannot be used with condoms.
    c. It does not protect against STIs, including HIV, and may actually increase the risk of HIV transmission.
    d. It protects against most STIs, including decreasing the risk of HIV transmission.

31. The contraceptive methods most popular among adolescents are:
    a. the birth control pill and the condom.
    b. abstinence and withdrawal (coitus interruptus).
    c. the Lea's shield and the cervical cap.
    d. the Ortho Evra transdermal system and spermicidal foam.

32. Amanda comes to the school nurse's office early in the morning, visibly upset. She tells the nurse that she and her boyfriend were having sexual relations last night and the condom broke. Amanda asks the nurse about a new pill she has read about that will keep her from becoming pregnant. She wants the nurse to give her more information about this pill. Which of the following statements made to Amanda provides the best information?
    a. "It is available without a prescription and must be taken within 24 hours of the unprotected sexual intercourse."
    b. "It is very effective but has side effects, so you will need to be out of school at least 1 day."
    c. "It contains estrogen, so you will need to have a pregnancy test before it can be administered."
    d. "It is available to adult women over the counter. It must be taken within 72 hours of the unprotected sexual intercourse."

33. The nurse is conducting a sexual education program. What technique has been found helpful when dealing with the subject of sexual abstinence?

34. Rape victims display a variety of manifestations. Which of the following might the nurse see in 16-year-old Sally as she arrives at the emergency department for treatment after being raped?
    a. Hysterical crying or giggling
    b. Calm and controlled behavior
    c. Anger and rage alternating with helplessness and agitation
    d. All of the above

35. The primary goal of nursing care for the adolescent rape victim is:
    a. not to inflict further stress on the victim.
    b. obtaining a complete history of the incident.
    c. assisting in the physical examination.
    d. notifying the police and the parents of the victim before proceeding with assessment.

36. Identify the following statements about STIs in adolescence as true or false.

    _____ The most prevalent STIs in adolescents are chlamydial infections and human papillomavirus (HPV) infections.
    _____ Adolescent females are at a lower risk for chlamydia and HPV infection because of the immature adolescent endocervix.
    _____ In the adolescent the immune system provides excellent localized antibody response to infectious agents at the cervical level.
    _____ Research has demonstrated that, as young women have more sexual partners, the use of hormonal contraception increases and the use of condoms declines.
    _____ Adolescents ages 15 to 19 have the highest overall incidence of gonococcal infection.
    _____ Symptoms of gonorrhea can occur 1 day to 2 weeks after sexual contact, or there may be no symptoms.
    _____ Treatment for uncomplicated gonorrhea is with a single dose each of cefixime 400 mg orally.
    _____ Conjunctival gonorrhea is always sexually transmitted.
    _____ Treatment for gonorrhea includes both the partner and the patient and provides life-long immunity.
    _____ Untreated chlamydial infections among adolescent females can result in infertility.
    _____ Long-term effects of PID include infertility because of tubal scarring.

37. Jeannie, age 18, has been diagnosed and treated for positive gonorrhea testing. Which of the following discharge instructions given to Jeannie is correct?
    a. "Be sure and come back for a test of cure in 2 weeks."
    b. "Be sure to abstain from sexual intercourse for 7 days after treatment."
    c. "Your vaginal discharge will clear up by tomorrow."
    d. "Make sure you do a vaginal douche tonight."

38. Therapeutic management for chlamydia includes:
    a. doxycycline 100 mg twice daily for 7 days in the pregnant adolescent and her partner.
    b. intramuscular injection of ceftriaxone (Rocephin) 125 mg for the patient and partner.
    c. intramuscular injection of penicillin 2.4 million international units for the patient and partner.
    d. azithromycin 1 g orally in a single dose for the patient and her partner.

39. Shirley, age 17, has been diagnosed with PID caused by gonorrhea. The nurse can expect treatment to include:
    a. Shirley will be admitted to the hospital immediately; outpatient treatment is not appropriate for PID.
    b. Shirley will be given ofloxacin 400 mg twice daily for 14 days, or levofloxacin 500 mg once daily for 14 days, with or without metronidazole 500 mg twice daily for 14 days.
    c. No treatment of Shirley's partner will be necessary.
    d. Shirley will be prescribed oral contraceptives.

40. The most common STI in the United States is _____ _____, which causes _____ _____. Individuals with this infection are at risk for development of _____ _____ and _____.

41. Human papillomavirus (HPV):
    a. has several types that are classified as high, medium, or low risk for causing cancer.
    b. can be treated by the patient using cryotherapy with liquid nitrogen every 1 to 2 weeks.
    c. can be treated by the patient using 80% to 90% trichloroacetic acid applied weekly.
    d. can be avoided through immunization of all girls at the 11- or 12-year-old well-child visit.

42. What are the current guidelines from the American Cancer Society regarding initiating Papanicolaou (Pap) screening?

43. New liquid-based cytologic screening techniques:
    a. have increased the sensitivity in the diagnosis of cervical dysplasia.
    b. are intended to replace the "gold standard" of yearly Pap smears.
    c. can test for HIV.
    d. are an excellent diagnostic tool to identify condyloma acuminatum.

44. One STI for which an immunization is recommended for all adolescents is:
    a. HIV.
    b. hepatitis B virus.
    c. syphilis.
    d. gonorrhea.

45. Connie, age 15 years, has requested information about prevention of STIs. As the nurse begins to discuss HIV and acquired immunodeficiency syndrome (AIDS), Connie tells the nurse to skip information on this topic. Based on knowledge about adolescents, which of the following is the most likely reason for Connie's response?
    a. Connie does not think she has at-risk behavior for AIDS.
    b. Connie already knows as much about AIDS as is necessary.
    c. Connie is not sexually active.
    d. Connie wants information about birth control but is afraid to ask.

CRITICAL THINKING—CASE STUDY

Bryan, age 14, has come to the clinic because he has started breaking out with acne on his face, chest, and shoulders. He says he is embarrassed to go out because his friends stare at him and girls avoid him. The physician has started medical treatment and sent him to you for further guidance.

46. Based on the information provided, what is a priority nursing diagnosis for Bryan at this time?
    a. Altered Family Process related to the adolescent with a skin problem
    b. Body Image Disturbance related to perception of acne lesions
    c. Bathing/Hygiene Self-Care Deficit related to skin care
    d. Altered Role Performance related to perceived peer separation

47. The best goal for Bryan would be:
    a. Bryan will have a positive body image.
    b. Bryan will receive appropriate education for hygiene.
    c. Bryan will have a reduction in dietary fat and calories.
    d. Bryan will receive appropriate referral to skin specialist.

48. Subjective data collection on Bryan should include:
    a. family history of acne.
    b. location and size of visible lesions.
    c. culture and sensitivity for identifying organism.
    d. All of the above

49. The nurse has established a care plan with Bryan. Which of the following would be an expected component of the plan to improve Bryan's body image?
    a. Help him find mechanisms to reduce emotional stress.
    b. Explain the disorder and therapy prescribed to increase family understanding.
    c. Emphasize the positive aspects, as well as the limited nature of the disorder, and assist Bryan with grooming to enhance appearance.
    d. Discourage peer relationships until Bryan's facial appearance has improved from medication.

Sixteen-year-old Jenny is pregnant and coming to the school-based clinic for prenatal care. Jenny and the baby's father, Doug, are still seeing each other, but their relationship has "cooled" since Jenny found out she was pregnant. Jenny is living at home. She is expecting her mother to help raise the infant while Jenny continues school.

50. The nurse is planning for prenatal and childrearing classes that both Jenny and Doug could attend. Based on knowledge of adolescent fathers, the nurse would:
    a. realize that adolescent fathers have little association with their infants.
    b. understand that Doug will want to start breaking the contact with Jenny and will refuse to go.
    c. realize that Doug is still most influenced by his male peer friends and is embarrassed about getting Jenny pregnant and will not go.
    d. realize that active participation in the pregnancy by Doug will have positive effects on Jenny's self-esteem and will decrease her level of distress and depression.

51. Which of the following does the nurse recognize as the best plan for Jenny and her infant?
    a. Have Jenny move out of her mother's house and care for the infant on her own.
    b. Have Jenny leave the care of the infant completely to her mother and get on with her life.
    c. Have Jenny go along with whatever her mother says to avoid open conflicts around the infant.
    d. Have Jenny care for her child even when other adults are involved.

52. Which of the following statements, if made by Jenny, would reflect the concept of a personal fable that could lead to risk-taking behaviors?
    a. "I don't want to get an STI, so it won't happen to me."
    b. "Only girls who are promiscuous get STIs."
    c. "Abstinence is the only way to prevent an STI."
    d. "All my friends have sex."

21 Behavioral Health Problems of Adolescence

1. Identify the following statements as true or false.

_____ The probability that overweight school-age children will become obese adults is estimated at 50%, whereas the likelihood that overweight adolescents will become obese adults is estimated at 70% to 80%.

_____ Gradual accumulation of adipose tissue during childhood establishes a pattern of eating that is difficult to reverse in adolescence.

_____ Obesity is the most common nutritional disturbance of children.

_____ Limiting television to no more than 4 hours daily is a recommended behavior to prevent obesity.

_____ *Obesity* refers to the state of weighing more than average for height and body build and may or may not include an increased amount of fat.

_____ Birth weight is an indicator of childhood obesity.

_____ In Prader-Willi syndrome, children exhibit characteristics of slow intellectual development, short stature, and obesity and go to great lengths to obtain food.

_____ Children with an age- and gender-specific body mass index (BMI) between the 85th and 94th percentiles should be considered overweight.

_____ Obese adolescents have been found to have higher total daily energy expenditure and resting energy expenditure than nonobese adolescents.

_____ Obesity in adolescence has been related to elevated blood cholesterol, high blood pressure, and an increase in type 2 diabetes mellitus.

_____ Obese children are often from families that emphasize large meals or scold children for leaving food on their plates.

_____ Obesity in childhood and adolescence is a significant risk factor for adult obesity.

_____ African-Americans, Hispanics, and Filipinos engage in less physical activity than non-Hispanic Caucasians.

_____ Institutional factors that encourage patterns of obesity include allowing students to leave school for lunch and allowing vending machines in schools that are filled with high-fat and high-calorie foods and soft drinks.

2. Increased obesity among children is related to:
   a. high birth weight.
   b. underlying disease.
   c. enzyme abnormalities and metabolic defects.
   d. overeating.

3. Physical inactivity has been linked with overweight children. Which of the following explain this decrease in childhood activity?
   i. Decrease in physical activity in secondary and elementary schools
   ii. Parental obesity and low levels of physical activity at home
   iii. Increased time spent with television, video games, computers, and the Internet
   iv. Lack of sidewalks, parks, and bike paths in low-income communities

   a. i, ii, and iii
   b. ii and iii
   c. i and iv
   d. i, ii, iii, and iv

4. Which of the following is not a complication of obesity in adolescents?
   a. Type 2 diabetes and insulin resistance
   b. Fatty liver disease
   c. Heart failure
   d. Sleep apnea

5. Psychologic and social findings in the obese adolescent include:
   a. negative self-image that persists into adulthood.
   b. same high school grade performance and college acceptance as nonobese adolescents.
   c. same rate of marriage and level of income as nonobese adolescents.
   d. higher prevalence of depression than in nonobese adolescents.

6. Gail, age 14, comes to the health provider's office for a yearly physical. Gail has always been overweight but has gained 50 lb since her last visit and now fits the criteria of obesity. The diagnostic evaluation of Gail should include all of the following except:
   a. history regarding the development of obesity.
   b. physical examination to differentiate simple obesity from increased fat that results from organic disease.
   c. family history, especially regarding obesity, diabetes, heart disease, and dyslipidemia.
   d. laboratory studies for anemia.

7. BMI measurement in adolescents:
   a. is currently considered the most reliable method to predict future obesity.
   b. varies in children and adolescents to accommodate age- and gender-specific changes in growth.
   c. is calculated based on skin thickness and muscle mass.
   d. requires determining total body density by total submersion in a water-filled tank.

8. Weight-reduction management in adolescents should include:
   a. significant caloric restriction.
   b. elimination of physical hunger cues.
   c. regular physical activity.
   d. appetite-suppressant drugs.

9. James has kept a diet history for the nurse, and the nurse has carefully reviewed this eating diary. Which of the following suggestions would best promote healthy eating habits in James?
   a. Limit fast-food consumption to no more than three times a week.
   b. Take second helpings of meat and vegetables only.
   c. Do not skip meals.
   d. Include more low-fat foods.

10. Janie, age 14, wants to discuss with the nurse how to modify her eating habits to reduce her weight. Which of the following methods does the nurse recognize as least helpful in assisting Janie to meet her goals?
    a. Have Janie keep a list of everything she eats.
    b. Request that Janie's parents remind Janie not to eat junk foods.
    c. Establish a system of rewards for changes in eating habits.
    d. Discuss with Janie methods other than eating than can be used to deal with emotional stress.

11. Obesity and overweight nutritional counseling is aimed at preventing an increase in body fat during growth. List the four aspects of changing eating habits that can best accomplish this.

12. The best approach to the management of obesity in children and adolescent is:
    a. prevention.
    b. pharmacologic agents sibutramine and orlistat.
    c. bariatric surgery
    d. behavior modification

13. When initiating a treatment plan for obesity, the nurse should:
    a. defer treatment until the family is ready to begin.
    b. proceed with the plan, regardless of the family's readiness, if the adolescent is ready.
    c. understand that the adolescent cannot take personal responsibility for dietary habits and physical activity.
    d. understand that adolescents who are forced by their parents to seek help can easily become motivated.

14. Which of the following least explains why a person with an eating disorder would hide the symptoms?
    a. Because of a lack of awareness of the effects on health
    b. Because of a fear of hospitalization and mandatory treatment
    c. Because of the shame of discussing the symptoms with others
    d. Because of an unwillingness to give up these harmful behaviors

15. Anorexia nervosa is characterized by:

16. Bulimia nervosa is characterized by:

17. Cindy, age 16, has been sent to the school nurse because her gym teacher has noticed a marked decrease in Cindy's weight since vacation. Which of the following does the nurse recognize as a common finding among adolescent girls with anorexia nervosa?
    a. Wears form-fitting clothes such as tank tops and jeans
    b. Has strong peer relationships with classmates and several best friends
    c. Has poor schoolwork performance because of little interest in school
    d. Is present at meals, selects foods, and appears to family and friends to be eating appropriately

18. Karen is suspected of being bulimic. Which of the following is clinically characteristic of this disease?
    a. Bulimia often begins with decreased dietary intake associated with poor relationships with family members.
    b. Once started, the binging decreases in frequency to only about once per day.
    c. Insulin production is decreased because of excessive self-induced vomiting.
    d. Impulse control and satiety regulation are problems in bulimic adolescents.

19. Which of the following diagnostic findings would most likely confirm the diagnosis of bulimia in Karen?
    a. Presence of distinctive lesions on the hands (Russell sign); that is, scars and cuts from repeated abrasions of the skin
    b. Hypertension, weakness, and cool skin
    c. Elevated potassium, magnesium, and erythrocyte sedimentation rate
    d. A heart murmur diagnosed as mitral valve prolapse

20. The patient with bulimia must be watched by the nurse for medical complications. Which of the following findings does the nurse recognize as needing immediate intervention?
    a. Osteoporosis
    b. Potassium depletion from diuretic abuse
    c. Erosion of teeth enamel from self-induced vomiting
    d. Chronic esophagitis from self-induced vomiting

21. Adolescents with anorexia nervosa are at risk for refeeding syndrome. Which of the following best describes refeeding syndrome?
    a. It reduces the risk for osteoporosis and returns the menses to normal.
    b. The risk for heart failure is greatest during the first 2 days of treatment.
    c. It occurs because of shifts in phosphate from extracellular to intracellular spaces in persons with total body phosphorus depletion.
    d. It causes mitral valve prolapse and significant electrolyte imbalance.

22. Which of the following does the nurse recognize as being an adolescent group at high risk for bulimia?
    a. Adolescents in the lower socioeconomic level
    b. Adolescents who want to be tough, muscular football players
    c. Adolescents who aspire to careers that require low weight
    d. Adolescents with good self-image

23. What are the three main focus goals for the therapeutic management of anorexia nervosa?

24. Cindy has been diagnosed with anorexia nervosa. Her therapeutic management plan includes dietary interventions combined with family psychotherapy. Which of the following would the nurse recognize as appropriate?
    a. Weight gain is a sign that the patient is not relapsing from the plan.
    b. The patient is only allowed to participate in setting up a food plan as a reward for weight gain.
    c. The plan needs to be firm but flexible.
    d. A reasonable goal for weight gain is about 4 lb/wk.

25. Which of the following is least appropriate when developing an outpatient contract between the patient with an eating disorder and the therapist?
    a. Begin the psychotherapy immediately before the contract is developed and before weight gain.
    b. Develop the contract so that the patient's feeling of control and responsibility toward recovery is established.
    c. Specify in the contract the weight at which tube feedings will be implemented.
    d. Specify in the contract when rewards for achievement will be implemented.

26. Cindy is about to be discharged after treatment for anorexia nervosa. The nurse has formulated a nursing diagnosis related to family coping, with a goal that the family will be prepared for home care. Which of the following interventions would best help meet this goal?
    a. Make certain both patient and family understand the therapeutic plan.
    b. Observe family interaction for assessment of family coping patterns.
    c. Explore feelings and attitudes of family members.
    d. Convey an attitude of caring and acceptance to family and patient.

27. In treating eating disorders:
    a. weight gain is a reliable sign of positive progress.
    b. when a therapeutic environment is removed, relapses seldom occur.
    c. antianxiety or antidepressant drug use has not been proven effective.
    d. psychotherapy is aimed at resolving adolescent identity crises and distorted body image.

28. Identify the following statements about substance abuse as true or false.

    _____ A person may be physically dependent on a narcotic without being addicted.

    _____ The adolescent abusing drugs has often adopted the use of a substance as a means of coping with feelings of depression, boredom, and emptiness.

    _____ Identification of the pattern of drug use in the adolescent is essential but offers little help in developing a successful approach to the problem.

    _____ The usual goal for the compulsive drug user is peer acceptance.

    _____ Adolescent drug users at greatest risk are those who report daily use of alcohol or marijuana during the past 30 days; those who report using illicit drugs such as heroin, crack cocaine, or Ecstasy within the past month; and those who used narcotics like oxycodone (OxyContin) in the past year.

    _____ Since 2000, increases have occurred in teenagers' use of most drugs, including alcohol, tobacco, and marijuana.

    _____ The absence of aldehyde dehydrogenase (ALDH), an enzyme that assists in the breakdown of ethanol in the body, reduces the likelihood that alcoholism will develop.

    _____ African-American youth are less likely to smoke cigarettes than Hispanic or Caucasian adolescents.

    _____ Cigarette smoking is the chief avoidable cause of death.

29. Which of the following adolescents does the nurse recognize as least likely to begin smoking?
    a. Johnny, age 16 years, whose father quit smoking 2 years ago
    b. Karen, age 15 years, whose older sister smokes
    c. Ted, age 17 years, who smoked a cigarette at home in front of his parents
    d. Lilly, age 12, who feels uncomfortable with her early maturing body

30. Johnny, age 16, has tried his first cigarette because of peer pressure to "look cool." In what stage of becoming a smoker is Johnny?
    a. Preparation
    b. Initiation
    c. Experimentation
    d. Regular smoking

31. The school nurse is planning an educational program centered on smoking prevention for high school adolescents. Which of the following methods does the nurse recognize as the most effective way to present this program?
    a. Ban smoking in the school.
    b. Teach methods of resistance to peer pressure.
    c. Use peer-led programs that emphasize social consequences.
    d. Use media, videos, and films on smoking prevention.

32. Which of the following statements is true?
    a. Smokeless tobacco is a safe alternative to cigarette smoking.
    b. Smokeless tobacco is often linked to periodontal disease and lesions in the oral soft tissue.
    c. Smokeless tobacco is not addictive.
    d. Smokeless tobacco users are not likely to become cigarette smokers.

33. Adolescent alcoholics:
    a. are often described as hard to live with and indecisive.
    b. are often described as good students with a strong desire to complete school.
    c. usually begin frequent, heavy drinking in middle school.
    d. have poor role models but excellent peer relations.

34. Certain protective factors have been identified as helping at-risk adolescents resist pressure to use drugs and alcohol. List five recognized protective factors.

35. The motivation phase of treatment and rehabilitation of young drug users is directed toward:
    a. assessing the drug habits and amount of drugs used.
    b. exploring the factors that influence drug use.
    c. preventing relapse into drug use.
    d. all of the above.

36. Complete the following statements about drug abuse.

    a. The form of cocaine known as the purer and more menacing form is _____.

    b. Cocaine taken by _____ is associated with the highest levels of dependence.

    c. Cocaine is a potent _____ _____, and the crash after a cocaine high usually

       consists of _____.

    d. Name five physical signs of narcotic abuse:

       _____

       _____

       _____

       _____

e. _____, also known as the "date rape drug," is 10 times more powerful than diazepam and produces short-term memory loss.

f. _____, with the street names of "crank" and "crystal," produces more stimulation than cocaine, and the user can remain "up" for hours. This drug is readily made from ephedrine and pseudoephedrine found in cold medications and diet pills.

g. Inhalant abuse usually gives the child an inexpensive euphoria but is extremely dangerous and can cause three serious consequences. List them below.

_____

_____

_____

h. The newer so-called date rape drug γ-hydroxybutyric acid (GHB) is usually administered by

_____

_____.

i. 3,4-Methylenedioxymethamphetamine (MDMA), also known as Ecstasy, is frequently used in dance club settings

and can lead to _____ and _____ after long hours of nonstop dancing.

j. Cannabis (marijuana), psilocybin mushrooms, and lysergic acid diethylamide (LSD) are examples of

_____.

37. The onset of suicide and depression during adolescence may be due to:
   a. expected low self-esteem among this population.
   b. the importance of peer pressure among this group.
   c. cognitive development and the ability to observe one's self and future orientation.
   d. higher rates of substance abuse among this group.

38. Jim, who has no history of previous suicide attempt, is talking with the school nurse about his feelings of despair and hopelessness about the future. He tells the nurse he would be better off dead. The nurse's best response is to:
   a. recognize that Jim is going through a common phase of adolescence.
   b. recognize that Jim is at low risk for suicide, because he has not previously attempted suicide.
   c. explain to Jim that suicide never solved anything and that he will feel better tomorrow.
   d. take Jim seriously, allow time for him to verbalize his feelings, and stay with him until referral.

39. The nurse has been asked to present an educational program on prevention of adolescent stress and suicide. In planning the program, the nurse should include:
   a. the importance of being supportive and establishing positive communication patterns between family and teens.
   b. the precipitating factors for suicide.
   c. effective coping mechanisms and problem-solving skills.
   d. all of the above.

40. Mark, age 14 years, has been rushed to the emergency department because of illegal drug ingestion at a party. Which of the following is most important for the nurse to collect to assist in the emergency treatment plan?
   i. The type and amount of drug taken
   ii. The time the drug was taken and mode of administration
   iii. Number of times Mark has previously overdosed
   iv. Why the drug was taken

   a. i and ii
   b. i, ii, and iii
   c. i only
   d. i, ii, iii, and iv

41. Match the term with its description.

    a. Suicidal ideation   d. Suicide
    b. Suicide attempt   e. Contagion suicide
    c. Self-harm

    _____ Behaviors that may not be direct suicide attempts but may occur along with suicidal thoughts or intent

    _____ Deliberate act of self-injury with death as result

    _____ Deliberate but unsuccessful act of self-injury

    _____ Preoccupation with thoughts about committing suicide

    _____ Phenomenon resulting from excessive media coverage after an adolescent suicide

42. Which of the following is the most common method of successful suicide among adolescents?
    a. Overdose of drugs
    b. Firearms
    c. Self-inflicted lacerations
    d. Hanging

CRITICAL THINKING—CASE STUDY

Kenny, 16 years of age, visits the clinic for follow-up of a recent infection he obtained while on a hunting trip. While talking with the nurse, he tells her that he has recently broken up with his girlfriend after going steady for 11 months. Kenny has a history of having a difficult home situation. His recent school performance has declined, and this has further upset Kenny's parents and their expectations for him. Physical examination of Kenny reveals an expressionless face with a slight smell of alcohol on his breath and signs consistent with depression.

43. The nurse suspects that Kenny might be suicidal. Which factors in the preceding data might support this assumption?
    i. Alcohol consumption
    ii. Recent breakup with girlfriend
    iii. History of difficult home situation
    iv. Depression
    v. Has a gun available to him

    a. i, ii, iii, and iv
    b. ii, iii, and iv
    c. ii, iv, and v
    d. i, ii, iii, iv, and v

44. On questioning by the nurse, Kenny admits to suicidal ideation. What should the nurse first assess to determine risk?
    a. History of suicide attempts within the family
    b. Past methods of coping with stress by the individual
    c. Whether Kenny has a plan for suicide
    d. How Kenny feels about suicide

45. Which of the following nursing diagnoses would the nurse develop to best deal with Kenny's suicide thoughts?
    a. High Risk for Injury related to feelings of rejection
    b. Sleep Pattern Disturbance related to inability to sleep
    c. Social Isolation related to withdrawal from friends
    d. High Risk for Self-Directed Violence related to excessive alcohol use

46. The most important goal in the nursing management for Kenny at this time should focus on:
    a. reestablishing Kenny's relationship with his girlfriend.
    b. teaching Kenny how to cope with the stress of being an adolescent.
    c. maintaining physical safety for Kenny.
    d. helping Kenny express his emotional pain and regain his ability to perform assigned tasks.

22 Family-Centered Care of the Child with Chronic Illness or Disability

1. Match each term with its description.

   a. Chronic illness
   b. Congenital disability
   c. Developmental delay
   d. Developmental disability
   e. Disability

   f. Handicap
   g. Impairment
   h. Technology dependent
   i. Home care
   j. Mainstreaming

   _____ A barrier imposed by society

   _____ A disability that has existed since birth but is not necessarily hereditary

   _____ Requiring the routine use of a medical device for support of a life-sustaining bodily function

   _____ A condition that interferes with daily functioning for more than 3 months

   _____ Any mental and/or physical disability that is manifested before age 22 years and is likely to continue indefinitely

   _____ A system of care with the goals to normalize the child's life, lessen disruption on the family, and maximize the child's growth and development

   _____ A maturational lag

   _____ The process of integrating children with special needs into regular classrooms and child care centers

   _____ A loss or abnormality of a structure or function

   _____ A long-term reduction in the child's ability to engage in day-to-day activities because of a chronic condition

2. Match each program with its description.

   a. Education for All Handicapped Children Act of 1975
   b. Individuals with Disabilities Education Act (IDEA)
   c. Individualized education program (IEP)
   d. Education of the Handicapped Act Amendments of 1986
   e. Individualized family service plan (IFSP)
   f. Americans with Disabilities Act (ADA)

   _____ The 1990 amendment to the Education for All Handicapped Children Act of 1975 that changed the name of the program

   _____ A program that requires daycare providers to make "reasonable modifications" for equal access to program participation

   _____ The approach in which a multidisciplinary team writes a plan that includes special education and therapeutic strategies and goals for each eligible child

   _____ A program developed jointly by families and professionals; includes information about the infant or toddler's present level of development, family strengths and needs related to enhancing development, major outcomes expected, services needed, identification of a case manager, and transition steps to preschool services

   _____ The public law that is largely responsible for the development of a variety of supplemental programs in the school system to accommodate children with special needs

   _____ The program that directs states to develop and implement statewide comprehensive, coordinated, multidisciplinary interagency programs of early intervention services for infants and toddlers with disabilities, as well as support services for their families

3. Match each term with its description.

a. Special Olympics
b. VSA arts
c. Coping Health Inventory for Parents (CHIPTS)
d. Approach behaviors
e. Avoidance behaviors
f. Trajectory model
g. Family management styles theory
h. Guilt

i. Anger, bitterness
j. Overprotection
k. Rejection
l. Denial
m. Gradual acceptance
n. Chronic sorrow
o. Functional burden
p. Programs for children with special health needs

_____ Offers disabled children an opportunity to celebrate and share their accomplishments in a variety of expressive activities such as art, music, poetry, dance, and drama

_____ An emotional response of parents manifested throughout the life span of the disabled or chronically ill child; includes elements of permanence with episodic surges during developmental or situational crises; may include resurgence of grief triggered by events that remind the parent of what could have been

_____ An 80-item checklist providing self-report information about how parents perceive their overall responsed to the management of family life with a child with a chronic illness

_____ A program that offers children with physical disabilities an opportunity to compete with their peers and to achieve athletic skill

_____ Those coping mechanisms that result in movement toward adjustment and resolution of the crisis

_____ A theory about chronic illness that acknowledges the condition has a course that varies and changes over time

_____ Self-accusation; a feeling that is often greatest when the cause of a disorder is directly traceable to the parent, as in cases of genetic disease

_____ A concept that considers the issues associated with caring for and living with the chronically ill or disabled child in relation to the family's resources and ability to cope

_____ Common and normal reactions of families to a chronic illness diagnosis; emotions that typically manifest in the parents, the ill child, and siblings (e.g., verbal self-degrading, arguments, withdrawal, complaints about nursing care)

_____ Characterized by parents acting as if the child's disorder does not exist or attempting to have the child overcompensate for the disability

_____ A theory about chronic illness that emphasizes the family's role in actively responding to a child's illness

_____ Behavior in which parents fear allowing the child to achieve any new skill, avoid all discipline, and cater to the child's desires to impede frustration

_____ Coping mechanism with the result of movement away from adjustment to the crisis

_____ Behavior in which parents detach themselves emotionally from the child but usually provide adequate physical care or constantly nag and scold the child

_____ Formerly called "crippled children's services"; provides financial assistance for children with various disabling conditions

_____ Characterized by parents placing necessary and realistic restrictions on the child, encouraging self-care activities, and promoting reasonable physical and social abilities

4. Which of the following diseases is the most common chronic childhood illness?
a. Asthma
b. Congenital heart disease
c. Cancer
d. Spina bifida

5. Which of the following is an example of how chronic illness and disability affect children's health, functional status, and family functioning?
   a. Families do not bring the disabled child for health care often.
   b. Siblings' routines are completely separated from those of the disabled child.
   c. Parents are usually not able to meet the child's normal developmental needs.
   d. Disabled children are often absent from school.

6. Emphasizing the characteristics that the disabled child has in common with other children, rather than viewing the disabilities within a pathologic framework, best describes:
   a. The chronologic approach to care of the disabled child.
   b. The developmental approach to care of the disabled child.

7. A goal that would be considered inappropriate for family-centered care would be to:
   a. maintain family routine in the hospital.
   b. empower the family members.
   c. support the family during stressful times.
   d. maintain a high level of professional control.

8. The individualized family service plan (IFSP) is:
   a. developed jointly by families and professionals.
   b. a comprehensive insurance plan for families with a disabled child.
   c. developed by a team of professionals for the disabled child.
   d. a plan that finances direct services for the disabled child.

9. When working with people of other cultural backgrounds who are caring for a child with a disability, the nurse should plan care that:
   a. uses a family member to translate into the family's language.
   b. incorporates the generalized culture of the United States.
   c. recognizes that culture fully defines how the child and family will react.
   d. remains consistent with the family's cultural practices when possible.

10. Match each developmental stage with the particular area of development in which a disability poses a challenge or risk.

    a. Infant   d. School-age child
    b. Toddler   e. Adolescent
    c. Preschooler

    _____ Self-concept and body image

    _____ Social development

    _____ Attachment

    _____ Mobility

    _____ Participation

11. A strategy that is recommended to promote normalization in children with special needs would be to:
    a. avoid discussing issues of appearance in the adolescent.
    b. focus on the areas of ability and competence.
    c. establish special family rules for the child with a disability.
    d. allow children with special needs to make all decisions about their care.

12. The child who is disabled tends to develop appropriate independence and achievement when the parents:
    a. protect the child from all dangers.
    b. establish reasonable limits.
    c. emphasize the child's limits.
    d. isolate the child to avoid peer rejection.

13. Which of the following strategies would be inappropriate for the nurse to use when teaching families with children who are disabled?
    a. Give information that meets the child's current needs.
    b. Give as much information as possible at the time of diagnosis.
    c. Answer the child's questions openly.
    d. Repeat information as often as needed.

14. The adolescent patient with a disability or chronic illness should be transferred to an adult provider:
    a. when the patient reaches the age of 18 years.
    b. when the patient reaches the age of 16 years.
    c. when the patient knows about the chronic condition and is prepared for the transition.
    d. None of the above; it is better not to change providers

15. The purpose of the initial assessment of the coping mechanisms of a child who is disabled is for the nurse to:
    a. determine help that the family may want or need.
    b. establish rapport with the child and family.
    c. provide care from stage to stage of development.
    d. provide care from phase to phase of the disorder.

16. Which of the following statements is false about family members' perceptions of a child's illness or disability?
    a. Children may interpret the illness or disability as a punishment.
    b. Family members are usually shocked to learn that their child has a serious illness or disability.
    c. Parents may interpret the illness or disability as a punishment.
    d. Family members usually have no knowledge about the disorder when they learn their child has it.

17. Which of the following statements about the time of diagnosis is false?
    a. Parents may not remember all that is said.
    b. Parents remember the tone of the communication.
    c. Parents cannot sense the tone of communication.
    d. Parents may not hear all that is said.

18. When initially informing the family of a child's serious condition, the nurse should:
    a. explain that, with time, everything will be all right.
    b. accept any emotional reaction without judgment.
    c. decide when and how to tell the child about the diagnosis.
    d. use therapeutic touch to stimulate free expression of feelings.

19. Describe at least three guidelines for the nurse to use when providing ongoing information to the family with a disabled or chronically ill child.

20. Parents in thriving families:
    a. stress normalcy and feel confident.
    b. have an enduring management style.
    c. feel competent but burdened.
    d. feel dominated by the illness.

21. The two most important environments for the child who is disabled or chronically ill are _____ and
    _____.

22. In adjusting to a child's chronic illness, the father is more likely than the mother to:
    a. suffer from isolation.
    b. use an emotional release.
    c. perceive he is coping poorly.
    d. view the child's temperament as influential.

23. To help siblings prepare for the changes in the disabled child, the nurse should:
    a. wait until questions are asked, because siblings often desire little or no involvement.
    b. recognize that permitting sibling hospital visits will increase stress in the whole family.
    c. reassure siblings that they will continue to be involved in the care whenever possible.
    d. help the sibling realize that the disabled child needs more parental attention.

24. Research indicates that, compared with their peers, siblings of a child with a disability exhibit:
    a. greater independence.
    b. more maturity.
    c. an increased sense of responsibility.
    d. all of the above.

25. Which of the following characteristics would most likely indicate that a sibling of a child with a disability is having difficulty?
    a. Sharing
    b. Withdrawal
    c. Competing
    d. Compromising

26. Describe how an extended family member may be a source of stress to the parents of the disabled or chronically ill child.

27. Identify each of the following coping behaviors as an approach behavior or an avoidance behavior.

    a. _____ A father stops at a friend's house and talks about his child's poor prognosis.

    b. _____ A father's alcohol use increases to the point of being excessive.

    c. _____ A mother tells the nurse that she is afraid to tell her child about his or her poor prognosis.

    d. _____ A mother never carries a glucose source for her toddler who takes insulin for type 1 diabetes mellitus.

    e. _____ A mother begins to cry in the nurse's office at school, saying that she always gets depressed at the beginning of the new year.

    f. _____ A father asks the nurse to explain a diagnosis again.

    g. _____ A mother asks her neighbor to watch her older child for a few hours while she is at the clinic.

28. Corbin and Strauss's chronic illness trajectory model is based on the idea that the:
    a. family understands the meaning of the illness situation.
    b. course of the illness changes over time.
    c. family member roles do not change with illness.
    d. coping patterns for the illness can be learned.

29. Nursing intervention that can encourage and empower families include:
    a. fostering normalization.
    b. teaching coping skills.
    c. assisting to define social support networks.
    d. all of the above.

30. If a family member reacts to the diagnosis of a chronic illness with denial, the nurse would recognize that denial is:
    a. an abnormal response to grieving this type of loss.
    b. preventing treatment and rehabilitation.
    c. necessary to prevent disintegration.
    d. necessary for the child's optimal development.

31. In regard to denial, it is imperative that health professionals:
    a. actively attempt to remove the denial behaviors.
    b. repeatedly give blunt explanations.
    c. label denial as maladaptive.
    d. understand the concept of denial.

32. Hope in the chronically ill child's family would be considered:
    a. a way to absorb stress in a manageable way.
    b. negative coping with a serious diagnosis.
    c. a maladaptive mechanism for dealing with the inevitable death.
    d. to have the same meaning for the nurse and the family.

33. Describe at least two effective methods of support that would help families manage their emotional response to the diagnosis of a disability or chronic illness in their child.

34. A strategy for the nurse to encourage parents to express their feelings about the diagnosis of a chronic illness in their child would be to:
    a. tell them that what they are going through is completely understandable.
    b. help them focus on their emotions.
    c. explain the policies and procedures regarding visiting hours.
    d. review the disease process with them.

35. Parents who provide adequate physical care but detach themselves emotionally from the child characterizes the type of parental reaction known as:
    a. overprotection.
    b. denial.
    c. gradual acceptance.
    d. rejection.

36. The nurse's response to anger in parents of the disabled child should be:
    a. reciprocal anger.
    b. disapproval.
    c. acceptance.
    d. avoidance.

37. List at least five characteristics of parental overprotection.

38. Nurses who provide support to parents of a child with a disability should develop an attitude that has all of the following characteristics except the belief that:
    a. every person has burdens to bear.
    b. trust is a foundation for good communication.
    c. parents are experts about their own child.
    d. parents and professionals are colleagues.

39. When the parents of a child with special needs experience chronic sorrow, the process:
    a. of grief is pronounced and self-limiting.
    b. involves social reintegration after grieving.
    c. is characterized by realistic expectations.
    d. is interspersed with periods of intensified grief.

40. Which of the following stressors can usually be predicted for a child with special needs?
    a. The approximate cost of the yearly medical bills
    b. The future needs for residential care
    c. The types of schooling and vocational training that will be needed
    d. The stress of developmental milestones and the start of school

41. Which of the following issues most influences the ability of the family to caring for and living with the child with special needs?
    a. functional burden.
    b. severity of the condition.
    c. complexity of the care.
    d. resources required for care.

42. The effectiveness of the family's support system depends on the:
    a. ability to match the best source of support for each need.
    b. diversity of the family's social network.
    c. extended family and their availability.
    d. extended family and their resources.

43. Which of the following is not necessarily a criterion to consider when selecting parents to offer support to other parents of children with disabilities?
    a. The parents should possess advocacy and problem-solving skills.
    b. The parents should have a child with the same diagnosis.
    c. The parents should have a nonjudgmental approach to problem solving.
    d. The parents should be good listeners.

44. Out-of-home placement of a child with a disability:
    a. may be the best option if the integrity of the family unit is in jeopardy.
    b. occurs if coping strategies are not employed within the home.
    c. is becoming increasingly difficult to accomplish.
    d. demonstrates that the family is maladjusted.

45. The program formerly known as "crippled children's services," which provides financial assistance for children with many disabling conditions, is now called:
    a. programs for children with special health needs.
    b. National Information Center for Children and Youth with Disabilities.
    c. Association for the Care of Children's Health.
    d. Alliance for Health, Physical Education, Recreation and Dance.

CRITICAL THINKING—CASE STUDY

Jerome is a 15-month-old infant who was born prematurely and was discharged from the hospital at age 3 months after multiple invasive procedures, including intubation, ventilation, and surgery. He is delayed in his motor development, but other areas of development are progressing as would be expected for a prematurely born infant of his age. Jerome has recently been diagnosed with cerebral palsy. He is at the physician's office for a routine health check. His mother is with him.

46. To assess the family's adjustment to the diagnosis, the nurse would gather more information. One area that could be deferred to a later date would be the assessment of the family's:
    a. goals for the future.
    b. available support system.
    c. coping mechanisms.
    d. perception of the disorder.

Jerome's mother has returned to work part-time as a partner in a computer consulting firm. Jerome's father is a marketing consultant in the food industry and travels frequently. The parents, who are in their late thirties, have hired a woman whom they trust with Jerome's many needs to come into the home. Jerome, who is an only child, goes out of the home several times a week for therapy.

47. Based on the information given, select the best nursing diagnosis for Jerome.
    a. High Risk for Injury
    b. Maladaptive Family Processes
    c. Delayed Growth and Development
    d. Disturbed Body Image

48. With the selected diagnosis in mind, what is the expected outcome with the highest priority for Jerome?
    a. Jerome will attain the physical development that is appropriate for any 15-month-old.
    b. Jerome will attain psychosocial and cognitive development that is appropriate for any 15-month-old.
    c. Jerome will attain physical, psychosocial, and cognitive development that is appropriate for his age and abilities.
    d. Jerome's parents will set realistic goals for themselves and Jerome.

49. An intervention that would address the issues involved with altered family process related to the birth of Jerome and the complexity of his care after birth would be to:
    a. teach safety precautions.
    b. help the family achieve a realistic view of Jerome's capabilities and limitations.
    c. stress the importance of sound health practices and frequent health supervision.
    d. encourage responsible use of equipment and appliances.

50. Between now and Jerome's next visit at 24 months of age, the nurse should provide anticipatory guidance to the parents about Jerome's growth toward developing:
    a. a sense of trust and attachment to his parents.
    b. mastery of self-care skills.
    c. a sense of body image.
    d. through sensorimotor experiences.

23 | Family-Centered End-of-Life Care

1. Match each term with its description.

   a. Euthanasia
   b. Assisted suicide
   c. Drug tolerance
   d. Addiction
   e. Palliative care

   f. Hospice
   g. DNR
   h. The Compassionate Friends
   i. Burnout
   j. Detached concern

   _____ Occurs when someone provides the patient with the means to end his or her life and the patient uses that means to do so

   _____ Psychologic dependence on the side effects of a drug; usually not a factor in pain management of terminally ill children

   _____ Active total care of patients whose disease is not responsive to curative treatment

   _____ The act of ending the life of a person who is suffering from a terminal condition; carried out by a person other than the suffering person; commonly referred to as "mercy killing"

   _____ One of the reasons for administering high doses of opioids for pain control in order to maintain the same level of pain relief

   _____ The level of involvement that allows sensitive, understanding care as a result of being sufficiently neutral to make objective rational decisions

   _____ A community health care organization that specializes in the care of dying patients and their families; combines the philosophy of dying as a natural process with palliative care

   _____ A state of physical, emotional, and mental exhaustion that occurs as a result of prolonged involvement with individuals in situations that are emotionally demanding; an occupational hazard to which nurses are susceptible

   _____ An indication to withhold cardiopulmonary resuscitation in response to cardiac arrest; "do not resuscitate"; no code

   _____ An international organization for bereaved parents and siblings

2. In children 5 to 9 years of age, the most common causes of death are:
   a. accidents, trauma, infectious illness, and suicide.
   b. injuries/trauma, cancer, and congenital anomalies.
   c. accidents/trauma, homicide, suicide, and cancer.
   d. prematurity, congenital birth defects, and infectious illness.

3. According to the American Nurses Association Code for Ethics, when caring for a terminally ill child, nurses are permitted to provide interventions that:
   a. actively aim to end a suffering child's life.
   b. relieve symptoms in a suffering child's life only if doing so poses a low risk for hastening death.
   c. offer relief to the dying child even if there is risk of hastening death.
   d. present the family with the means to end the dying child's life.

4. List three strategies nurses can use to communicate with families of children with life-threatening illness.

5. A nurse is about to present facts to parents about the possible death of their child. In this case, which of the following techniques would be most effective in promoting communication?
   a. Acknowledging denial in the parents whenever it occurs
   b. Using only medical terms for all explanations
   c. Using body language to communicate caring
   d. Recognizing feelings and reactions but not acknowledging them

6. When communicating with dying children, the nurse should remember that:
   a. older children tend to be concrete thinkers.
   b. when children can recite facts, they understand the implications of those facts.
   c. if children's questions direct the conversation, the assessment will be incomplete.
   d. games, art, and play provide a good means of expression.

7. When assisting parents in supporting their dying child, the nurse should stress the importance of honesty; if parents are honest and openly discuss their fears, the child is more likely to:
   a. discuss his or her fears.
   b. ask fewer distressing questions.
   c. lose his or her sense of hope.
   d. do all of the above.

8. Fear of the unknown is one of the greatest threats to seriously ill children of which age-group?
   a. Toddlers
   b. Preschoolers
   c. School-age children
   d. Adolescents

9. Separation is one of the greatest threats to seriously ill children of which age-group?
   a. Toddlers
   b. Preschoolers
   c. School-age children
   d. Adolescents

10. Fear of punishment is one of the greatest threats to seriously ill children of which age-group?
    a. Toddlers
    b. Preschoolers
    c. School-age children
    d. Adolescents

11. Inability to use their parents for emotional support is one of the greatest threats to seriously ill children of which age-group?
    a. Toddlers
    b. Preschoolers
    c. School-age children
    d. Adolescents

12. Which one of the following age-groups is most likely to suffer negative reactions to an altered body image as a result of a life-threatening illness?
    a. Young children
    b. School-age children
    c. Adolescents
    d. All age groups affected equally

13. Describe at least three benefits of implementing the hospice concept in the child's home environment.

14. Which of the following interventions is most important for the dying child?
    a. Emotional support
    b. Preparing parents to deal with fears
    c. Relief from pain
    d. Control of pain

15. When the parent of a child who is dying tells the nurse the child is in pain, even when the child appears comfortable, the nurse should be sure that:
    a. as-needed pain control measures are instituted.
    b. pain control is administered on a regular preventive schedule.
    c. parents understand that pain is a physical process.
    d. parents understand that the child is probably in less pain than the parents think.

16. Interventions to help the family prepare for the care of a terminally ill child include:
    a. educating the family about complications of overfeeding or overhydration.
    b. providing a supply of medications to alleviate discomfort.
    c. encouraging fun and memorable activities.
    d. all of the above.

17. The sibling of a dying child may feel:
    a. displaced.
    b. isolated.
    c. resentful.
    d. all of the above.

18. List at least five physical signs of approaching death.

19. Methods to support grieving families at the time of death and in the grieving period after death include:
    a. encouraging family members to avoid upsetting each other by keeping their feelings to themselves.
    b. consoling with phrases such as "I know how you feel."
    c. emphasizing that the painful grieving usually lasts less than a year.
    d. allowing the family time to stay with the child after the death.

20. List at least three behaviors that are characteristic in children as death approaches.

21. The extended phase of mourning:
    a. usually takes about a year.
    b. is accompanied by support of the family at the funeral.
    c. may extend over years.
    d. can be eliminated if the family is well prepared.

22. Which of the following strategies would be best for the nurse to use to support the family's spiritual needs when their child's death is imminent and a clergy member is unavailable?
    a. Pray appropriately with the family.
    b. Implement relaxation techniques.
    c. Make an appointment for the family to speak with an expert.
    d. Review the physical signs of death with the family.

23. When a child dies suddenly, which of the following interventions would be least beneficial?
    a. Avoid having the family view the body of a disfigured child.
    b. Inform the family of what to expect when they see the disfigured body of their child.
    c. Offer the parents the opportunity to see the child's body even after resuscitation was performed.
    d. Arrange to have a health care worker with bereavement training meet with the family.

24. Identify each of the following statements as true or false.

    _____ Children with cancer, chronic disease, or infection or who have suffered prolonged cardiac arrest are excellent candidates for organ donation.

    _____ The nurse should never inquire whether organ donation was discussed with the child but should allow the family to come forward with this information on their own.

    _____ If organs are donated, the family will most likely need to choose a closed-casket funeral service.

    _____ Most families choose not to donate organs because of the high cost.

    _____ Many body tissues and organs can be donated, but their removal may cause mutilation of the body.

25. In regard to whether a child should attend the funeral of a loved one, the nurse should consider:
    a. the child's age.
    b. that it will be a frightening experience.
    c. the nurse's responsibility to protect the child from distressing events.
    d. that attending the funeral may be beneficial to the child.

26. Current research supports the notion that:
    a. involvement in the experiences of the dying sibling is beneficial.
    b. siblings of children who died in the hospital reported readiness for the death.
    c. protecting the sibling of the dying child from the death rituals is beneficial.
    d. it is better for the sibling to remember the dying child as he or she was when alive.

27. Which of the following techniques would be considered an example of the most therapeutic communication to use with the bereaved family?
    a. Cheerfulness
    b. Interpretation
    c. Validating loss
    d. Reassurance

28. Which of the following helping statements would be least therapeutic for the nurse to use with the bereaved family shortly after the time of death?
    a. "You can stay with him and hold him if you wish."
    b. "It must be painful for you to return to the doctor's office without her."
    c. "Fortunately his suffering is over now."
    d. "Will your husband return to be with you soon?"

29. Which of the following symptoms would be considered normal grief behavior?
    a. Depression
    b. Anger
    c. Hearing the dead person's voice
    d. All of the above

30. The resolution of grief usually:
    a. occurs in sequential phases.
    b. is completed in about 2 years.
    c. is completed in about 3 years.
    d. is a timeless process that is never completed.

31. Reorganization after the death of a child means that the:
    a. loved one is forgotten.
    b. pain is gone.
    c. survivors have "let go."
    d. survivors have recovered from their loss.

32. List at least three of the reactions that nurses have when caring for children with fatal illnesses.

33. Intervening therapeutically with terminally ill children and their families requires:
    a. only self-awareness.
    b. nursing practice that is based on a theoretical foundation.
    c. years of experience.
    d. all of the above.

CRITICAL THINKING—CASE STUDY

Julie is a 6-year-old child with leukemia. She has undergone a bone marrow transplant with associated complications and has had several remissions. After the last remission she deteriorated rapidly. Her parents tell the nurse that they believe Julie is now in the final stages of her illness. Her parents also express their feelings of discouragement and depression.

34. How should the nurse approach the parents in regard to their feelings about Julie's impending death?
    a. The nurse should begin by assessing the reason for the depression.
    b. The nurse should be certain that Julie's parents know that repeated relapses with remissions are associated with a better prognosis.
    c. The nurse should begin to help the parents work through their depression.
    d. The nurse should use heavy sedation to help Julie and her parents cope with this phase.

35. As Julie's parents express their concerns, it becomes clear that pain control is a fear for Julie and her parents. What strategy should the nurse use to help them deal with this fear?
    a. The nurse should assure the parents that all of Julie's pain will be eliminated.
    b. The nurse should use heavy sedation to help Julie and her parents cope with this phase.
    c. A regular preventive medication schedule should be adopted as pain develops.
    d. The pain medications should be given only intravenously when Julie is near death.

36. After Julie's death in late December, which of the following evaluation strategies is most likely to help support and guide the family through the resolution of their loss?
    a. A written questionnaire
    b. A telephone call placed in early January
    c. A meeting with the family at the time of death
    d. A telephone call placed in early February

37. Which of the following would be the best expected outcome for the nursing diagnosis of Fear/Anxiety when planning care for Julie in this terminal stage?
    a. Julie will discuss her fears without evidence of stress.
    b. Julie will exhibit no evidence of loneliness.
    c. Julie's parents are actively involved in Julie's care.
    d. Julie's parents demonstrate ability to provide care for her.

24 The Child with Cognitive, Sensory, or Communication Impairment

1. Match each cognitive impairment term with its description.

a. Cognitive impairment
b. Mild intellectual disability
c. Moderate intellectual disability
d. Bayley Scales of Infant Development
e. Wechsler Intelligence Scale for Children, fourth edition
f. Vineland Adaptive Behavior Scale
g. Primary prevention strategies

h. Secondary prevention activities
i. Tertiary prevention strategies
j. Task analysis
k. Trisomy 21
l. Translocation of chromosome 21
m. Mosaicism
n. Atlantoaxial instability
o. Fragile site

_____ Identification and early treatment to avert cerebral damage; includes prenatal diagnosis or carrier detection of disorders such as Down syndrome and newborn screening for treatable inborn errors of metabolism such as congenital hypothyroidism, phenylketonuria, and galactosemia

_____ A general term that encompasses any type of intellectual disability (a term increasingly used instead of "mental retardation")

_____ Comprises about 10% of the intellectually disabled population

_____ Comprises about 85% of all people with intellectual disability

_____ Standardized test used most often during the school years to make the diagnosis of cognitive impairment

_____ Standardized test used most commonly for making the diagnosis of cognitive impairment in infants; the Mullen Scales of Early Learning is also used

_____ Used, along with the AAMR Adaptive Behavior Scale, to assess adaptive behaviors

_____ Treatment to minimize long-term consequences, including identification of conditions and provision of appropriate therapies and rehabilitation services; medical treatment of coexisting problems such as hearing and visual impairment in Down syndrome; and programs for infant stimulation, parent training, preschool education, and counseling services to preserve the integrity of the family unit

_____ Strategies designed to avoid conditions that cause cognitive impairment, including avoidance of prenatal rubella infection; maintenance of current immunizations; genetic counseling, especially regarding risk of Down or fragile X syndrome; and use of folic acid supplements during pregancy to avoid neural tube defects

_____ Refers to a condition in which a person has cell populations with both normal and abnormal chromosomes; associated with 1% to 3% of persons with Down syndrome; degree of impairment related to the percentage of cells with the abnormal chromosome makeup

_____ The process used to delineate the components for each step so that each step can be taught completely before proceeding to the next activity

_____ A genetic aberration that is usually hereditary and associated with 3% to 6% of Down syndrome cases

_____ An extra chromosome 21 (group G); the genetic pattern present in approximately 97% of Down syndrome cases

_____ Occurs in 15% to 20% of children with Down syndrome; instability of the first and second cervical verebrae; includes symptoms of neck pain, weakness, and torticollis, although most affected children are asymptomatic

_____ A region on the chromosome that fails to condense during mitosis; characterized by a nonstaining gap or narrowing

2. Match each hearing impairment term with its description.

a. Severe to profound hearing loss
b. Slight to moderately severe hearing loss
c. Conductive hearing loss
d. Sensorineural hearing loss
e. Mixed conductive-sensorineural hearing loss
f. Central auditory imperception
g. Organic type of central auditory imperception
h. Aphasia
i. Agnosia

j. Dysacusis
k. Functional type of hearing loss
l. Decibel (dB)
m. Hearing threshold
n. Cochlear implants
o. Closed captioning
p. Acoustic feedback
q. ASL/BSL
r. Telecommunication devices (TDD)

_____ Refers to a person whose hearing disability precludes successful processing of linguistic information through audition, with or without a hearing aid

_____ Middle-ear hearing loss; results from the interference of transmission of sound to the middle ear; most common of all types of hearing loss; frequently a result of recurrent serous otitis media; mainly involves interference with loudness of sound

_____ Describes a person who has residual hearing sufficient to enable successful processing of linguistic information through audition, generally with the use of a hearing aid

_____ Includes all hearing losses that do not demonstrate defects in the conductive or sensorineural structures; divided into organic and functional classifications

_____ Involves damage to the inner ear structures or the auditory nerve; commonly caused by congenital defects of inner ear structures, kernicterus, infection, administration of ototoxic drugs, or exposure to excessive noise; results in distortion of sound and problems in auditory discrimination; child hears some but sounds are distorted, which severely affects discrimination and comprehension

_____ Results from interference with transmission of sound in the middle ear and along neural pathways; frequently caused by recurrent otitis media and its complications

_____ Defect involving the reception of auditory stimuli along the central pathways and the expression of the message into meaningful communication (e.g., aphasia, agnosia, dysacusis)

_____ Hearing loss with no organic lesion; may occur in conversion disorder (an unconscious withdrawal from hearing to block remembrance of a traumatic event)

_____ Inability to express ideas in any form, either written or verbal

_____ The method used to classify hearing impairment; measured by an audiometer

_____ Inability to interpret sound correctly

_____ Difficulty in processing details or in discriminating among sounds

_____ A unit of loudness measured in frequencies; cycles per second

_____ Surgically implanted prosthetic devices that convert sound to electrical impulses and feed them directly to the auditory nerve

_____ Visual-gestural languages that use hand signals and concepts in the English language that roughly correspond to specific words; commonly referred to as "signing"

_____ A special decoding device that translates the audio portion of a television program into subtitles that appear written on the television screen

_____ An annoying whistling sound usually caused by improper fit of the ear mold of the hearing aid

_____ Special equipment that helps hearing-impaired people communicate over the telephone

3. Match each visual impairment term with its description.

a. Legal blindness
b. Partially sighted
c. Visual impairment
d. Refraction
e. Myopia
f. Hyperopia
g. Penetrating wound of the eye
h. Nonpenetrating wound of the eye
i. Tapping method

j. Guides
k. Self-stimulatory activities
l. Braille
m. Braillewriter
n. Braille slate/stylus
o. Library of Congress
p. Finger spelling
q. Tadoma method
r. John Tracy Clinic

_____ Trauma to the eye that is most often a result of sharp instruments such as sticks, knives, or scissors

_____ Portable systems for written communication used by the blind person

_____ A human or dog used to help a person who is visually impaired move around in the environment and avoid obstacles

_____ A general term that includes both partial sight and legal blindness

_____ Condition in which light rays enter the lens and, rather than falling directly on the retina, fall in front of it

_____ A system that uses raised dots to represent each letter and number

_____ Condition in which light rays enter the lens and, rather than falling directly on the retina, fall beyond it

_____ May be a result of foreign objects in the eye, lacerations, a blow from a blunt object such as a baseball or fist, or thermal or chemical burns

_____ Communication system where words are spelled letter by letter into the hearing and visually impaired child's hand, and the child spells out ideas to the other person

_____ Defined as visual acuity better than 20/200 but worse than 20/70 in the better eye with correction

_____ Use of a cane to survey the environment for direction and avoid obstacles

_____ The bending of light rays as they pass through the lens of the eye

_____ Used to compensate for inadequate stimulation; body rocking, finger flicking, or arm twirling; delay the child's social acceptance; often reduced or eliminated through behavior modification

_____ A small typewriter-like device that enables the blind child to write a message

_____ Offers programs for combined auditory and visual impairments with a home correspondence course for parents

_____ Publishes a reference circular titled *Deaf-Blindness: National Resources and Organizations*

_____ Defined as visual acuity of 20/200 or less and/or a visual field of 20 degrees or less in the better eye

_____ A type of tactile communication that involves the child placing the hand over the speaker's face and neck to monitor facial movements associated with speech production

4. Match each communication impairment term with its description.

a. Language
b. Receptive language
c. Expressive language
d. Speech
e. Developmental language disorder
f. Articulation errors
g. Dysfluencies
h. Stuttering, stammering
i. Block

j. Voice disorders
k. Blissymbols
l. Direct observation
m. Indirect assessment
n. Denver Articulation Screening Examination
o. Early Language Milestone (ELM) Scale
p. Denver II
q. Peabody Picture Vocabulary Test III

_____ A standardized screening instrument for assessing language development in children less than 3 years of age

_____ A method of assessing speech and language development that uses spontaneous language interaction between the child and nurse for children less than 3 years of age

_____ Speaking verbal signals

_____ A communication impairment that occurs without impairment in other developmental realms

_____ Understanding the spoken word

_____ Rhythm disorders; usually consist of repetitions of sounds, words, or phrases

_____ Primarily refers to the symbol system used to convey thoughts or feelings to others

_____ The oral production of language, including articulation of sounds, rhythm, and tone

_____ One of the most common and potentially serious dysfluencies, characterized by tense repetition of sounds or complete blockages of sound or words; a normal characteristic of language development during the preschool years

_____ Sounds that a child makes incorrectly or inappropriately

_____ A highly stylized communication system consisting of graphic symbols that represent words, ideas, and concepts

_____ A useful screening instrument to measure receptive (hearing) vocabulary for verbal ability giftedness and cognitive impairment in English-speaking individuals

_____ A reliable, effective screening test to measure speech development that takes about 10 minutes to administer

_____ A stutter that is characterized by no sound coming out when the person tries to speak

_____ A revision of the Denver Developmental Screening Test that includes an expanded section with language items

_____ Characterized by differences in pitch, loudness, and/or quality

_____ A method of evaluating speech and language development that relies on parental information obtained through a history

5. Match each level of cognitive impairment–intelligent quotient (IQ) range with its appropriate example of maturation or development.

a. Mild (50-55 to about 70)
b. Moderate (36-49)

c. Severe (20-35)
d. Profound (below 20)

_____ A preschool-age child with noticeable delays in motor development and in speech

_____ An adolescent who may walk but needs complete custodial care

_____ A school-age child who is able to walk and who can profit from systematic habit training

_____ A preschool-age child who may not be noticed as cognitively impaired but is slow to walk, feed self, and talk

6. The American Association on Intellectual and Developmental Disabilities' definition of intellectual disability includes:
a. an IQ that is lower than 50.
b. an emphasis on function.
c. only intelligence and no other criteria.
d. an age limit of 12.

7. List at least four early behavioral signs that are suggestive of cognitive impairment.

8. When teaching a child with a cognitive impairment, the nurse's best strategy to present symbols in an exaggerated, concrete form is:
   a. singing.
   b. memorizing.
   c. verbal explanation.
   d. ignoring the child.

9. Define the term *fading*.

10. Define the term *shaping*.

11. Acquiring social skills for the child who is intellectually disabled includes:
    a. learning acceptable sexual behavior.
    b. being exposed to strangers.
    c. learning to greet visitors appropriately.
    d. all of the above.

12. Describe the pros and cons involved in a marriage between two individuals with significant cognitive impairment.

13. Which of the following strategies would best help the intellectually disabled child acquire social skills?
    a. Use discipline and negative reinforcement.
    b. Provide information about the importance of socialization skills.
    c. Use active rehearsal with role-playing and practice sessions.
    d. Use all of the above.

14. For the child who is cognitively impaired, the contraceptive choice that requires little compliance, produces amenorrhea, and provides long-term protection from pregnancy is:
    a. the intrauterine device.
    b. Depo-Provera.
    c. the diaphragm.
    d. oral contraception.

15. Define *task analysis* and describe its use when teaching a child who is intellectually disabled.

16. The primary purpose of record keeping for 7 days before toilet-training an intellectually disabled child is to:
    a. determine the child's patterns of behavior and parents' response.
    b. determine the amount of urinary output and usual times the child urinates.
    c. assess the child's physical and psychologic readiness to use the toilet.
    d. determine all of the above.

17. Describe the conditions necessary for a child with cognitive impairment to begin learning how to dress.

18. The mutual participation model of care for the child who is cognitively impaired and needs hospitalization would include:
    a. isolating the child from others to avoid conflicts.
    b. allowing parents to room in and participate in the care.
    c. having the parents perform all activities of daily living.
    d. having the nurse perform all activities of daily living.

19. Another name for trisomy 21 is:
    a. phenylketonuria.
    b. Turner syndrome.
    c. Down syndrome.
    d. galactosemia.

20. Testing of the parents is necessary to identify the carrier and offer genetic counseling when Down syndrome is caused by:
    a. mosaicism.
    b. translocation.
    c. maternal age over 40.
    d. paternal age over 40.

21. List five physical features that are found in the infant with Down syndrome.

22. Some research has shown that families who keep the child with Down syndrome at home report having:
    a. negative feelings for the child.
    b. a more accepting attitude toward others.
    c. higher divorce rates.
    d. more sibling problems.

23. Decreased muscle tone in the infant with Down syndrome:
    a. indicates inadequate parenting.
    b. is a sign of infant detachment.
    c. compromises respiratory expansion.
    d. predisposes the infant to diarrhea.

24. Fragile X syndrome is:
    a. the most common inherited cause of cognitive impairment.
    b. the most common inherited cause of cognitive impairment next to Down syndrome.
    c. caused by an abnormal gene on chromosome 21.
    d. caused by a missing gene on the X chromosome.

25. In regard to fragile X syndrome, the fragile site is caused by:
    a. 5 to 40 repeats of nucleotide base pairs.
    b. gene mutation.
    c. infection.
    d. all of the above.

26. The correct term to use for a person whose hearing disability precludes successful processing of linguistic information through audition without the use of a hearing aid is:
    a. deaf-mute.
    b. slight to moderate hearing loss.
    c. severe to profound hearing loss.
    d. deaf and dumb.

27. Conductive hearing loss in children is most often a result of:
    a. the use of tobramycin and gentamicin.
    b. the high noise levels from ventilators.
    c. congenital defects.
    d. recurrent serous otitis media.

28. At what decibel level would a hearing loss be considered profound?
    a. Less than 30 dB
    b. 55-70 dB
    c. 71-90 dB
    d. More than 91 dB

29. One behavior associated with hearing impairment in the infant is:
    a. a monotone voice.
    b. consistent lack of the startle reflex to sound.
    c. a louder than usual cry.
    d. inability to form the word "da-da" by 6 months.

30. In assessing a child for the development of a hearing impairment, the nurse would look for:
    a. a loud monotone voice.
    b. consistent lack of the startle reflex.
    c. a high level of social activity.
    d. attentiveness, especially when someone is talking.

31. All of the following strategies will enhance communication with a child who is hearing impaired except:
    a. touching the child lightly to signal presence of a speaker.
    b. speaking at eye level or a 45-degree angle.
    c. using facial expressions to convey the message better.
    d. moving and using animated body language to communicate better.

32. To best promote socialization for the child with a hearing impairment, teachers should:
    a. discourage hearing-impaired children from playing together.
    b. use frequent group projects to promote communication.
    c. use audiovisual-assisted instruction as much as possible.
    d. minimize background noise.

33. Care for the hearing-impaired child who is hospitalized should include:
    a. supplementing verbal explanations with tactile and visual aids.
    b. communicating only with parents to ensure accuracy.
    c. discouraging parents from rooming in.
    d. sending nonvocal communication devices home to avoid loss.

34. Which of the following situations would be considered abnormal?
    a. A neonate who lacks binocularity
    b. A toddler whose mother says he looks cross-eyed
    c. A 5-year-old who has hyperopia
    d. Presence of a red reflex in a 7-year-old

35. If a child has a penetrating injury to the eye, the nurse should:
    a. apply an eye patch.
    b. attempt to remove the object.
    c. irrigate the eye.
    d. use strict aseptic technique to examine the eye.

36. Match each type of visual impairment with its description or characteristics.

    a. Astigmatism
    b. Anisometropia
    c. Amblyopia

    d. Strabismus
    e. Cataract
    f. Glaucoma

    _____ Increased intraocular pressure

    _____ Squint or cross-eye; malalignment of eyes

    _____ Different refractive strength in each eye

    _____ Unequal curvatures in refractive apparatus

    _____ Opacity of crystalline lens

    _____ Lazy eye; reduced visual acuity in one eye

37. List at least eight strategies the nurse can use during hospitalization of a child who has lost his sight.

38. Which of the following statements is correct about eye care and sports?
    a. Glasses may interfere with the child's ability in sports.
    b. Face mask and helmet should be required gear for softball.
    c. Contact lenses provide less visual acuity than glasses for sports.
    d. It is usually difficult to convince children to wear their glasses to play sports.

39. The method of communication used with combined auditory and visual impairments that involves spelling into the child's hand is called:
    a. finger spelling.
    b. the Tadoma method.
    c. blindism.
    d. the tapping method.

40. To help families with children who are hearing and vision impaired, the nurse should teach the parents to establish communication by:
    a. always placing the child in the same place in the room to help identify surroundings.
    b. selecting a cue that is always used to help the child discriminate one person from another.
    c. limiting the cues that are sent and received.
    d. limiting stimulation to allow the child to feel safe.

41. Which of the following examples would be most indicative of a language disorder?
    a. A 22-month-old child who has not uttered his first word
    b. A 38-month-old who has not uttered his first sentence
    c. An 18-month-old who uses short "telegraphic" phrases
    d. A 4-year-old who stutters

42. Which of the following statements about stuttering is correct?
    a. Stuttering is normal in the school-age child.
    b. Stuttering occurs because children do not know what they want to say.
    c. Undue emphasis on a stutter may cause an abnormal speech pattern.
    d. Chances for reversal of stuttering are good until about age 3 years.

43. One of the clinical manifestations associated with the speech sounds known as *articulation errors* is the:
    a. omission of consonants at the end of words.
    b. deviation in pitch or quality of the voice.
    c. pauses within a word.
    d. frequent use of circumlocutions.

44. Diagnostic criteria for autism include symptoms related to:
    a. social interactions.
    b. impairments in communication.
    c. repetitive behavior patterns.
    d. all of the above.

45. Strategies to use when caring for the hospitalized child with autism include:
    a. maintaining direct eye contact when explaining procedures.
    b. using holding and touch to comfort the child.
    c. decreasing stimulation.
    d. all of the above.

46. The parents of a child who is stuttering should be encouraged to:
    a. have the child start again more slowly.
    b. give the child plenty of time.
    c. show concern for the hesitancy.
    d. reward the child for proper speech.

47. Define the term *situated approach*.

48. Detecting communication disorders during early childhood:
    a. adversely affects the child's social relationships.
    b. increases the child's difficulty with academic skills.
    c. increases the child's ability to correct deficit skills.
    d. adversely affects the child's emotional interactions.

49. Following assessment and detection of a language problem, the nurse should advise the family to:
    a. wait and see what happens.
    b. wait because the child will grow out of it.
    c. obtain a specialized evaluation.
    d. repeat words so that the child will learn more language.

50. Which of the following findings would indicate a need for referral regarding communication impairment?
    a. A 5-year-old who stutters
    b. A 3-year-old who omits word endings
    c. A 2-year-old with unintelligible speech
    d. A 3-year-old who substitutes easier sounds for difficult ones

CRITICAL THINKING—CASE STUDY

Paula Larson, a 9-month-old infant with Down syndrome (DS) who is also blind and hearing impaired, is admitted to the hospital with pneumonia. She holds her head steady but cannot sit without support or pull up on the furniture. Paula squeals and laughs but does not imitate speech sounds or have any words, not even "da-da" or "ma-ma." She can shake a rattle but cannot pass a block from one hand to the other. She smiles spontaneously and holds her own bottle, but she does not play "pattycake" or wave "bye-bye."

Along with the developing developmental deficits, Paula has congenital heart anomalies and has been hospitalized many times for pneumonia and bronchiolitis. Paula's parents knew that she would be born with DS. They have chosen to care for Paula at home. Paula's care has become increasingly time-consuming. During the admission assessment interview, Mr. and Mrs. Larson state they are both exhausted.

51. The nurse determines that Paula's developmental lag is least pronounced in the area of:
    a. gross motor skills.
    b. language skills.
    c. fine motor skills.
    d. personal-social skills.

52. Paula's parents have cared for her at home since her birth. Mrs. Larson expresses concern that she is not doing a good enough job and that perhaps it is time to consider placement out of the home for Paula. The nurse responds based on the knowledge that:
    a. the potential for development varies greatly in DS.
    b. every available source of assistance to help Mr. and Mrs. Larson with the care of Paula should be explored.
    c. the nurse's responses may influence Mr. and Mrs. Larson's decisions.
    d. all of the above are true.

53. Which of the common nursing diagnoses used in planning care for intellectually disabled children should take priority in Paula's current situation?
    a. Altered Growth and Development
    b. Risk for Interrupted Family Processes
    c. Anxiety related to the hospitalization
    d. Impaired Social Interaction

54. Mr. and Mrs. Larson make the decision to explore residential care for Paula. The best expected outcome during this time for Paula Larson would be for the parents to:
    a. demonstrate acceptance of Paula.
    b. express feelings and concerns regarding the implications of Paula's birth.
    c. make a realistic decision based on Paula's needs and capabilities as well as their own.
    d. identify realistic goals for Paula's future home care.

25 Family-Centered Home Care

1. Match each term with its description.

   a. Home care
   b. Hospice
   c. Home care implementation areas
   d. Cost of care

   e. Individualized home care plan
   f. Care coordination
   g. Nurse case manager
   h. American Nurses Credentialing Center

   i. Hospice and Palliative Nurses Association
   j. Collaborative caring

   _____ The approach to nursing practice that allows the nurse and family to work together and share outcomes in a deep and meaningful way

   _____ Offers certification in hospice nursing

   _____ One person who works with the family to accomplish the many tasks and responsibilities involved; should have a minimum of a baccalaureate degree in nursing and 3 years of experience; needs to be knowledgeable about community resources

   _____ Care provided for children and families with complex health care needs in the place of residence; for the purpose of promoting, maintaining, or restoring health or for maximizing the level of independence while minimizing the effects of disability and illness, including terminal illness

   _____ Intermittent skilled nursing visits and private-duty nursing

   _____ A subsidiary of the American Nurses Association; offers generalist and clinical specialist certification in both home health and community health

   _____ A program of palliative and supportive care services that provides physical, psychologic, social, and spiritual care for dying persons, their families, and their loved ones

   _____ A critical factor that influences the numbers of technology-dependent children who are returned home more quickly than ever

   _____ The concept of linking children who have special home needs (and their families) to services and resources in a effort to provide the child with optimal care

   _____ A general plan developed before discharge, ideally with multidisciplinary input; should address the range of needs identified as part of the comprehensive predischarge assessment

2. Name at least two major reasons why care for complex medical conditions has moved from the hospital to the home setting.

3. Private-duty nursing is the area of pediatric home care nursing most likely to be used to care for:
   a. a child at risk, such as one with nonorganic failure to thrive.
   b. a medically stable child with multiple skilled nursing needs.
   c. a technology-dependent (e.g., ventilator-dependent) child requiring direct care.
   d. all of the above.

4. The cost of home care for children dependent on medical technology is usually more than the cost of hospital care for:
   a. third-party payers.
   b. the government.
   c. the family.
   d. all of the above.

5. Pediatric home care is planned based on assessment of:
   a. parental ability.
   b. safety and support systems in the home.
   c. actual health care practices in the home environment.
   d. all of the above.

6. Which of the following situations would be of most concern to the nurse who was evaluating a family for the possibility of a discharge with home care?
   a. The preterm infant who will be managed with home care is stable after surgery for his congenital heart anomaly.
   b. The family of a child who will be on a ventilator at home has no telephone.
   c. The parents are asking about the availability of respite care.
   d. The mother plans to stop working outside the home to be with the infant.

7. List four major areas of predischarge assessment for the child who is dependent on medical technology.

8. List the elements of a high-quality home care agency.

9. The best strategy to use when planning for transition from hospital to home for the child with complex home care requirements is to:
   a. give the parents a trial period at home during which they provide some of the care.
   b. teach a family member all aspects of the child's care.
   c. allow the parents to provide total care in the hospital with support from the staff as needed.
   d. arrange a predischarge visit during the hospitalization by the home care nurse.

10. Ideally, home care of the child who is technology dependent should be based on the concept of:
    a. traditional case management.
    b. independent care.
    c. primary care management.
    d. case management with care coordination.

11. According to the American Nurses Association, the qualifications of the nurse case manager should include:
    a. a baccalaureate degree in nursing.
    b. 3 years of experience.
    c. knowledge about community resources.
    d. all of the above.

12. List the responsibilities involved in pediatric home care coordination.

13. The pediatric home care nurse's practice includes all of the following except:
    a. consultation with peers to make most daily decisions.
    b. a high level of technical clinical expertise.
    c. knowledge of child development.
    d. the ability to support family autonomy.

14. The pediatric nurse in home care practice is expected to be guided by:
    a. the World Health Organization Standards for Pediatric Home Care.
    b. written standards of practice developed for pediatric patients.
    c. the American Association of Colleges of Nursing Standards.
    d. the National League for Nursing Pediatric Standards.

15. Strategies that promote the central goal of family-centered home care would include all of the following except:
    a. emphasizing family strengths.
    b. identifying family coping mechanisms.
    c. developing unidirectional communication.
    d. promoting family empowerment.

16. List five characteristics of collaborative caring.

17. Basic principles used to communicate with the family include all of the following except:
    a. informing families who will have access to the information.
    b. assuring families that they have the right to confidentiality.
    c. collecting all information firsthand.
    d. restricting communications with other professionals to clinically relevant information.

18. The nurse should use all of the following guidelines for communication with family members except:
    a. giving information slowly and repeating it as necessary.
    b. sharing complete and unbiased information.
    c. using medical terminology.
    d. showing respect for families' knowledge.

19. When conflict occurs between the family and the nurse about the child's treatment, the nurse should first:
    a. call the physician and negotiate a change.
    b. contact the home care supervisor.
    c. respect parental preferences if no danger is posed.
    d. explain the correct way and have the family return a demonstration.

20. The nursing process in home care nursing practice integrates:
    a. normalization.
    b. various disciplines.
    c. family priorities.
    d. all of the above.

21. In home nursing practice the nurse allows the family members to maintain control over:
    a. their home.
    b. their child's care.
    c. their personal lives.
    d. all of the above.

22. When a family chooses not to pursue developmental intervention, the nurse should:
    a. develop an individualized family service plan.
    b. ensure that developmental needs have been explained in a meaningful way.
    c. notify child protective services.
    d. perform all of the above.

23. Describe at least three of the general guidelines a nurse should use when the nurse and family members disagree about the care of the child at home.

24. The school-age child who is physically able may be expected to participate in his or her own care by:
    a. doing no more than holding equipment and discarding used supplies.
    b. administering his or her own medicines with supervision.
    c. assuming responsibility for scheduling home visits.
    d. none of the above; the school-age child is too young to participate in his or her own care.

25. When a child requiring special medical care enters an education setting, the school personnel should:
    a. develop parent advocacy skills.
    b. train staff and caregivers.
    c. coordinate the educational plan.
    d. carry out all of the above.

26. A safety issue specific to the home care child who is dependent on electrical equipment is the need to:
    a. have a telephone on site.
    b. be cared for by trained individuals.
    c. notify the telephone and electric companies that the family needs to be placed on a priority service list.
    d. have someone in the house at all times who knows how to perform cardiopulmonary resuscitation.

27. At night, the care of the child dependent on medical technology presents safety concerns because:
    a. the child may become frightened from the strange noises.
    b. accidental strangulation on equipment wires can occur during sleep.
    c. the lights must be kept brightly lit all night so that procedures can be performed correctly.
    d. All of the above

28. Family-to-family support:
    a. promotes family strength through shared experiences.
    b. replaces professional sources of support.
    c. meets the specific emotional needs of all families.
    d. accomplishes all of the above.

CRITICAL THINKING—CASE STUDY

William Patterson, who is now 18 months old, was born with Werdnig-Hoffmann disease, a congenital neuromuscular disorder. His disease has developed to the point that he is unable to breathe for more than a few hours without ventilator assistance. William's older brother, George, died 2 years ago from complications of the same disease. His parents took care of George at home until his death. William's parents are preparing for a similar progression of the disease, which means that William will probably be maintained at home on a ventilator for many months until his death.

The case manager assigned to William is the same nurse who was assigned to his brother 2 years ago. This nurse, Ruth, was instrumental in helping the family cope with the technical issues of home ventilator management and total parenteral nutrition, as well as the stressors of caring for their dying child.

29. Ruth is concerned about crossing the boundary between collaborating with the Patterson family and becoming enmeshed in the family system, as she did when George was dying. Ruth knows that the family is able to care technically for William, but she feels as if she also needs to be involved again in some way. Ruth has consulted her supervisor for advice. Based on the preceding information, the supervisor is most likely to suggest:
    a. reassignment.
    b. psychologic counseling for Ruth.
    c. assessment of the therapeutic relationship.
    d. psychologic counseling for the Pattersons.

30. If William suddenly becomes less active and demonstrates regressive behavior, the nurse should implement a plan that addresses William's stage of development and use strategies to better promote:
    a. oral-motor development.
    b. mobility and exploration.
    c. self-care.
    d. independence in home management.

31. The quality of William's home care would best be evaluated by asking:
    a. Ruth to review the goals.
    b. the Pattersons to review the goals.
    c. Ruth and the Pattersons to jointly review the goals.
    d. the Pattersons to complete an evaluation questionnaire.

26 Family-Centered Care of the Child During Illness and Hospitalization

1. The following terms are related to children's reactions to hospitalization. Match each term with its description.

   a. Nursing admission history
   b. Anaclitic depression
   c. Protest
   d. Despair

   e. Detachment
   f. Dramatic play
   g. Anger, guilt
   h. Fear, anxiety, frustration

   i. Depression
   j. Family-centered care
   k. Self-care

   _____ The practice of activities that individuals initiate and perform on their own behalf to maintain life, health, and well-being

   _____ The philosophy of care that recognizes the integral role of the family in a child's life and acknowledges the family as an essential part of the child's care and illness experience

   _____ Usually occurs when the acute crisis is over; may be related to concerns for the child's future well-being, including negative effects produced by hospitalization and financial burden incurred

   _____ Common feelings expressed by parents as they respond to their child's illness; may be related to the seriousness of the illness and the type of medical procedures involved

   _____ Reactions that parents may have following the realization of their child's illness; they may resist admitting to such feelings because they expect others to disapprove of behavior that is less than perfect

   _____ Well-recognized technique for emotional release, allowing children to reenact frightening or puzzling hospital experiences; use of puppets and replicas or actual hospital equipment to allow children to act out the situations

   _____ Also called *denial*; the uncommon third phase of separation anxiety, in which superficially the child appears to have finally adjusted to the loss; behavior that is a result of resignation and not a sign of contentment

   _____ The phase of separation anxiety in which the child stops crying, is much less active, and withdraws from others

   _____ A phase of separation anxiety in which children react aggressively; cry loudly, scream for parents, refuse the attention of anyone else, and are inconsolable in their grief

   _____ Separation anxiety; the major stress from middle infancy throughout the preschool years

   _____ Systematic collection of data about the child and family that allows the nurse to plan individualized care

2. Match each hospitalization term with its description.

   a. Play therapy
   b. Therapeutic play

   c. Child life specialists
   d. Interdisciplinary approach

   _____ An effective nondirective modality for helping children deal with their concerns and fears; often helps the nurse gain insights into the child's needs and feelings

   _____ All members of the health care team working together with the patient and family

   _____ Technique used as an interpretive method with emotionally disturbed children by trained and qualified therapists

   _____ Health care professionals with expertise in child development; promote effective coping and adjustment during potentially stressful situations through play, psychologic preparation, education, and support

3. Separation anxiety would be most expected in the hospitalized child at age:
   a. 3 to 6 months.
   b. 16 to 30 months.
   c. 30 months to 2 years.
   d. 2 to 4 years.

4. Match each phase of separation anxiety with the behaviors that are typical of that phase.

   a. Protest

   b. Despair

   c. Detachment

   _____ Withdraws from others; is inactive, depressed, sad, uninterested in environment, uncommunicative, regressive

   _____ Shows increased interest in surroundings; interacts with caregivers; appears happy; forms new but superficial relationships (rarely seen in hospitalized children)

   _____ Cries continuously; screams; attacks stranger physically and verbally; attempts to escape

5. One difference between toddlers and school-age children in their reactions to hospitalization is that most school-age children:
   a. do not experience separation anxiety.
   b. show less fright or overt resistance to pain.
   c. rely on family more.
   d. experience separation anxiety to a greater degree.

6. A toddler is most likely to react to short-term hospitalization with feelings of loss of control that are manifested by:
   a. regression.
   b. withdrawal.
   c. formation of new superficial relationships.
   d. self-assertion and anger.

7. The technique that is most appropriate to prepare a toddler for a painful procedure is to:
   a. encourage the child to act grown up.
   b. demonstrate the procedure.
   c. verbally instruct the child.
   d. allow structured choices.

8. Which of the following statements about getting a cold is most characteristic of the toddler?
   a. "I got this cold because I did not wear my hat."
   b. "I got this cold by breathing in bacteria."
   c. "I got this cold because I feel sick."
   d. "I got this cold from harmful germs."

9. The most consistent indicator of distress in infants is:
   a. initial cry.
   b. heart rate.
   c. facial expression.
   d. uncooperativeness.

10. School-age children with chronic illness are most likely to be concerned about:
    a. Pain
    b. Physical symptoms
    c. Strange surroundings
    d. Privacy

11. Which of the following risk factors would make a child more vulnerable to the stresses of hospitalization?
    a. Urban dwelling
    b. Strong will
    c. Female gender
    d. Passive temperament

12. Complex care of the pediatric population in the hospital today differs from the pediatric population of 10 years ago in that the usual length of stay has:
    a. decreased and the acuity has increased.
    b. increased and the acuity has decreased.
    c. increased and the acuity has increased.
    d. decreased and the acuity has decreased.

13. Describe at least one of the possible psychologic benefits a child might gain from hospitalization.

14. Which of the following factors, according to Craft's 1993 framework, would be considered most likely to negatively influence the reactions of siblings to the hospitalized child?
    a. The sibling is an adolescent.
    b. Care providers are not relatives.
    c. The sibling has received information about the ill child.
    d. The ill child is cared for in the home.

15. Which of the following statements is true in regard to parent participation in the hospitalized child's care?
    a. The parents need 24-hour responsibility to help maintain their feeling of importance to the child.
    b. Fathers and mothers need the same kind of support during the hospitalization of their child.
    c. Nurses may express support of parent participation but may not foster an environment that encourages parental involvement.
    d. Mothers feel comfortable assuming responsibility for their child's care.

16. List three strategies nurses can use to minimize stresses for the parents of the hospitalized child.

17. To help the parents deal with issues related to separation while their child is hospitalized, the nurse should not suggest:
    a. using associations to help the child understand time frames.
    b. ways to explain departure and return.
    c. quietly leaving while the child is distracted or asleep.
    d. short frequent visits over an extended stay if rooming in is impossible.

18. Which of the following strategies should the nurse use to help the hospitalized child adjust to the strange environment?
    a. Discontinue school lessons.
    b. Evaluate stimuli from the adult point of view.
    c. Send personal items home to prevent loss.
    d. Combine familiar sights with the unfamiliar.

19. Strategies used to minimize the hospitalized child's feelings of loss of control include attempts to:
    a. alter the child's schedule to match the hospital schedule.
    b. establish a daily schedule for the hospitalized child.
    c. eliminate rituals that have been used at home.
    d. perform all of the above.

20. The Joint Commission recommends that children's rights and responsibilities during hospitalization be:
    a. the same as those of adults.
    b. the same throughout the agency.
    c. different from those of adults.
    d. prominently displayed as a "Bill of Rights" for parents.

21. When performing a painful procedure on a child, to minimize fear of bodily injury, the nurse should attempt to:
    a. perform the procedure in the playroom.
    b. standardize techniques from one age-group to the next.
    c. perform the procedure quickly with the parent present.
    d. have the parents leave during the procedure.

22. After administering an intramuscular injection, the nurse would best reassure the young child with poorly defined body boundaries by:
    a. telling the child that the bleeding will stop after the needle is removed.
    b. using a large bandage to cover the injection site.
    c. using a small bandage to cover the injection site.
    d. using a bandage but removing it a few hours after the injection.

23. One way to evaluate whether a child fears mutilation of body parts is to:
    a. explain the procedure.
    b. ask the child to draw a picture of what will happen.
    c. stress the reason for the procedure.
    d. investigate the child's individual concerns.

24. Which of the following reactions to surgery is most typical of an adolescent's reaction of fear of bodily injury?
    a. Concern about the pain
    b. Concern about the procedure itself
    c. Concern about the scar
    d. Understanding explanations literally

25. List three functions of play in the hospitalized child.

26. When helping parents select activities for their hospitalized child, the nurse should recommend:
    a. simpler activities than would normally be chosen.
    b. new toys and games to help distract the child.
    c. challenging new games to keep the child engaged.
    d. games that can be played with adults.

27. List at least two ways that drawing or painting can be used by the nurse in caring for the hospitalized child.

28. The nurse can foster the hospitalized child's feelings of self-mastery by:
    a. acknowledging uncooperative behavior.
    b. acknowledging negative behavior.
    c. emphasizing aspects of the child's competence.
    d. providing emotional support to the family.

29. Preparation for hospitalization reduces stress in which of the following age-groups?
    a. Adolescents
    b. Toddlers
    c. Preschoolers
    d. All of the above

30. Define the role of a child life specialist.

31. Questions related to activities of daily living at the time of admission are:
    a. inappropriate and should be saved for later.
    b. directed toward evaluation of the child's preparation for hospitalization.
    c. asked directly and in the order provided on the assessment form.
    d. designed to help the nurse develop appropriate routines for the hospitalized child.

32. Describe at least three strategies that can be used in the intensive care unit to support the child and family.

33. The question "How does your child act when annoyed or upset?" would be asked on admission to assess the child's:
    a. health perception–health management pattern.
    b. cognitive-perceptual pattern.
    c. activity-exercise pattern.
    d. self-perception/self-concept pattern.

34. The question "How does your child usually handle problems or disappointments?" would be asked on admission to assess the child's:
    a. role-relationship pattern.
    b. sexuality-reproductive pattern.
    c. coping–stress tolerance pattern.
    d. value-belief pattern.

35. The advantages of a hospital unit specifically for adolescents include:
    a. exclusive group membership.
    b. fewer preparation requirements.
    c. increased socialization with peers.
    d. all of the above.

36. The benefit of the ambulatory/outpatient setting is reduction of:
    a. stressors.
    b. infection risk.
    c. cost.
    d. all of the above.

37. Discharge instructions from the ambulatory setting should always include all of the following except:
    a. guidelines for when to call.
    b. dietary restrictions.
    c. activity restrictions.
    d. referral to a home health agency.

38. When caring for the child in isolation, the nurse should:
    a. spend as little time as possible in the room.
    b. teach the parents to care for the child to decrease the risk for spreading infection.
    c. let the child see the nurse's face before donning the mask.
    d. perform all of the above.

39. Describe the process for counseling after an event has occurred.

40. The most ideal way to support parents when they first visit the child in the intensive care unit is:
    a. for the nurse to accompany them to the bedside.
    b. to use picture books of the unit in the waiting area.
    c. to limit the visiting hours so that parents are encouraged to rest.
    d. to expect parents to stay with their child continuously.

41. Transfer from the intensive care unit to the regular pediatric unit can be best facilitated by:
    a. discussing the details of the transfer at the bedside, where the child can listen.
    b. establishing a schedule that mimics the child's home schedule.
    c. assigning a primary nurse from the regular unit who visits the child before the transfer.
    d. explaining to the family that there are fewer nurses on the regular unit.

42. Transitional care, which is a trial period for the family to assume the child's care with minimal supervision, may take place:
    a. on the nursing unit.
    b. during a home pass.
    c. in a motel near the hospital.
    d. All or during any of the above

CRITICAL THINKING—CASE MANAGEMENT

Peter Chen is an 8-year-old child who is admitted to the pediatric unit for an appendectomy. He is in the third grade and is very active in after-school activities. Recently he began to take karate lessons, and he also plays baseball. Peter loves school, particularly when he is able to read. He awakens every morning at 6 AM to read, and reading is the last thing he does before he falls asleep.

Peter's parents are with him during the admission interview. His mother works, but she has made arrangements to take some time off after surgery and during his hospital stay to be available to him.

43. Based on the preceding information, the nurse should expect:
    a. a normal response to hospitalization.
    b. more anxiety than would normally be seen.
    c. difficulty with the parents.
    d. cultural factors to take precedence.

44. Which of the following nursing diagnoses after Peter's surgery is correct?
    a. Powerlessness related to the environment
    b. Activity Intolerance related to pain or discomfort
    c. Anxiety/Fear related to distressing procedures
    d. Any of the above

45. One reasonable expected outcome for Peter's diagnosis of powerlessness would be:
    a. Peter will tolerate increasing activity.
    b. Peter will remain injury-free.
    c. Peter will play and rest quietly.
    d. Peter will help plan his care and schedule.

46. Which of the following interventions would be best for the nurse to incorporate into Peter's plan related to the diagnosis of activity intolerance?
    a. Organize activities for maximum sleep time.
    b. Keep side rails up.
    c. Choose an appropriate roommate.
    d. Assist with dressing and bathing.

27 Pediatric Variations of Nursing Interventions

1. The following terms are related to pediatric procedures. Match each term with its description.

a. Medically emancipated conditions
b. Emancipated minor

c. Assent
d. Adherence
e. Organizational strategies

f. Teaching principles
g. Treatment strategies
h. Behavioral strategies

_____ Interventions that are designed to modify behavior directly, with the goal of improving compliance (e.g., positive reinforcement and contracting)

_____ Usually a verbal agreement; requires that the child be informed about the proposed treatment or research and that the child concurs with the decisions made by the person who gives consent

_____ One who is legally under the age of majority but is recognized as having the legal capacity of an adult under circumstances prescribed by state law

_____ Conditions determined by the state legislatures that entitle adolescents to consent to treatment without their parents' knowledge; used by adolescents to obtain treatment for conditions such as sexually transmitted infections and alcohol and drug abuse, as well as to seek contraceptive advice; statutes vary from state to state

_____ Interventions that are related to the child's refusal or inability to take a prescribed medication or follow a prescribed treatment regimen; used to improve compliance

_____ May enhance compliance; concerned with instructing the child and family about the treatment plan

_____ Interventions that are concerned with the care setting and the therapeutic plan; used to improve compliance

_____ Another term for *compliance;* refers to the extent to which the patient's behavior coincides with the prescribed regimen

2. The following terms are related to general hygiene and care. Match each term with its description.

a. Pressure ulcers
b. Pressure reduction device
c. Pressure relief device
d. Friction
e. Shear

f. Epidermal stripping
g. Set point
h. Fever
i. Hyperthermia
j. Chill phase

k. Plateau
l. Defervescence
m. Reactive hyperemia

_____ Flush; the earliest sign of tissue compromise and pressure-related ischemia

_____ Hyperpyrexia; an elevation in set point such that the body temperature is regulated at a higher level; may be arbitrarily defined as temperature above 38° C (100° F)

_____ The point in the febrile state in which shivering and vasoconstriction generate and conserve heat and raise the central temperatures to a level of the new set point

_____ The point during the febrile state in which the temperature stabilizes at the higher range

_____ Can develop when the pressure on the skin and underlying tissues is greater than the capillary closing pressure, causing capillary occlusion; results in tissue anoxia and cellular death; most commonly occurs over a bony prominence

_____ The result of the force of gravity pulling down on the body and friction of the body against a surface; occurs, for example, when a patient is in the semi-Fowler position and begins to slide to the foot of the bed

_____ A product used to decrease the pressure that occurs with a regular hospital bed or chair; usually consists of an overlay that is placed on top of the regular mattress

_____ Occurs when the surface of the skin rubs against another surface, such as the sheets on a bed

_____ A product that maintains pressure below the level that would cause capillary closing; usually consists of a high-technology bed used for patients who have multiple problems and cannot be turned effectively

_____ A situation in which body temperature exceeds the set point; usually occurs when the body or external conditions create more heat than the body can eliminate, such as in heat stroke, aspirin toxicity, or hyperthyroidism

_____ The point when the temperature is greater than the set point or when the pyrogen is no longer present

_____ Results when the epidermis is unintentionally torn away when tape is removed

_____ The temperature around which body temperature is regulated by a thermostat-like mechanism in the hypothalamus

3. The following terms are related to safety and collection of specimens. Match each term with its description.

a. Nosocomial
b. Standard Precautions
c. Transmission-Based Precautions
d. Airborne Precautions
e. Droplet Precautions
f. Contact Precautions
g. Direct contact transmission
h. Indirect contact transmission
i. Bladder catheterization
j. Suprapubic aspiration
k. Allen test
l. Gastric washings
m. Nasal washings

_____ Lavage; used to collect a sputum specimen from infants and small children who are unable to follow directions to cough effectively and who may swallow sputum produced when they do

_____ Designed to reduce the risk for transmission of infectious agents that are spread when large particles generated during coughing, sneezing, or talking come into contact with the conjunctiva or the mucous membrane of the nose or mouth of a susceptible person; suctioning or bronchoscopy generate these particles

_____ Designed to reduce the risk of transmission of microorganisms transmitted by direct or indirect contact

_____ Interventions that synthesize the major features of universal (blood and body fluid) precautions and body substance isolation; involve the use of barrier protection; designed for the care of all patients to reduce the risk for transmission of microorganism from both recognized and unrecognized sources of infection

_____ A sterile procedure in which a feeding tube or Foley catheter is inserted into the urethra to obtain a sterile urine specimen when the child is unable to void or otherwise provide an adequate specimen

_____ Also referred to as *hospital acquired*

_____ Involves skin-to-skin contact and physical transfer of microorganisms to a susceptible host from an infected or colonized person

_____ Designed for patients documented or suspected to be infected or colonized with highly transmissible or epidemiologically important pathogens for which interventions beyond Standard Precautions are needed to interrupt transmission in hospitals

_____ Involves contact of a susceptible host with a contaminated intermediate object, usually an inanimate object in the patient's environment

_____ A procedure that involves aspirating bladder contents by inserting a needle in the midline above the symphysis pubis and vertically downward into the bladder; used to obtain a urine specimen when the child is unable to void or otherwise provide an adequate specimen, when the bladder cannot be accessed through the urethra, and/or when use of a catheter poses too high a risk for contamination; useful in clarifying the diagnosis of suspected urinary tract infection in acutely ill infants

_____ A procedure in which 1 to 3 ml of sterile normal saline are instilled into one nostril and then aspirated; usually performed to diagnose an infection of respiratory syncytial virus

_____ A procedure that assesses the circulation of the radial, ulnar, or brachial arteries

_____ Designed to reduce the transmission of infectious agents that remain suspended in air or by dust particles containing the infectious agent

4. The following terms are related to administration of medication and feeding techniques. Match each term with its description.

a. Body surface area
b. West nomogram
c. Needleless injection system
d. Subcutaneous injections

e. Intradermal injection
f. Orogastric or nasogastric gavage
g. Enteral gavage
h. Gastrostomy

i. Jejunostomy
j. Skin-level device
k. Familial adenomatous polyposis

_____ A long-term gastrostomy feeding device consisting of a small, flexible silicone tube that protrudes slightly from the abdomen (e.g., MIC-KEY, Bard Button, Gastroport); advantages—affords increased comfort and mobility to the child, is easy to care for, is fully water immersible, has a one-way valve to minimize reflux, and eliminates the need for clamping; disadvantages—requires a well-established gastrostomy site and is expensive

_____ Administered to the lateral side of the volar surface of the forearm

_____ The most reliable basis to use for calculating children's drug dosages from a standard adult dose

_____ Feeding by a tube inserted directly into the stomach

_____ Feeding by way of a tube inserted orally or nasally into the duodenum-jejunum

_____ Usually used to determine body surface area

_____ Condition that may require a colectomy with ileoanal reservoir to prevent or treat carcinoma of the colon

_____ Biojector; delivers intramuscular or subcutaneous injections without the use of a needle; eliminates the risk for accidental needle puncture

_____ Feeding by way of a tube inserted orally or nasally into the stomach

_____ Common injection sites include the center third of the lateral aspect of the upper arm, the abdomen, and the center third of the anterior thigh

_____ Feeding by a tube inserted directly into the jejunum

5. An informed consent is required for:
a. an emergency appendectomy.
b. a cutdown for intravenous medications.
c. release of medical information.
d. all of the above.

6. When parents are divorced, who is eligible to consent to medical treatment of their child?
a. Usually, the custodial parent consents.
b. Only the noncustodial parent may consent.
c. Both parents must consent.
d. The child is the responsible party.

7. The statutes for the mature minors doctrine vary from state to state. Based on the doctrine, a minor may be permitted to consent for:
a. elective surgery.
b. treatment for any kind of health problem.
c. treatment for sexually transmitted infections.
d. routine physical examinations only.

8. Although statutes vary from state to state, minors are usually recognized as having the legal capacity of an adult in all matters after they:
   a. have acquired a sexually transmitted infection.
   b. use contraceptives.
   c. use drugs or alcohol.
   d. become pregnant.

9. When preparing a child for a procedure, the nurse should:
   a. use abstract terms.
   b. teach based on the child's developmental level.
   c. use phrases with dual meanings.
   d. introduce anxiety-laden information first.

10. If a child needs support during an invasive procedure, the nurse should:
    a. insist that the parents participate in distraction techniques.
    b. instruct parents to stand quietly in back of the room and maintain eye contact with the child.
    c. respect parents' wishes and coach the parents about what to do.
    d. instruct parents to stay close by to console the child immediately after the procedure.

11. To prepare a toddler for an invasive procedure, the best strategy for the nurse to use would be to:
    a. give one direction at a time.
    b. prepare the child a day in advance.
    c. set up the equipment while the child watches.
    d. expect the child to sit still and cooperate.

12. Which of the following words or phrases is considered nonthreatening?
    a. "A little stick"
    b. "An owie"
    c. Die
    d. Deaden

13. Which of the following strategies is a powerful coping method that can be used with a small child during painful procedures?
    a. Ask the child whether he or she wants to take the pain medicine.
    b. Administer medication in the playroom.
    c. Give a comprehensive explanation of what will occur.
    d. Use distraction techniques for a painful procedure.

14. List at least five strategies the nurse can use to support the child during and after a procedure.

15. Describe at least one play activity for each of the following procedures.
    a. Ambulation:

    b. Range-of-motion exercises:

c. Injections:

d. Deep breathing:

e. Extending the environment:

f. Soaks:

g. Fluid intake:

16. The most effective method of preoperative preparation is:
    a. consistent supportive care.
    b. systematic preparation at specific stress points.
    c. offering parents the option of attending the induction of anesthesia.
    d. a single session of preparation.

17. One strategy to provide atraumatic care for pediatric patients undergoing surgery is:
    a. restrict fluids in infants for at least 10 hours.
    b. always use a face mask during induction.
    c. allow child to wear regular clothing into surgery.
    d. remove parents from the child's sight.

18. To prepare a breast-fed infant physically for surgery, the nurse would expect to:
    a. permit breast-feeding up to 4 hours before surgery.
    b. withhold breast-feeding from midnight the night before surgery.
    c. permit breast-feeding up to 6 hours before surgery.
    d. replace breast milk with formula and permit feeding up to 2 hours before surgery.

19. Preoperative sedation in children is best accomplished by:
    a. oral transmucosal fentanyl.
    b. intravenous midazolam.
    c. intravenous opioids.
    d. oral analgesics.

20. Early symptoms of malignant hyperthermia include:
    a. anemia.
    b. enlarged lymph nodes.
    c. tachycardia.
    d. elevated temperature.

21. Fear of induction of anesthesia by mask can be minimized by applying:
    a. the mask quickly and with assurance.
    b. an opaque mask.
    c. the mask while the child is sitting.
    d. the mask while the child is supine.

22. A change in vital signs of the young child in the postanesthesia recovery room that demands immediate attention is:
    a. increased temperature.
    b. tachypnea.
    c. muscle rigidity.
    d. all of the above.

23. Noncompliant families:
    a. share typical characteristics.
    b. have less education than compliant families.
    c. often have complex medical regimens.
    d. often have an increased loss of control.

24. An example of an organizational strategy to improve compliance would be for the nurse to:
    a. incorporate teaching principles that are known to enhance understanding.
    b. encourage the family to adapt hospital medication schedules to their home routine.
    c. evaluate and reduce the time the family waits for their appointment.
    d. all of the above are organizational strategies.

25. In planning strategies to improve the child's compliance with the prescribed treatment, the nurse knows that:
    a. an every-8-hour schedule should be implemented.
    b. an every-6-hour schedule should be implemented.
    c. the child may not be able to swallow pills.
    d. the family usually does not remember or understand the instructions given.

26. General guidelines for care of a child's skin includes:
    a. covering the fingers of the extremity used for an intravenous line.
    b. lifting the child under the arms to transfer the child from the bed to a stretcher.
    c. placing a pectin-based skin barrier directly over excoriated skin.
    d. keeping the skin moist at all times.

27. A stage III pressure ulcer usually manifests as:
    a. full-thickness tissue loss.
    b. an abrasion.
    c. nonblanchable erythema.
    d. reactive hyperemia.

28. To prevent injuries from shearing, the nurse should avoid:
    a. using sheepskin over the elbows.
    b. pulling the patient up in bed without a lift sheet.
    c. pulling the patient up in bed with a lift sheet.
    d. using Montgomery straps.

29. When bathing an uncircumcised boy over the age of 3 years, the nurse should:
    a. gently remind the child to clean his genital area.
    b. not retract the foreskin.
    c. gently retract the foreskin.
    d. avoid cleansing between the skinfolds of the genital area.

30. To braid the hair of a child with curly hair, braid the hair:
    a. when it is damp.
    b. tightly.
    c. when it is dry.
    d. after petroleum jelly is applied.

31. To prevent a child from becoming dehydrated from diarrhea, the nurse should:
    a. use gentle persuasion.
    b. force fluids.
    c. awaken the child to offer fluids.
    d. allow only high-quality, nutritious liquids.

32. The best example of adequate documentation of a child's food intake would be:
    a. "Child ate one bowl of cereal with milk."
    b. "Child ate an adequate breakfast."
    c. "Child ate 80% of the breakfast served."
    d. "Parent states that child ate an adequate breakfast."

33. During the chill phase of the febrile state:
    a. heat is generated and conserved.
    b. the temperature stabilizes at a higher range.
    c. a crisis of the temperature is occurring.
    d. the temperature is greater than the set point.

34. Of the following, the most effective intervention for the treatment of fever in a 4-year-old child is to administer:
    a. a tepid sponge bath.
    b. ibuprofen.
    c. an alcohol sponge bath.
    d. acetaminophen.

35. Of the following, the best intervention for the treatment of hyperthermia in a 4-year-old child is to administer:
    a. a tepid sponge bath.
    b. acetaminophen.
    c. an alcohol sponge bath.
    d. aspirin.

36. In which of the following strengths are ibuprofen oral drops available?
    a. 100 mg/1.25 ml
    b. 100 mg/5 ml
    c. 50 mg/1.25 ml
    d. 50 mg/5 ml

37. Standard Precautions involve the use of barrier protection to prevent contamination from:
    a. blood.
    b. body fluids.
    c. mucous membranes.
    d. all of the above.

38. To prevent spread of contamination from one patient to another after procedures, the most important strategy the nurse can use is to:
    a. follow disease-specific infection control guidelines.
    b. wear vinyl gloves.
    c. avoid wearing nail polish.
    d. wash the hands routinely after each patient contact.

39. List three acceptable methods to transport infants and children.

40. List five nursing interventions for the child who is restrained.

41. After mouth or lip surgery, the nurse would choose to restrain the child using:
    a. arm and leg restraints.
    b. elbow restraints.
    c. a jacket restraint.
    d. a mummy restraint.

42. The best strategy to use when performing venipuncture on a toddler is to:
    a. give simple instructions for the child to hold still.
    b. extend the neck and maintain head alignment to expose the jugular vein.
    c. place the child prone with legs in a frog position to expose the groin area.
    d. hold the child's upper body to prevent movement.

43. The best positioning technique for a lumbar puncture in a neonate is a:
    a. side-lying position with neck flexion.
    b. sitting position.
    c. side-lying position with modified neck extension.
    d. side-lying position with knees to chest.

44. The most frequently used site for bone marrow aspiration in children is the:
    a. femur.
    b. sternum.
    c. tibia.
    d. iliac crest.

45. To facilitate urination in a 12-month-old infant, the nurse could:
    a. wipe the abdomen with alcohol and fan it dry.
    b. elicit the Perez reflex.
    c. apply a urine collection device.
    d. wash and dry the genitalia thoroughly.

46. When applying a urine specimen bag to an infant boy, it is sometimes necessary to:
    a. oil the surface of the skin.
    b. place the scrotum inside the bag.
    c. remove and replace the bag often.
    d. restrain all four extremities tightly.

47. When necessary, suprapubic aspiration is used:
    a. to access the bladder through the urethra.
    b. to obtain sterile specimens from young infants.
    c. even though it may increase the risk for contamination.
    d. All of the above

48. Suprapubic aspiration has a _____ success rate than catheterization of the bladder through the urethra.
    a. Higher
    b. Lower

49. To collect a blood culture specimen from a central venous line or peripheral lock, the nurse should:
    a. use the first sample of blood.
    b. discard the first sample of blood.
    c. irrigate the device with D_5W first.
    d. use a heparinized collection tube.

50. Of the following venipuncture techniques, the most important to use to avoid the complication of necrotizing osteochondritis would be to:
    a. warm the site with moist compresses.
    b. cleanse the site with alcohol.
    c. puncture no deeper than 2 mm.
    d. use the inner aspect of the heel.

51. After a venipuncture is performed in the young child, the nurse should:
    a. use a "spot" bandage for the day.
    b. extend the arm while pressure is applied.
    c. avoid the use of any bandage.
    d. flex the arm while pressure is applied.

52. To obtain a sputum specimen to test for tuberculosis or respiratory syncytial virus in an infant, the nurse may need to:
    a. stimulate the infant's cough reflex.
    b. obtain mucus from the throat.
    c. insert a suction catheter into the back of the throat.
    d. perform gastric lavage.

53. The most accurate method for determining the safe dosage of a medication for a child is to use:
    a. the body surface area formula.
    b. Clark's rule.
    c. Wright's rule.
    d. milligrams per kilogram.

54. The form of medication that is best to administer to a young child is the:
    a. intravenous preparation.
    b. intramuscular preparation.
    c. solid oral preparation.
    d. liquid oral preparation.

55. To administer 1 teaspoon of medication at home, the parent should use the:
    a. household soup spoon.
    b. household measuring spoon.
    c. hospital's molded plastic cup.
    d. household teaspoon.

56. All of the following techniques for medication administration in the infant are acceptable except:
    a. adding the medication to the infant's formula.
    b. allowing the infant to sit in the parent's lap during administration.
    c. allowing the infant to suck the medication from a nipple.
    d. inserting a needleless syringe into the side of the mouth while the infant nurses.

57. Which of the following intramuscular injection sites is generally reserved for children who have been walking for more than a year?
    a. Deltoid muscle
    b. Vastus lateralis
    c. Dorsogluteal
    d. Ventrogluteal

58. When administering intramuscular medications to infants and small children, the nurse should:
    a. depress the plunger at the same time the needle is inserted.
    b. use the dorsogluteal muscle in infants.
    c. instruct the small child to stand and lean against his or her parent for support.
    d. inject the medication slowly.

59. When administering intravenous medication to an infant, the nurse should:
    a. check site for patency before each dose.
    b. administer medications along with blood products.
    c. combine antibiotics to avoid fluid overload.
    d. use the maximum dilution of the drug permitted by the manufacturer.

60. When administering medications to a child through a gastric tube, the nurse should:
    a. use oily medications to ease passage through the tube.
    b. mix the medication with the enteral formula.
    c. use a syringe with the plunger in place to administer the drug.
    d. flush the tube well between each medication administration.

61. The rectal route of medication administration is used in children when the child:
    a. is not responding to oral antiemetic preparations.
    b. needs a reliable route of administration.
    c. is constipated.
    d. all of the above.

62. To instill eyedrops in an infant whose eyelids are clenched shut, the nurse should:
    a. apply finger pressure to the lacrimal punctum.
    b. place the drops in the nasal corner where the lids meet and wait until the infant opens the lid.
    c. administer the eyedrops before nap time.
    d. use any of the above techniques.

63. During continuous enteral feedings, the nurse should:
    a. use the same pole as used for the intravenous line.
    b. use a burette to calibrate the feeding times.
    c. give the infant a pacifier for sucking.
    d. all of the above.

64. In the small infant, a feeding tube is usually inserted through the:
    a. nose.
    b. mouth.

65. When administering an enema to a small child, the nurse should use:
    a. a pediatric Fleet enema.
    b. a commercially prepared solution.
    c. an isotonic solution.
    d. plain water.

66. A young child with an ostomy pouch may need to:
    a. wear one-piece outfits.
    b. begin toilet training at a later than usual age.
    c. use an alcohol-based skin sealant.
    d. use a rubber band to help the appliance fit.

CRITICAL THINKING—CASE STUDY

Janis is a 6-year-old child admitted to the hospital for an emergency appendectomy. Her parents have been divorced for 4 years, and her mother accompanies her to the hospital. Janis has a sister who is 7 years old.

67. Based on Janis's developmental characteristics, the nurse's plan for preparing the girl for surgery should include:
    a. an emphasis on privacy.
    b. the correct scientific medical terminology.
    c. ways to help Janis accept new authority figures.
    d. teaching sessions that last no longer than 5 minutes.

68. One of the nursing diagnoses identified by the nurse for Janis is High Risk for Injury related to the surgical procedure and anesthesia. During the assessment interview, which of the following sets of facts would be most pertinent to this diagnosis?
    a. The nurse auscultated vesicular breath sounds.
    b. Janis's mother tells the nurse that the child's father is 27 years old and in good health but had some heart problems related to anesthesia after a minor surgical procedure last year.
    c. Janis's mother tells the nurse not to expect the child's father to participate in the preoperative preparation because he lives in another state.
    d. The nurse determines that the child has moist mucous membranes and no tenting of the skin.

69. The nursing diagnosis of Anxiety related to the surgery and hospitalization is identified by the nurse. Which of the following strategies is the best to incorporate into the surgical care plan to address this diagnosis?
    a. Encourage Janis's mother to be present as much as possible.
    b. Administer analgesics around the clock.
    c. Teach Janis to use the incentive spirometer.
    d. Help Janis ambulate as early as possible.

70. Which of the following findings represents the most appropriate measurable data to evaluate the care plan in regard to the nursing diagnosis of High Risk for Fluid Volume Deficit?
    a. The child has vesicular breath sounds.
    b. The child's father, who is 27 years old and in good health, had some heart problems with anesthesia after a minor surgical procedure last year.
    c. The child's father lives in another state.
    d. The child has moist mucous membranes and no tenting of the skin.

Balance and Imbalance of Body Fluids

1. Match each term with its description or function.

a. Total body water
b. Intracellular fluid
c. Extracellular fluid
d. Renin-angiotensin system
e. Dehydration
f. Aldosterone
g. Antidiuretic hormone

h. Intravascular fluid
i. Interstitial
j. Transcellular fluid
k. Insensible water loss
l. Third-spacing
m. Peripheral edema
n. Ascites

o. Pulmonary edema
p. Oral rehydration solution
q. Acidosis (acidemia)
r. Alkalosis (alkalemia)
s. pH
t. Infiltration
u. Extravasation

_____ Constitutes about half of the total body water at birth

_____ Fluid within the cells

_____ Constitutes 45% to 75% of body weight

_____ Inadvertent administration of a nonvesicant parenteral solution or medication into surrounding tissue as a result of catheter dislodgment.

_____ Inadvertent administration of vesicant solution or medication into surrounding tissue as a result of catheter dislodgement.

_____ Enhances sodium reabsorption in renal tubules

_____ Released from the posterior pituitary gland in response to increased osmolality and decreased volume of intravascular fluid

_____ Diminished blood flow to the kidneys stimulates secretion, which reacts with plasma globulin to generate a vasoconstrictor

_____ Occurs whenever the total output of fluid exceeds the total intake

_____ Fluid loss through the skin and respiratory tract

_____ Pooling of body fluids in a body space

_____ Localized or generalized swelling of the interstitial space

_____ Used to treat infants with dehydration

_____ Surrounding the cell and the location of most extracellular fluid

_____ Accumulation of fluid in the abdomen

_____ Fluid contained within the body cavities (e.g., cerebrospinal fluid)

_____ Occurs when there is an increase in the interstitial volume

_____ Fluid contained within the blood vessels

_____ Represents the concentration of hydrogen in solution and indicates only whether the imbalance is more acidic or more alkaline

_____ Results from either accumulation of base or loss of acid

_____ Results from either accumulation of acid or loss of base

2. Which of the following conditions would produce an increased fluid requirement?
   a. Heart failure
   b. High intracranial pressure
   c. Mechanical ventilation
   d. Tachypnea

3. Which of the following individuals has the least water content in relation to weight?
   a. Obese adolescent female
   b. Thin adolescent female
   c. Obese adolescent male
   d. Thin adolescent male

4. Infants and young children are at high risk for fluid and electrolyte imbalances. Which of the following factors contributes to this vulnerability?
   a. Decreased body surface area
   b. Lower metabolic rate
   c. Mature kidney function
   d. Increased extracellular fluid volume

5. Chloe, age 4 weeks, is brought to the clinic by her mother. When asking about Chloe's feeding schedule, the nurse learns that the mother has been adding twice the required amount of dry formula powder to water in Chloe's bottles for the past 2 days. The mother thinks that this will help Chloe gain weight faster. Which of the following does the nurse recognize as true about this practice?
   a. The infant's kidneys are functionally mature at birth and able to handle this concentration of formula.
   b. The infant's kidneys are functionally immature at birth, and this concentration of formula can cause Chloe to be dehydrated.
   c. The infant's kidneys are functionally immature at birth, and this concentration of formula will cause Chloe to become overhydrated.
   d. The infant's kidneys are functionally mature at birth, but because of her greater body surface area and longer gastrointestinal tract, Chloe would need the formula diluted.

6. _____ dehydration occurs when electrolyte and water deficits are present in balanced proportion.

7. _____ dehydration occurs when the electrolyte deficit exceeds the water deficit. There is a greater proportional loss of extracellular fluid, and plasma sodium concentration is usually _____ than 130 mEq/L.

8. _____ dehydration results from water loss in excess of electrolyte loss. This is often caused by a large _____ of water and/or a large _____ of electrolytes. Plasma sodium concentration is _____ than 150 mEq/L.

9. In infants and young children, the most accurate means of describing dehydration or fluid loss is:
   a. as a percentage.
   b. by milliliters per kilogram of body weight.
   c. by the amount of edema present or absent.
   d. by the degree of skin elasticity.

10. An infant with moderate dehydration has clinical signs of:
    a. mottled skin color, decreased pulse and respirations.
    b. decreased urinary output, tachycardia, and fever.
    c. tachycardia, oliguria, capillary filling within 2 to 4 seconds.
    d. tachycardia, bulging fontanel, decreased blood pressure.

11. Diagnostic evaluation of dehydration to initiate a therapeutic plan includes:
    i. serum electrolytes.
    ii. acid-base imbalance determination.
    iii. physical assessment to determine degree of dehydration.
    iv. type of dehydration based on pathophysiology.

    a. i and ii
    b. i, ii, and iii
    c. i, ii, iii, and iv
    d. iii and iv

12. Which of the following instructions for treating the child with mild dehydration is not correct?
    a. Administer 2 to 5 ml of oral rehydration solution (ORS) by syringe or small medication cup every 2 to 3 minutes until the child is able to tolerate larger amounts.
    b. Oral administration of ondansetron (Zofran) to the child with acute gastroenteritis and vomiting may prevent the need for intravenous (IV) therapy.
    c. ORS management consists of replacement of fluid loss over 4 to 6 hours.
    d. ORS should not be started until after all vomiting has stopped.

13. Johnny, age 13 months, is being admitted for parenteral fluid therapy because of excessive vomiting. Which of the following is most essential in implementing care for Johnny?
    a. Give Johnny oral fluids until the parenteral fluid therapy can be established.
    b. Question the physician's order for parenteral fluid therapy of 0.9% sodium chloride.
    c. Withhold the ordered potassium additive until Johnny's renal function has been verified.
    d. Replace half of Johnny's estimated fluid deficit over the first 24 hours of parenteral fluid therapy.

14. Rapid fluid replacement is contraindicated in dehydration that is:
    a. isotonic.
    b. hypotonic.
    c. hypertonic.

15. Water intoxication can occur in children from:
    i. excessive intake of electrolyte-free formula.
    ii. administration of inappropriate hypotonic solutions.
    iii. dilution of formula with water.
    iv. isotonic dehydration.
    v. vigorous hydration with water following a febrile illness.
    vi. fluid shifts from intracellular to extracellular spaces.

    a. i, ii, iii, and iv
    b. i, ii, iii, and v
    c. ii, iii, and iv
    d. ii, iii, v, and vi

16. Severe generalized edema in all body tissues is called _____.

17. Edema formation can be caused by:
    a. Decreased venous pressure
    b. Alteration in capillary permeability
    c. Increased plasma proteins
    d. Increased tissue tension

18. How does the nurse assess for pitting edema?
    a. Measure abdominal girth.
    b. Observe for fluid retention in the lower extremities.
    c. Press fingertip against bony prominence for 5 seconds.
    d. Observe for loss of normal skin creases.

19. Match each term with its description.

    a. Respiratory acidosis   c. Metabolic acidosis
    b. Respiratory alkalosis   d. Metabolic alkalosis

    _____ Occurs when there is a reduction of hydrogen ion concentration or an excess of base bicarbonate

    _____ Caused by any process that reduces base bicarbonate concentration or increases metabolic acid formation

    _____ Results from factors that depress the respiratory center, factors that affect the lung, and factors that interfere with the bellows action of the chest wall

    _____ Results primarily from central nervous system stimulation

20. Which of the following results does the nurse recognize as respiratory acidosis (partially compensated)?
    a. Increased plasma pH, decreased plasma P_{CO_2}, decreased plasma HCO_3^-
    b. Decreased plasma pH, increased plasma P_{CO_2}, increased plasma HCO_3^-
    c. Decreased plasma pH, decreased plasma P_{CO_2}, decreased plasma HCO_3^-
    d. Increased plasma pH, increased plasma P_{CO_2}, increased plasma HCO_3^-

21. To obtain relevant information from the parents of a child with fluid and electrolyte disturbances, the nurse should question the parents about:
    a. the type and amount of the child's intake and output.
    b. the child's general appearance.
    c. the child's weight over the past month.
    d. whether they have taken the child's temperature within the past 24 hours.

22. In measuring intake and output, the nurse often has to weigh the diaper. As a rule, what is the wet diaper weight equivalent to in milliliters of urine?

23. Which symptoms would the nurse expect in a child with hypocalcemia?
    a. Abdominal cramps, oliguria
    b. Muscle cramps, neuromuscular irritability, tetany
    c. Thirst, low urine specific gravity
    d. Flushed, mottled extremities and weight gain

24. Joan, age 3 years, is admitted for fluid and electrolyte disturbances. The nurse's assessment should include:
    i. general appearance observation.
    ii. vital signs.
    iii. intake and output measurements.
    iv. daily weights.
    v. review of laboratory results.

    a. i, ii, iii, and iv
    b. ii, iii, and iv
    c. iii, iv, and v
    d. i, ii, iii, iv, and v

25. Johnny, age 2, is seen with moderate dehydration from diarrhea. What would you expect to be the recommendation for oral rehydration therapy (ORT)?

26. The American Academy of Pediatrics no longer advises withholding food and fluids for 24 hours after the onset of diarrhea or administering the BRAT diet (bananas, rice, applesauce, and tea or toast).
    a. True
    b. False

27. Billy, age 3 years, has just been ordered to take nothing by mouth (NPO). To prevent intake of fluids, the nurse should:
    a. place an NPO sign over his bed and remove fluids from the bedside.
    b. place him in a private room away from other children.
    c. apply an elbow restraint jacket to keep Billy from being able to drink by himself.
    d. provide ice chips every 30 minutes.

28. In starting an IV infusion in most children, the nurse recognizes the care plan should include:
    a. Interruptions during the procedure are kept to a minimum.
    b. Use of a 20-gauge over-the-needle catheter is preferred.
    c. Allow the child to handle the equipment before the procedure.
    d. Before the procedure begins, prepare the IV fluid and tubing, set to deliver 20 drops/ml.

29. Identify the following statements as true or false.

    _____ Glucose 10% in water is a hypotonic solution.

    _____ One molecule of glucose has half the osmolality of one molecule of sodium chloride.

    _____ IV solutions given to infants and young children should contain at least 0.2% sodium chloride to prevent brain edema.

    _____ For IV infusion for children, an over-the-needle 24- to 22-gauge catheter may be used if therapy will last less than 5 days.

    _____ Pediatric patients receiving IV fluids via continuous infusion pumps need less monitoring.

    _____ The IV infusion must be monitored every 4 hours for proper infusion rate and for site assessment.

    _____ Chloraprep is approved for patients above the age of 2 months as a skin antisepsis before initiating a peripheral IV.

    _____ Over-the-needle safety catheters and the needleless system help prevent needlestick injuries.

    _____ Peripherally placed catheters are associated with fewer complications than centrally placed catheters.

    _____ When using safety catheters, the nurse reinserts the needle into the catheter after it is removed for inspection and before insertion.

    _____ When securing a peripheral IV line, the nurse should not immobilize the thumb because of the danger of development of contractures and limited movement.

    _____ The initial signs of phlebitis are always erythema and pain at the insertion site.

    _____ The peripheral lock should be flushed with saline before and after administration of medication.

    _____ Heavy cutaneous colonization of the insertion site is the single most important predictor of catheter-related infection with all types of short-term, percutaneously inserted catheters.

    _____ IV infusion for children is given with an apparatus that delivers a microdrop factor of 60 drops/min and contains a calibrated volume control chamber.

    _____ The IV pump's occlusion alarm is completely reliable for detecting infiltration.

30. What are intraosseous infusions, and when are they used?

31. The nurse has orders to start an IV infusion in 4-year-old Martha. Which of the following does the nurse include in the plan?
    a. Gather supplies in Martha's room so that she will not have to be moved after the procedure.
    b. Gather supplies in the treatment room, because this is not a "safe place" for Martha.
    c. Realize that Martha will need to be restrained before the procedure begins.
    d. Start at the proximal site of the vein and move to a more distal site if the first attempt fails.

32. What nursing action should be included in the care plan for 10-year-old Debbie, who requires IV fluid therapy?
    a. Position the extremity in a natural anatomic position, with the fingers and thumb immobilized.
    b. Use an Ace bandage and completely encircle the extremity with tape to secure the IV line, insertion site, and extremity.
    c. Allow Debbie to help select the IV site.
    d. For the IV placement, use Debbie's dominant hand or the same extremity where her identification bracelet is located.

33. The nurse is starting a peripheral IV infusion in the scalp of 6-month-old Bennett. Which of the following is correct?
    a. This site should be used only when attempts at other sites have failed.
    b. Shave the site of the scalp for IV insertion before the needle is placed.
    c. The needle should be inserted in the opposite direction of blood flow or toward the head.
    d. The occipital area of the scalp is the site of choice.

34. Which of the following is not correct when securing a peripheral IV line?
    a. The catheter hub is firmly secured at the puncture site with a transparent dressing.
    b. The IV House site protector is used over the site.
    c. The connector tubing or extension tubing is looped and placed under the protective cover.
    d. A plastic medicine cup is cut in half with edges taped and placed over the site and connector tubing.

35. The nurse is removing the peripheral IV line from 10-year-old Debbie. Which of the following strategies is correct for this procedure?
    a. Exert firm pressure at the IV site while removing the catheter.
    b. Turn off the IV pump after removal of the catheter.
    c. Allow Debbie to help remove the tape from the site.
    d. Cut the tape with bandage scissors to facilitate its removal on the lateral aspect (opposite to the thumb side) of the extremity.

36. Which of the following alerts the nurse to a potential problem in a child receiving IV fluids?
    a. Edema, blanching, and cool skin are evident at the IV insertion site.
    b. The IV tubing is not changed or replaced for 16 hours.
    c. Blood appears in the tubing when the IV bag is held below the IV site level.
    d. There is unrestricted flushing of the catheter.

37. The nurse has started a peripheral IV on 12-month-old Jessica. What should the nurse document about the IV insertion?

38. What should the nurse document about the IV fluid in Jessica's case (see question 37)?

39. The nurse has orders to discontinue Jessica's IV therapy after completion. What should be included in the charting?

40. An infiltration or extravasation is observed. The nurse should do all of the following except:
    a. stop the infusion immediately.
    b. remove the IV catheter immediately.
    c. elevate the extremity.
    d. notify the practitioner.

41. Joey, age 12 years, has developed phlebitis related to IV therapy. Identify the three causes of phlebitis, and describe the initial sign of phlebitis at the insertion site.

42. The nurse is starting an IV. Which of the following steps in insertion is least likely to prevent infection at the site?
    a. Wash hands before starting.
    b. Rigorously clean skin with povidone solution in a back-and-forth motion from the outside inward.
    c. Palpate the area for the vein before skin prep.
    d. Allow the antiseptic area to dry before insertion.

43. When IV infusion continues for several days, it is important to prevent infection.
    a. What is the time frame for changing the IV tubing and the solution administration set?

    b. What is the time frame for changing parenteral nutrition fluids?

    c. What is the time frame for changing pure intralipid infusions?

44. Match each device with its description or safety guideline. (A device may be used more than once.)

    a. Peripheral intermittent infusion device (peripheral lock)
    b. Short-term or nontunneled catheters (subclavian, femoral, jugular)
    c. Peripherally inserted central catheters
    d. Long-term central venous tunneled catheters and implanted ports

_____ Most contact sports prohibited while using this device (e.g., implanted infusion ports)

_____ Placed by specially trained nurses in the antecubital area using the median, cephalic, or basilic veins into superior vena cava.

_____ A chest radiograph taken to verify placement of the catheter tip before administration of medication or fluids; device used in acute care, intensive care, and emergency departments

_____ Used for infusion when extended access is necessary without the need for continuous fluid

_____ If catheter is threaded midline, total parenteral nutrition (TPN) is not administered because it irritates the vessel

_____ Implanted with patient under local or general anesthesia via small cut-down site

45. Describe the best technique of flushing any venous access device, peripheral or central.

46. Discuss ways to prevent catheter-related bloodstream infections.

47. The drug alteplase is:
   a. used to treat large thrombi formed by the central venous catheter rubbing against the vessel wall.
   b. used to prevent small thrombi at the tip of the catheter.
   c. a tissue plasminogen activator, which initiates fibrinolysis and clot dissolution, but is not used in children because of its safety profile.
   d. recognized as the common drug used to treat catheter-related thrombi occlusion in children.

48. A patient's central venous catheter is accidentally cut. Which of the following is the correct action for the nurse to take at this time?
   a. Apply pressure at the exit site on the skin.
   b. Use a padded clamp and clamp the catheter proximal to the exit site.
   c. Remove the catheter immediately to prevent blood loss.
   d. Order a repair kit for the catheter so that it can be saved and further surgery to replace the cut catheter can be avoided.

49. Which of the following discharge instructions is correct for the nurse to give to the parents of 14-year-old Edward, who has a central venous catheter?
   a. It is okay for Edward to continue being on the football team.
   b. Signs of localized infection are fever, chills, general malaise, and an ill appearance.
   c. If the catheter leaks, tape it above the leak and then clamp the catheter at the taped site.
   d. Edward will need to avoid tub baths and take only showers.

50. A patient's central venous catheter is accidentally removed. Where is pressure applied?
   a. Exit site on the skin
   b. Entry site to the vein

51. Jamie, age 12 years, is receiving parenteral hyperalimentation. Which of the following serum levels must be carefully monitored?
   a. White blood cell
   b. Calcium
   c. Bicarbonate
   d. Glucose

52. The practitioner has ordered cyclic TPN. The nurse understands that:
    a. the child will be off the machine at night.
    b. the child will have increased risk for TPN-induced liver damage.
    c. the child will be off the machine for a number of hours during the day.
    d. the child will have decreased blood glucose levels.

53. Which of the following is the most prevalent gastrointestinal complication associated with TPN administration in pediatric populations?
    a. Liver disease
    b. Pancreatitis
    c. Intestinal obstruction
    d. Peptic ulcers

54. Pediatric TPN has a higher concentration of calcium and phosphorus. Knowing this, the nurse watches closely for:
    a. increased infection rate at the site.
    b. solution precipitation.
    c. pneumothorax.
    d. cholecystitis.

55. Before the nurse initiates home TPN, what factors should be assessed?

CRITICAL THINKING—CASE STUDY

Jennifer, age 4 months, is admitted to the hospital because of dehydration caused by diarrhea. Her mother has been giving her electrolyte-free solutions for volume replacement. Parenteral fluids have been ordered for Jennifer.

56. What type of dehydration does Jennifer most likely have?
    a. Isotonic
    b. Hypertonic
    c. Hypotonic
    d. Water intoxication

57. Diarrhea most commonly causes:
    a. Respiratory acidosis
    b. Respiratory alkalosis
    c. Metabolic acidosis
    d. Metabolic alkalosis

58. Which of the following data about Jennifer should the nurse obtain during the admission history?
    a. Type and amount of food and fluid intake
    b. Urinary output amount or frequency
    c. Number and consistency of stools in the past 24 hours
    d. All of the above

59. Which of the following observations does the nurse recognize as the best indicator that Jennifer's dehydration is becoming more severe?
    a. Jennifer's cry is whining and low-pitched.
    b. Jennifer's activity level is increased.
    c. Jennifer's appetite is diminished.
    d. Jennifer is becoming more irritable and lethargic.

60. A priority goal in the management of acute diarrhea is:
    a. determining the cause of the diarrhea.
    b. preventing the spread of the infection.
    c. rehydrating the child.
    d. managing the fever associated with the diarrhea.

61. The nurse's most critical responsibility when administering IV fluids to Jennifer is to:
    a. prevent IV infiltration.
    b. ensure sterility.
    c. prevent cardiac overload.
    d. maintain the fluid at body temperature.

62. Tim is a 1-month-old infant admitted for uncontrolled vomiting. The nurse will observe Tim for signs of:
    a. alkalosis.
    b. acidosis.
    c. hypocalcemia.
    d. hemodilution.

63. An infant is to receive 500 ml of IV fluid per 24 hours. The drop factor of the microdropper is 60 gtts/ml. The nurse should regulate the IV to run at:
    a. 15 gtts/min.
    b. 60 gtts/min.
    c. 21 gtts/min.
    d. 27 gtts/min.

29 Conditions That Produce Fluid and Electrolyte Imbalance

1. Acute diarrhea:
   a. can be caused by celiac disease.
   b. can be related to hyperthyroidism.
   c. can be caused by viral, bacterial, and parasitic pathogens.
   d. is an increase in stool frequency and increased water content with a duration of more than 14 days.

2. Chronic diarrhea:
   a. can be caused by viral, bacterial, and parasitic pathogens.
   b. is an increase in stool frequency and increased water content with a duration of more than 14 days.
   c. is a leading cause of illness in children younger than 5 years of age.
   d. is often associated with upper respiratory or urinary tract infections.

3. What type of diarrhea occurs in the first few months of life, persists for longer than 2 weeks with no recognized pathogens, and is refractory to treatment?

4. Which of the following is most likely to cause acute diarrhea?
   a. Food allergy
   b. Malabsorption syndromes
   c. Parasitic infections
   d. Immunodeficiency

5. Which of the following is most likely to develop acute diarrhea?
   a. The 2-month-old infant who attends daycare each day
   b. The 18-month-old infant who stays at home each day with his mother
   c. The 6-year-old child who attends public school
   d. The 24-month-old infant with two older brothers, ages 5 years and 8 years

6. Identify the following statements as true or false.

   _____ Rotavirus is the most important cause of serious gastroenteritis among children and a significant nosocomial pathogen.

   _____ Acute diarrhea in children may be associated with respiratory tract infections, otitis media infections, and urinary tract infections.

   _____ Chronic nonspecific diarrhea, also known as "irritable colon of childhood" and "toddlers' diarrhea," is a common cause of chronic diarrhea in children 6 to 54 months of age.

   _____ Antibiotics are seldom associated with diarrhea in children because of their lower specific gravity.

   _____ *Clostridium difficile* produces a protective mechanism against diarrhea because it alters the intestinal flora, increasing absorption surfaces.

   _____ Infants are more susceptible to frequent and severe bouts of diarrhea because their immune system has not been exposed to many pathogens and has not acquired protective antibodies.

   _____ Continuing to feed breast milk to an infant during diarrhea illness results in reduced severity and duration of the illness.

7. Which of the following is not a serious and immediate physiologic disturbance associated with severe diarrheal disease?
   a. Dehydration
   b. Acid-base imbalance
   c. Circulatory status impairment
   d. Decreased growth rate

8. Johnny, age 2 years, is diagnosed with uncomplicated diarrhea with no signs of dehydration. Diagnostic evaluation should include:
   a. cultures of the stool.
   b. presence of associated symptoms.
   c. complete blood count.
   d. urine specific gravity.

9. Listed below are subjective and objective findings associated with diarrhea. For each finding, identify the suspected cause of diarrhea.

   a. _____ Administration of cefaclor for 1 month for recurrent ear infections

   b. _____ Neutrophils or red blood cells in the stool

   c. _____ Watery, explosive stools

   d. _____ Foul-smelling, greasy, bulky stools

   e. _____ High numbers of eosinophils in the stools

10. Which of the following laboratory values, often found in acute diarrhea with dehydration, will return to normal after hydration of the patient?
    a. Elevated hemoglobin, hematocrit, blood urea nitrogen (BUN), and creatinine
    b. Decreased hemoglobin, hematocrit, BUN, and creatinine
    c. Red blood cells in stool
    d. Decreased white blood cell count, decreased hemoglobin, elevated BUN, and creatinine

11. What are the four major goals in the management of acute diarrhea?

12. What is the most appropriate therapeutic management for rehydration of Jenny, age 8 months, who has been diagnosed with acute diarrhea and has evidence of mild dehydration?
    a. Beginning oral rehydration therapy of 40 to 50 ml/kg within 4 hours
    b. Restarting lactose-free formula
    c. Encouraging oral intake of clear fluids, such as fruit juices and gelatin
    d. Feeding the BRAT diet, which consists of bananas, rice, apples, and toast or tea

13. Drug therapy for acute infectious diarrhea in young children should include:
    a. bismuth subsalicylate (Kaopectate) administered until the diarrhea has stopped.
    b. continuation of antibiotics for the presence of *C. difficile*.
    c. administration of sedatives to decrease bowel motility.
    d. antibiotic therapy in patients with persistent disease.

14. Early reintroduction of nutrients (normal diet) in the patient with diarrhea:
    a. is delayed until after the diarrhea has stopped except in the case of breast-fed infants.
    b. has adverse effects and actually prolongs diarrhea.
    c. should be limited to formula-fed infants being given lactose-free formula.
    d. has no adverse effects, lessens the severity and duration of the illness, and improves weight gain when compared to gradual reintroduction of foods.

15. Which of the following dietary instructions given by the nurse to the parents of a pediatric patient with acute diarrhea without dehydration is correct?
    a. Follow the BRAT diet for the first 24 hours.
    b. Give clear fluid diet for the first 24 hours.
    c. Give fluids and a normal diet during diarrhea illness.
    d. Keep the patient NPO (nothing by mouth) until stool output slows.

16. Which of the following nursing interventions is not appropriate for 6-month-old Terry, who was admitted to the pediatric unit with acute diarrhea and vomiting?
    a. Ongoing assessment of Terry's intake and output and physical appearance
    b. Education of the parents about the necessity of administering oral rehydration solution
    c. Rectal temperatures at least every 4 hours to monitor fever elevations
    d. Gentle cleansing of perianal areas and application of protective topical ointments

17. Prevention measures for diarrhea in children include all of the following except:
    a. wash hands, utensils, and work area with hot, soapy water after contact with raw meat.
    b. proper disposal of soiled diapers.
    c. during travel to areas where water may be contaminated, allow the child to drink only bottled water from the container through a straw supplied from home.
    d. administration of vaccines and medications to prevent traveler's diarrhea before travel.

18. The major emphasis of nursing care for the vomiting infant or child is:
    a. determining prior treatments used for the vomiting.
    b. preventing the spread of the infection.
    c. managing the fever associated with the vomiting.
    d. observing and reporting vomiting behavior and associated symptoms.

19. Fill in the blanks to identify the type of shock described in each of the following statements.

    a. _____ shock follows a reduction in circulating blood volume, plasma volume, or extracellular fluid loss.

    b. _____ shock results from impaired cardiac muscle function, resulting in reduced cardiac output.

    c. _____ shock results from a vascular abnormality that produces maldistribution of blood supply throughout the body.

    d. _____ shock is characterized by a hypersensitivity reaction, causing massive vasodilation and capillary leak.

    e. _____ shock is characterized by decreased cardiac output and derangements in the peripheral circulation in response to a severe, overwhelming infection.

    f. _____ shock is characterized by massive vasodilation resulting from the loss of sympathetic nervous system tone, which can occur with spinal cord injuries.

20. The following terms are related to shock. Match each term with its description.

a. Compensated shock
b. Decompensated shock
c. Irreversible shock
d. Colloids
e. Acidosis

f. Isotonic crystalloid solution
g. Dopamine
h. Diuretics (e.g., furosemide [Lasix])
i. Hydrostatic edema
j. Permeable edema

_____ Improves cardiac output, circulation, and renal perfusion in the shock patient

_____ Condition that results from shock and may be corrected by sodium bicarbonate administration

_____ Normal saline or lactated Ringer solution

_____ Cardiovascular efficiency diminished; microcirculatory perfusion marginal despite compensatory adjustments; tissue hypoxia, metabolic acidosis, and impairment of organ systems function

_____ Occurs from elevation of pulmonary microvascular pressure as a result of left ventricular dysfunction

_____ Protein-containing fluids, often administered to children in shock; albumin

_____ Cause a reduction in ventricular filling pressures without changing cardiac output or heart rate, and promote sodium and water excretion by the kidneys in cases in which pulmonary congestion is a problem

_____ Condition in which vital organ function is maintained by intrinsic compensatory mechanism, and blood flow is usually normal or increased but generally uneven or maldistributed in the microcirculation

_____ Occurs when damage to alveolar cells and pulmonary capillary epithelium causes fluid to leak into the interstitial space, resulting in acute respiratory distress syndrome

_____ Condition in which actual damage to vital organs occurs and death ensues even if measurements return to normal with therapy

21. Clinical manifestations of pronounced tachycardia, narrowed pulse pressure, poor capillary filling, and increased confusion would suggest:
a. compensated shock.
b. decompensated shock.
c. irreversible shock.

22. The position of choice for the child in shock is:
a. Trendelenburg.
b. head-down with feet straight.
c. flat with the legs elevated.
d. semi-Fowler.

23. List the three major efforts in the treatment of shock.

24. Match each stage of septic shock with its characteristics.

a. Hyperdynamic stage
b. Normodynamic stage
c. Hypodynamic stage

_____ Progressive deterioration of cardiovascular function, hypothermia, cold extremities, weak pulses, and hypotension

_____ Warm, flushed skin with tachypnea, chills, fever, and normal urinary output

_____ Duration of only a few hours; cool skin, normal pulses and blood pressure, decreased urinary output, and depressed mental state

25. Which of the following describes the most common initial signs of anaphylaxis?
   a. Cutaneous signs and complaint of feeling warm
   b. Bronchiolar constriction with wheezing
   c. Vasodilation and hypotension
   d. Laryngeal edema and stridor

26. The sudden development of high fever, vomiting and diarrhea, profound hypotension, shock, oliguria, and an erythematous macular rash with subsequent desquamation are clinical signs of:
   a. anaphylaxis.
   b. irreversible shock.
   c. *C. difficile* infections.
   d. toxic shock syndrome.

27. What should be included in the teaching plan for adolescent females to prevent toxic shock syndrome associated with tampon use?

28. Name the five causes of burns.

29. Burn injury from child abuse is seen most often in children under 3 years of age and includes injury most often caused by _____ burns and _____ burns.

30. Identify the following statements as true or false.

   _____ Thirty percent of children suffering recurrent burn injury are eventually mortally injured.

   _____ Because electric current travels through the body on the path of least resistance, the area surrounding the long bones would be expected to experience the most damage.

   _____ An area of concern for electrical burns in the very young child is the possibility of the child chewing on electrical cords.

   _____ The physiologic responses, therapy, prognosis, and disposition of the injured child with burns are all directly related to the amount of tissue destroyed.

   _____ Children playing with matches or other ignition devices account for 1 in 10 residential fire deaths.

   _____ The severity of injury in chemical burns is related to the chemical agent and the duration of contact.

   _____ In general, the more intense the heat source and the longer the contact, the deeper the resulting burn injury.

   _____ Children younger than 2 years of age have significantly higher mortality rates than older children with burns of a similar magnitude.

31. The standard adult "rule of nines" cannot be used to determine the total body surface area of a burn in a child because:
   a. the child has different body proportions than the adult.
   b. the child has different fluid body weight than the adult.
   c. the child's trunk and arm proportions are larger than the adult's.
   d. as the infant grows, the percentage allotted for the head increases while the percentages for the arms decrease.

32. Brock, 12 years old, has burns involving the epidermis and part of the dermis. Blister and edema formation are present, and the burns are extremely sensitive to temperature changes, exposure to air, and light touch. Brock has:
    a. superficial first-degree burns.
    b. partial-thickness second-degree burns.
    c. full-thickness third-degree burns.
    d. fourth-degree burns.

33. The severity of burn injury is determined by:
    i. pain associated with the burn, measured on a scale of 1 to 10.
    ii. percentage of body surface area burned.
    iii. level of consciousness of the victim.
    iv. depth of the burn.
    v. vital sign measurements.

    a. i, ii, and iii
    b. i, ii, iii, and v
    c. i, iii, iv, and v
    d. ii and iv

34. The expected predominant symptom of a superficial burn is:
    a. pain.
    b. significant tissue damage.
    c. absence of protective functions of the skin.
    d. blister formation.

35. Which of the following pediatric patients is at higher risk for complications from burn injury?
    a. The 12-month-old infant who pulled a pan of hot water over on his chest
    b. The 12-month-old infant who is burned on his chest by gasoline
    c. The 9-month-old infant who is burned on the hands and feet with scalding water as a punishment
    d. The 12-year-old child who is burned on one side of the face as a result of playing with cigarettes

36. Jordan, age 12 years, has suffered severe burns, and now his chest appears constricted. The nurse should prepare for:
    a. intubation.
    b. chest tube insertion.
    c. escharotomy.
    d. hydrotherapy.

37. Systemic response to thermal injury would include:
    a. hypoglycemia.
    b. increased capillary permeability.
    c. myoglobinuria.
    d. decreased metabolic rate.

38. Decrease in cardiac output in the postburn period is caused by:
    a. circulating myocardial depressant factor.
    b. fluid losses through denuded skin.
    c. vasodilation and increased capillary permeability.
    d. All of the above

39. In the first few days after a major thermal burn injury, the nurse observes oliguria. What is the most likely cause for this finding?
    a. Acute renal failure
    b. Inadequate fluid replacement
    c. BUN and creatinine elevations
    d. All of the above

40. The metabolic rate is affected in burn patients. Using knowledge about this systemic response, which of the following is correct?
    a. Blood glucose levels may be elevated because of insulin resistance.
    b. Temperature may be elevated even in absence of infection.
    c. Medications may be used to help restore muscle mass, increase weight gain, and promote wound healing.
    d. All of the above.

41. Thermally injured children have an immediate threat to life related to _____
    _____ and _____ During healing,
    _____ is the primary complication.

42. Systemic responses to severe burns may include:
    i. blood flow decreases to the gastrointestinal system by one third even though cardiac output is maintained by resuscitation fluids.
    ii. adrenal activity decrease.
    iii. hematocrit decrease.
    iv. loss of circulating red blood cells.
    v. metabolic acidosis.

    a. ii, iii, and iv
    b. i, iv, and v
    c. i, iii, and v
    d. ii and iv

43. A common cause of respiratory failure in the pediatric population after severe burns is:
    a. bacterial pneumonia.
    b. pneumothorax.
    c. pulmonary edema.
    d. restriction of chest wall as a result of edema and inelastic eschar formation.

44. A gram-negative organism that is commonly found on the burn wound surface on the third day after burn and is responsible for wound sepsis is:
    a. *Staphylococcus aureus.*
    b. *Pseudomonas aeruginosa.*
    c. group B streptococci.
    d. *Haemophilus influenzae.*

45. What should be included in the plan for emergency care of the burned child?
    a. Apply large amounts of cold water over denuded areas.
    b. Apply ointments to the burned area.
    c. Remove jewelry and metal.
    d. Apply neutralizing agents to the skin of chemical burn areas.

46. Bobby, age 2 years, has suffered a minor burn injury. Expected management would include:
    a. redressing the wound with a gauze dressing every 5 days.
    b. soaking stuck dressings in hydrogen peroxide before removal.
    c. watching wound margins for redness, edema, or purulent drainage.
    d. administering narcotics for pain.

47. In major burn injuries of children weighing less than 30 kg (66 lb), adequate fluid replacement during the emergent phase is best assessed by:
    a. urinary output of 30 ml/hr.
    b. urinary output of 1 to 2 ml/kg/hr.
    c. increasing hematocrit.
    d. normal blood pressure.

48. To maintain adequate nutrition and promote healing in the child with a major burn injury, the nurse would recommend a:
    a. diet high in proteins and calories.
    b. diet high in calories and low in proteins.
    c. diet high in fats and carbohydrates.
    d. diet high in vitamins A and D.

49. Johnny, age 8 years, suffered partial-thickness second-degree burns of his chest, abdomen, and upper legs while on a recent camping trip. He is scheduled for hydrotherapy each morning for 20 minutes followed by débridement. The best nursing action to assist Johnny at this time is to:
    a. ensure that pain medication is given before treatment.
    b. hold Johnny's breakfast until he returns from treatment.
    c. offer sedation after the procedure to promote rest.
    d. reassure Johnny that hydrotherapy and débridement are not painful.

50. Which of the following is a temporary graft obtained from human cadavers and used in burn treatment?
    a. Allograft
    b. Xenograft
    c. Autograft
    d. Isograft

51. Topical antimicrobial agents in burn therapy:
    a. eliminate organisms from the wound.
    b. do not eliminate organisms from the wound but can effectively inhibit bacterial growth.
    c. are not used because they encourage strains of resistant bacteria.
    d. are used on full-thickness wounds.

52. In caring for the donor site following split-thickness skin graft, the nurse expects:
    a. the dressing to be changed daily.
    b. the dressing not to be changed for 10 to 14 days.
    c. the area to be washed daily with soap and water.
    d. the application of an antibiotic ointment daily.

53. Which of the following statements about Integra, an artificial skin used in burn treatment, is correct?
    a. It is applied only to full-thickness burns.
    b. The second layer is pulled off after the dermis is formed.
    c. It replaces the need for additional skin grafting.
    d. It prepares the burn wound to accept an ultrathin autograft.

54. Prevention of burn injury in children includes education of parents and caregivers. Which of the following is not included in the educational program?
    a. Importance of adequate supervision and establishment of safe play area in the home
    b. Teaching children at an early age how to "stop, drop, and roll" to extinguish a fire
    c. Placing microwave ovens higher than children's faces
    d. Setting hot water heater thermostats no higher than 54° C (130° F)

CRITICAL THINKING—CASE STUDY

Kenny, age 5 years, is brought to the emergency department after his clothes caught on fire while he was playing with matches in the family garage. He has partial-thickness second-degree burns and full-thickness third-degree burns on his anterior chest, anterior abdomen, upper right arm, both shoulders, and right hand. Singed nasal hair is evident on physical examination, and some minor burns are apparent on his face. A Foley catheter is inserted, and a small amount of clear urine is obtained. Two IV routes are established for fluid replacement.

55. In conducting the physical examination of Kenny's burns, the nurse calculates the extent of body surface area involvement. How would the nurse best assess whether circulation to the area is intact?
    a. Touch the area to see whether Kenny feels pain.
    b. Test injured surfaces for blanching and capillary refill.
    c. Inspect the burns for eschar formation.
    d. Watch for edema of the affected part.

56. Based on the information given, the nurse should be careful to watch Kenny for immediate signs of:
    a. inhalation injury.
    b. facial deformities.
    c. sepsis.
    d. renal failure related to formation of myoglobin.

57. During the acute phase of Kenny's burn management, the nursing plan indicates a need to administer pain medication by the IV route rather than by the intramuscular route. What is the rationale for this decision?
    a. Relieves pain more effectively
    b. Bypasses the impaired peripheral circulation
    c. Prevents further damage to sensitive tissue
    d. Reduces the risk for skin irritation and infection

58. Kenny has normal bowel sounds 24 hours after admission and is placed on a high-calorie, high-protein diet, of which he eats very little. Kenny's hydrotherapy is scheduled right after breakfast and before supper. Which of the following interventions by the nurse would most likely increase Kenny's dietary intake?
    a. Show Kenny a feeding tube and explain to him that if he does not eat more, the tube will need to be inserted.
    b. Maintain the current meal schedule and stay with Kenny until he eats all of his meal.
    c. Rearrange his meal and hydrotherapy schedule to prevent conflicts.
    d. Insist that Kenny stop snacking between meals.

59. Considering the extent and distribution of Kenny's burns, which of the following nursing diagnoses would be recognized as the highest priority for Kenny during the management phase of his illness?
    a. Impaired Gas Exchange related to inhalation injury
    b. High Risk for Altered Nutrition: Less Than Body Requirements related to loss of appetite
    c. Fluid Volume Deficit related to edema associated with burn injury
    d. High Risk for Infection related to denuded skin, presence of pathogenic organisms, and altered immune response

60. Kenny has progressed well with skin grafts and healing and is now ready for discharge. The nurse will know that Kenny's parents understand discharge instructions if they state:
    a. "Kenny will only need to wear this elastic support bandage for 1 month."
    b. "Kenny will not be able to participate in any sports until the grafts have taken hold firmly."
    c. "We will visit the teacher and Kenny's peers before Kenny returns to school to prepare them for his appearance."
    d. "We will need to protect Kenny from normal activities until he requires no further surgery."

61. Harry, age 2 years, is being admitted for a 5-day history of acute diarrhea. As the admitting nurse, what history should you include related to this chief complaint?

The Child with Renal Dysfunction

1. Identify the following statements as true or false.

_____ The primary responsibility of the kidney is to maintain the composition and volume of body fluids in excess of body needs.

_____ The kidney functions in the production of erythropoietin and thus in the formation of red blood cells.

_____ Renin is secreted by the kidney in response to reduced blood volume, decreased blood pressure, or increased secretion of catecholamines.

_____ Approximately half of the total cardiac output makes up the blood flow to the kidneys.

_____ Protein is a normal finding in urine because it is too large a molecule to be reabsorbed in the proximal tubule.

_____ Glucose is reabsorbed in the proximal tubule and returned directly to the blood.

_____ Because there is a limit to the concentration gradient against which sodium can be transported out, when larger than normal amounts of sodium remain in the tubules, water is obliged to remain with the sodium.

_____ An end product of protein metabolism is urea.

_____ The newborn is unable to dispose of excess water and solute rapidly or efficiently because glomerular filtration and absorption do not reach adult values until the child is between 1 and 2 years of age.

_____ The loop of Henle, the site of urine-concentrating mechanism, is short in the newborn, thus reducing the ability to reabsorb sodium and water and produce concentrated urine.

_____ Newborn infants are unable to excrete a water load at rates similar to those of older persons.

_____ *Escherichia coli* is responsible for 80% of urinary tract infections.

_____ Extrinsic factors that can cause functional bladder neck obstruction and contribute to urinary stasis are pregnancy and chronic and intermittent constipation.

_____ Research studies conducted on cranberry products have proven their effectiveness in prevention of urinary tract infections.

_____ Renal or bladder ultrasound is an invasive procedure that allows visualization of renal pelvis.

2. What are the three factors that must function normally for urinary continence to be achieved and maintained?

3. Jordan is a 2-year-old who has had a clean-catch urinalysis done as part of a diagnostic work-up. The results of Jordan's urinalysis are listed below. Identify whether each result is normal (mark with an N) or abnormal (mark with an A).

_____ +1 glucose

_____ Specific gravity 1.020

_____ RBC 3-4

_____ WBC greater than 10

_____ Occasional casts

_____ Negative protein

_____ Positive nitrites

4. Match each term with its description.

a. Bacteriuria
b. Efflux
c. Reflux
d. Glomerular filtration rate
e. Creatinine
f. Cystitis
g. Urethritis
h. Pyelonephritis
i. Urosepsis

j. Vesicoureteral reflux
k. Azotemia
l. Chronic renal function
m. Uremia
n. Hemodialysis
o. Peritoneal dialysis
p. Hemofiltration
q. Anasarca

_____ Backward flow of urine

_____ Inflammation of the bladder

_____ Inflammation of the upper urinary tract and kidneys

_____ Retrograde flow of bladder urine into the ureters

_____ Accumulation of nitrogenous waste within the blood, resulting in elevated blood urea nitrogen (BUN) and creatinine levels.

_____ Forward movement of urine from the kidney to the bladder

_____ Measure of the amount of plasma from which a substance is cleared in 1 minute

_____ Febrile urinary tract infection coexisting with systemic signs of bacterial illness; blood culture reveals presence of urinary pathogen

_____ An end product of protein metabolism in muscle

_____ Inflammation of the urethra

_____ Presence of bacteria in the urine

_____ Toxic symptoms caused by retention of nitrogenous products in the blood

_____ Begins when the diseased kidneys can no longer maintain the normal chemical structure of body fluids under normal conditions

_____ Condition in which the abdominal cavity acts as a semipermeable membrane through which water and solutes of small molecular size move by osmosis and diffusion according to their respective concentrations

_____ Process by which blood is circulated outside the body through artificial cellophane membranes that permit a similar passage of water and solutes

_____ Process by which blood filtrate is circulated outside the body by hydrostatic pressure exerted across a semipermeable membrane and replaced simultaneously by electrolyte solution

_____ Severe generalized edema

5. The nurse, in preparing the child for a diagnostic test, explains that which one of the following tests provides direct visualization of the bladder through a small scope?
a. Cystoscopy
b. Voiding cystourethrogram
c. Intravenous pyelogram
d. Renal biopsy

6. Preprocedural preparation of the child who is scheduled to have a cystourethrography includes:
a. keeping the child NPO (nothing by mouth) for 8 hours before the test.
b. assessing for an allergy to iodine.
c. administering a Fleet enema before the examination.
d. preparing the child for catheterization.

7. For children with renal conditions, the most significant ongoing assessments conducted by the nurse are:
   a. weight, intake and output, and blood pressure.
   b. intake and output, height, and weight.
   c. weight, temperature, and creatinine clearance.
   d. daily urinalysis, weight, and output.

8. Which of the following does not predispose the patient to urinary tract infections?
   a. The short urethra in the young girl
   b. Urinary stasis
   c. Urinary reflux
   d. Lowering of urine pH

9. Symptoms of urinary tract infection often observed in children over age 2 years include:
   i. incontinence in a child previously toilet trained.
   ii. abdominal pain.
   iii. strong or foul odor to the urine.
   iv. frequency of urination.
   v. diarrhea.

   a. i, ii, and iii
   b. iii and iv
   c. iii, iv, and v
   d. i, ii, iii, and iv

10. Three-year-old Ivy is brought to the clinic because of a suspected urinary tract infection. Which of the following is the correct method for collecting the urine specimen?
    a. Encourage large amounts of water because Ivy is unable to void at this time.
    b. Set Ivy on the toilet facing the tank to decrease likelihood of contamination.
    c. Wait until the first morning voided specimen can be collected.
    d. Bag Ivy with the bag covering the entire peritoneal area.

11. The treatment objectives for children with urinary tract infections include:

    a.

    b.

    c.

    d.

12. Which symptom suggests pyelonephritis in a 3-year-old child?
    a. Flank pain and tenderness
    b. Foul-smelling urine
    c. Dysuria or urgency
    d. Enuresis or daytime incontinence

13. The nurse is asked to obtain a urine specimen from 5-year-old Anne. Which of the following is the correct procedure?
    a. Place a urine bag on Anne to collect the next specimen.
    b. Obtain a catheterized specimen.
    c. Encourage Anne to drink large volumes of water in an attempt to obtain a specimen.
    d. Obtain a midstream specimen, preferably the first morning specimen.

14. Justin, age 8 years, has been diagnosed with pyelonephritis. The nurse would expect medical management to include:
    a. administration of oral nitrofurantoin.
    b. admission to the hospital with intravenous antibiotics administered for the first 24 hours.
    c. radiographic evaluation before antibiotic therapy.
    d. urine cultures repeated every month for 3 months.

15. Common antiinfective agents used for urinary tract infections in children include all of the following except:
    a. quinolones.
    b. penicillins.
    c. sulfonamides.
    d. cephalosporins.

16. The nurse is developing a preventive teaching plan for Tracy, a sexually active 16-year-old who has been diagnosed with a urinary tract infection. Which of the following should be included in the plan?
    a. Promote perineal hygiene by wiping back to front.
    b. Urinate as soon as possible after intercourse.
    c. Douche as soon as possible after intercourse to flush out bacteria.
    d. Eliminate all carbonated and caffeinated beverages because they irritate the bladder.

17. Vesicoureteral reflux (VUR) is closely associated with:
    a. acute glomerulonephritis.
    b. nephrotic syndrome.
    c. renal scarring and kidney damage.
    d. high alkaline content in the urine.

18. A minimally invasive endoscopy option called *subtrigonal injection* (STING) is available to treat children with less severe VUR. Describe this procedure, and explain why it is an attractive alternative to other treatment options.

19. Acute poststreptococcal glomerulonephritis (APSGN):
    i. is the least common of the noninfectious renal diseases in children.
    ii. can occur at any age but primarily affects school-age children, the peak age of onset being 6 to 7 years.
    iii. is an immune complex disease related to a reaction that occurs as a by-product from certain strains of group A β-hemolytic streptococcus.
    iv. follows a latent period of 10 to 14 days between the infection of the throat or skin and the onset of symptoms for APSGN.
    v. most commonly occurs in fall and spring.

    a. i, ii, iii, iv, and v
    b. ii, iii, and iv
    c. i, iii, and iv
    d. ii, iii, and v

20. Which of the following clinical manifestations are associated with acute glomerulonephritis?
    a. Normal blood pressure, generalized edema, oliguria
    b. Periorbital edema, hypertension, dark-colored urine
    c. Fatigue, elevated serum lipid levels, elevated serum protein levels
    d. Temperature elevation, circulatory congestion, normal BUN and creatinine serum levels

21. The major complications that may develop during the acute phase of glomerulonephritis are:

22. Nursing interventions in caring for the child with acute glomerulonephritis include:
    a. enforced bed rest.
    b. daily weights.
    c. keeping the child NPO.
    d. high-sodium diet.

23. Chronic glomerulonephritis (CGN) describes a variety of different disease processes that may be distinguished from one another by:
    a. renal biopsy.
    b. cystoscopy.
    c. blood cultures.
    d. serologic tests, including ASO titers.

24. Which of the following diagnostic findings would suggest failing renal function?
    a. Decreased creatinine and elevated BUN
    b. Elevated BUN, creatinine, and uric acid levels
    c. Elevated potassium, phosphorus, and calcium
    d. Proteinuria and decreased creatinine and BUN

25. Clinical manifestations of nephrotic syndrome include:
    a. hyperlipidemia, hypoalbuminemia, edema, and proteinuria.
    b. hematuria, hypertension, periorbital edema, and flank pain.
    c. oliguria, hypolipidemia, and hyperalbuminemia.
    d. hematuria, generalized edema, hypertension, and proteinuria.

26. Which child is most at risk for minimal-change nephrotic syndrome?
    a. A 4-year-old recovering from viral upper respiratory tract infection
    b. A 7-year-old after a group A β-hemolytic streptococcus throat infection
    c. A 6-year-old with acquired immunodeficiency syndrome (AIDS)
    d. A 2-year-old who recently received several bee stings

27. The diet requirement for minimal-change nephrotic syndrome includes:
    a. water restriction.
    b. low-protein diet during both acute and remission stages.
    c. salt restriction during periods of edema.
    d. high-protein diet during both acute and remission stages.

28. Therapeutic management in nephrotic syndrome includes the administration of prednisone. Which of the following is a correct administration guideline?
    a. Corticosteroid therapy is begun after BUN and serum creatinine elevation.
    b. Prednisone is administered orally once daily for 3 weeks.
    c. The drug is given daily for 6 weeks, then decreased on alternate days for 6 more weeks.
    d. The drug is discontinued as soon as the urine is free from protein.

29. Drug side effects associated with cyclophosphamide (Cytoxan) are:
    i. leukopenia.
    ii. azoospermia.
    iii. effects on gonadal function in females.
    iv. hypertension.
    v. cognitive impairment.

    a. i, ii, and iii
    b. i, iv, and v
    c. ii, iii, and v
    d. i, ii, iii, iv, and v

30. Which of the following urine tests is conducted daily while the child is receiving medicine for nephrotic syndrome?
    a. Glucose
    b. Specific gravity
    c. Albumin
    d. pH

31. Identify the following statements as true or false.

    _____ Renal tubular disorders are seen with clinical manifestations of edema, hypertension, and elevated BUN levels.

    _____ Renal tubular acidosis is caused by impaired bicarbonate reabsorption in the proximal tubule.

    _____ Proximal tubular acidosis is caused by the inability of the kidney to establish a normal pH gradient between tubular cells and tubular contents.

    _____ Primary functions of the distal renal tubules are acidification of urine; potassium secretion; and selective and differential reabsorption of sodium, chloride, and water.

    _____ Treatment of both proximal and distal disorders consists of administration of sufficient bicarbonate or citrate to balance metabolically produced hydrogen ions and maintain the plasma bicarbonate level within normal range.

    _____ In nephrogenic diabetes insipidus, the distal tubules and collecting ducts are insensitive to the action of antidiuretic hormone and vasopressin.

    _____ Nephrogenic diabetes insipidus is associated with a Y-linked defect of the vasopressin receptor and appears in the newborn period with vomiting, fever, failure to thrive, dehydration, and hypernatremia.

    _____ Hemolytic uremic syndrome is characterized by acute renal failure, hemolytic anemia, and thrombocytopenia.

    _____ Alport syndrome is a condition of chronic hereditary nephritis, which consists of hematuria, high-frequency sensorineural deafness, ocular disorders, and chronic renal failure.

    _____ Transient proteinuria generally indicates renal disease.

32. Multiple cases of hemolytic uremic syndrome caused by enteric infection of the *E. coli* O157:H7 serotype have been traced to:
    i. undercooked meat, especially ground beef.
    ii. unpasteurized apple juice.
    iii. alfalfa sprouts.
    iv. public pools.
    v. unwashed grapes.

    a. i, iv, and v
    b. i and ii
    c. i, ii, iii, and iv
    d. ii, iii, and v

33. Diagnostic evaluation results for hemolytic uremic syndrome include:
    a. Proteinuria, hematuria, urinary cast, elevated BUN and serum creatinine, low hemoglobin and hematocrit, and a high reticulocyte count
    b. High potassium, low sodium, high hemoglobin and hematocrit, and proteinuria
    c. High number of urinary casts, low serum BUN and creatinine, and decreased sedimentary rates
    d. Urine negative for protein but positive for red blood cells, normal hemoglobin and hematocrit, and elevated serum BUN and creatinine

34. In evaluation of the child with possible renal trauma, which of the following are usually indicative of kidney damage?
    a. Flank pain and hematuria
    b. Dysuria, proteinuria, and nausea
    c. Abdominal ascites, nausea, and hematuria
    d. Proteinuria and bladder spasms

35. What is the most common cause of prerenal failure in infants and children?
    a. Nephrotoxic agents
    b. Obstructive uropathy
    c. Dehydration related to diarrhea and vomiting
    d. Burn shock

36. The primary manifestation of acute renal failure is:
    a. edema.
    b. oliguria.
    c. metabolic acidosis.
    d. weight gain and proteinuria.

37. The most immediate threat to the life of the child with acute renal failure is:
    a. hyperkalemia.
    b. anemia.
    c. hypertension crisis.
    d. cardiac failure from hypovolemia.

38. Which drug therapy is used in the removal of potassium from the body?
    a. Mannitol
    b. Sodium bicarbonate
    c. Kayexalate
    d. Calcium gluconate

39. The major nursing task in the care of the infant or child with acute renal failure is:

40. Which of the following manifestations of chronic renal failure can have the most social consequences for the developing child?
    a. Anemia
    b. Growth retardation
    c. Bone demineralization
    d. Septicemia

41. Dietary regulation in the child with chronic renal failure includes:
    a. increasing dietary phosphorus.
    b. providing protein of high biologic value in the diet.
    c. restricting potassium when creatinine clearance falls below 50 ml/min.
    d. adding vitamin A, E, and K supplements.

42. The treatment for the pediatric patient with anemia related to chronic renal failure includes all of the following except:
    a. ferrous sulfate supplements.
    b. ascorbic acid supplements.
    c. vitamin B_{12} supplements.
    d. administration of erythropoietin.

43. Bobby, age 12 years, was diagnosed with chronic renal failure at the age of 6 years. He has reached end-stage renal failure. Which of the following nursing care management interventions should not be included in Bobby's care plan?
    a. Assist Bobby in adjusting to the fact that he will always be different from his peers. He will be shorter, more tired at times, and unable to participate in all activities.
    b. Prepare Bobby for acceptance of the need for dialysis.
    c. Explain to Bobby that he will no longer be able to go to school.
    d. Assist the parents in exploring the financial drain the disease will have on the family resources and provide information on assistance that is available.

44. Fill in the blanks in the following statements as they relate to dialysis for renal care.

    a. Methods of dialysis for management of renal failure are _____, _____

       _____, and _____.

    b. _____ is the preferred method for treating children with life-threatening hyperkalemia.

    c. In peritoneal dialysis, _____ _____ is greater than with hemodialysis.

    d. _____ is not recommended for small children because of the rapid changes in blood volume and systemic blood pressure and the difficulty of placing vascular access devices.

    e. The major complication associated with peritoneal dialysis is _____.

    f. The nurse can expect to see the child undergoing dialysis to have improved _____ _____

       and _____ _____ but not to recover to _____ _____.

    g. Continuous venovenous hemofiltration (CVVH) is an ideal form of dialysis for children with _____

       _____ from _____ _____.

45. Amy, age 14 years, is scheduled to receive hemodialysis. She will need to have a vein and artery surgically connected for blood access. Which of the following is the correct name for this type of blood access?
    a. Graft
    b. Fistula
    c. Percutaneous catheter

46. Johnny, age 12, had a renal transplant 5 months ago. He now comes to the hospital outpatient clinic with fever, tenderness over the graft area, decreased urinary output, and slightly elevated blood pressure. The nurse's priority at this time is:
    a. to recognize that Johnny is probably undergoing acute rejection and to notify the physician immediately.
    b. to recognize that this is an episode of increased inflammation within the donor kidney because Johnny has probably been noncompliant with his immunosuppressant drugs. The nurse should educate Johnny regarding drug compliance and notify Johnny's physician when he makes rounds.
    c. to obtain a urine specimen for culture and sensitivity and a blood count to quickly identify Johnny's infection before alerting the physician.
    d. to recognize that Johnny is in chronic rejection and that no present therapy can halt the progressive process.

47. An immunosuppression drug used to prevent kidney transplant rejection is cyclosporine. Which of the following can be a side effect of this drug?
    a. Cataracts
    b. Linear growth decline
    c. Gastric ulcer
    d. Hypertension

CRITICAL THINKING—CASE STUDY

Dean, age 3 years, is brought to the clinic by his mother. He has a history of a recent fever of 37.8 ° C (100.2 ° F), sore throat, and slight cough approximately 8 days ago that lasted about 3 days. Yesterday morning Dean's mother noticed "puffiness around his eyes" when he got up and then "swelling of his lower legs and scrotal area." Dean's appetite and activity level have decreased. This morning Dean's mother noticed that his urine was "darker in color" and "seemed to be less than usual." Physical examination of Dean reflects a child who does not appear acutely ill but who is irritable and seems fatigued, with pale skin color. His blood pressure, pulse, and temperature are within normal limits. He has generalized edema. Laboratory findings of Dean's urine specimen include large amounts of protein and microscopic hematuria. Serum protein levels are very low with elevated lipid levels.

48. Based on the information given, which of the following conditions should be suspected?
    a. Acute poststreptococcal glomerulonephritis
    b. Minimal-change nephrotic syndrome
    c. Acute renal failure
    d. Hemolytic uremic syndrome

49. Dean is diagnosed by the health care provider as having nephrotic syndrome. Identify goals for restoring renal function in Dean.
    i. Urine is protein free.
    ii. Edema is resolved.
    iii. Fluid and electrolyte balance are restored.
    iv. Nutritional needs have returned to a state of positive nitrogen balance.

    a. i, ii, and iii
    b. i, ii, and iv
    c. ii and iii
    d. i, ii, iii, and iv

50. Which of the following nursing diagnoses is of least benefit in planning for Dean's care?
    a. Impaired Skin Integrity related to edema, lowered body defenses
    b. Altered Nutrition: Less Than Body Requirements related to decreased appetite
    c. Altered Patterns of Elimination related to obstruction
    d. Fluid Volume Excess related to fluid accumulation in tissues and third space

51. Which nursing intervention is appropriate for Dean's nursing diagnosis of Impaired Skin Integrity?
    a. Administer corticosteroids on time with careful monitoring for infections.
    b. Monitor for complications, strict intake and output, daily checks of urine for protein, daily weight, and abdominal girth.
    c. Enforce bed rest during the edema phase of the disease.
    d. Support scrotum on small pillow.

52. Dean has progressed well and is being discharged. What teaching interventions will be necessary to prepare the family for discharge?

53. Darlene, age 15 years, has been diagnosed with chronic renal failure. She is being discharged and will need peritoneal dialysis at home. Describe the teaching interventions the nurse would include in the discharge plan for Darlene.

54. The nurse has developed the nursing diagnosis of Altered Nutrition: Less Than Body Requirements related to the restricted diet based on Darlene's diagnosis of chronic renal failure. Discuss expected nursing interventions to be used with this nursing diagnosis.

55. BUN and serum creatinine are both blood tests for renal function. Which one, if elevated, would be the best indicator of renal dysfunction? Why?

31 The Child with Disturbance of Oxygen and Carbon Dioxide Exchange

1. The following terms are related to respiratory tract structure. Match each term with its description.

a. Respiratory tract
b. Thoracic cavity
c. Mediastinum
d. Parietal pleura
e. Visceral pleural sac
f. Pneumothorax
g. Pleural effusion
h. Hydrothorax
i. Hemothorax

j. Empyema
k. Barrel chest
l. Nasal structures
m. Upper airway
n. Pharynx
o. Larynx
p. Glottis
q. Epiglottis
r. Cricoid cartilage

s. Lower airway
t. Trachea
u. Carina
v. Bronchioles
w. Compliance
x. Generations
y. Alveoli
z. Septa
aa. Lung growth

_____ The disease state in which there is fluid in the space between the visceral and the parietal pleura

_____ Encased in the bony framework provided by the ribs, vertebrae, and sternum; consists of three major partitions: the three-lobed lung on the right, the two-lobed lung on the left, and the space between them—the mediastinum

_____ The disease state in which there is blood in the space between the visceral and the parietal pleura

_____ Consists of many complex structures with the primary responsibility to distribute air and exchange gases so that cells are supplied with oxygen while carbon dioxide is removed

_____ Structure that encases each lung by only enough fluid to lubricate the surface for painless movement during filling and emptying of the lungs

_____ Pyothorax; the disease state in which there is pus in the space between the visceral and the parietal pleura

_____ Adheres to the ribs and superior surface of the diaphragm

_____ The condition in severe obstructive lung disease in which the anteroposterior measurement approaches the transverse (side to side) measurement

_____ Contains the esophagus, trachea, large blood vessels, and the heart; located in the thoracic cavity between the right and left lungs

_____ Affected by numerous pathologic conditions, such as kyphoscoliosis, coxsackievirus, hormone level changes, and biochemical substances

_____ Rigid passageways for air that warm and moisten the air, filter impurities, and destroy microorganisms

_____ Composed of smooth muscle supported by C-shaped rings of cartilage; ensures an open airway

_____ Oronasopharynx, pharynx, larynx, and upper part of the trachea; shared by both the respiratory and alimentary tracts; dilates during inspiration; constricts during exhalation

_____ The branch levels of the bronchioles that are divided into the two categories: the conducting airways and the terminal respiratory units

_____ The dividing point of the trachea into two primary bronchi

_____ A passageway for the entry and exit of air; plays a role in phonation; helps to produce vowel sounds

_____ The disease state in which there is serum in the space between the visceral and the parietal pleura

_____ The process of elasticity of the lungs, which allows the lungs to expand and recoil; complemented by the concept of resistance, which affects the flow through the airways

_____ The part of the respiratory system one generation below the bronchi

_____ At the upper end of the trachea; constructed of a rigid circular framework of cartilage; contains the epiglottis and the glottis (vocal cords)

_____ The disease state in which there is air in the space between the visceral and the parietal pleura

_____ Airsacs; gas exchange occurs through these thin-walled sacs

_____ Vibrates to produce voice sounds; located closer to the head in infancy than in later childhood; very active reflexes in infancy

_____ Prevents solids or liquids from entering the airway during swallowing; is longer and projects further posteriorly in infants

_____ The term for the shared walls of the alveoli

_____ A structure located at the narrowest portion of the larynx

_____ Consists of the lower trachea, mainstem bronchi, segmental bronchi, subsegmental bronchioles, terminal bronchioles, and alveoli

2. The following terms are related to respiratory function. Match each term with its description.

a. Respiratory movements
b. Ventilation
c. Artificial ventilation
d. Positive pressure breathing devices
e. Negative pressure ventilator
f. Pneumotaxic center
g. Acid-base balance
h. Alveolar surface tension

i. Surfactant
j. Elastic recoil
k. Resistance
l. Partial pressures
m. Millimeters of mercury
n. Fraction of inspired air
o. Oxyhemoglobin
p. Oxyhemoglobin saturation

q. Oxyhemoglobin dissociation curve
r. Neural system
s. Chemical system
t. Neural control
u. Proprioceptive vagal impulses
v. Central chemoreceptors
w. Peripheral chemoreceptors

_____ One of the major factors determining compliance; lowered by surfactant

_____ The exchange of gases in the lungs; results from changes in pressure gradients created by changes in the size of the thoracic cavity

_____ A lipoprotein at the air-fluid interface that allows alveolar expansion and prevents alveolar collapse

_____ Based on the concept of air moving from higher pressure into the lungs, which have a lower pressure

_____ The tendency of the lungs to return to the resting state after inspiration; a major factor in determining compliance

_____ Fio_2; the term used for inspired oxygen; expressed as 1.0 for 100%, 0.21 for ambient air at 21%

_____ First evident at about 20 weeks of gestation when amniotic fluid is exchanged in alveoli

_____ Determined primarily by airway size; caused during breathing by the chest wall, lungs, and flow in the airways; determined by flow rate velocity, gas viscosity, length of the airway, and airway diameter

_____ The neutral center that modulates respiratory depth and frequency

_____ The oxygen that is carried by hemoglobin; a large portion of oxygen is transported throughout the body this way

_____ Artificial respiratory devices that increase the pressure entering the air passages

_____ Unit of measure used to express tensions; partial pressures of individual gases in the blood

_____ A process in which the lungs play an important role by acting as a chemical buffer; adjusts pH by eliminating or retaining Pco_2, acting within 1 to 3 minutes

_____ Units in which partial pressures are expressed

_____ Arterial oxygen saturation (Sao_2); hemoglobin saturation

_____ Located in a pneumotaxic center, apneustic center, and the medullary respiratory centers

_____ Artificial respiratory device that lowers the atmospheric pressure around the body

_____ Nerve cells located in the medulla that mediate respiratory changes by responding to changes in pH, P_{CO_2}, and P_{O_2}

_____ The nonlinear relationship between P_{aO_2} and S_{aO_2}

_____ Located in the great vessels (e.g., the carotid bodies); nerve cells that mediate respiratory changes by responding to changes in pH, P_{CO_2}, and P_{O_2}

_____ A signal that is generated by stretching of the lungs and is then transmitted to the respiratory center, which inhibits further inflation and prevents overdistention (e.g., the Hering-Breuer reflex); one of the categories that control respiration; maintains a coordinated, rhythmic respiratory cycle and regulates the depth of respiration

_____ Neurohumoral system that regulates alveolar ventilation and maintains normal blood gas pressure

_____ Maintains the coordinated rhythmic respiratory cycles and regulates the depth of respiration

3. The following terms are related to defenses of the respiratory tract. Match each term with its description.

a. Lymphoid tissues   d. Cough   g. Lymphatics
b. Mucous blanket   e. Tracheobronchial dynamics   h. Humoral defenses
c. Ciliary action   f. Position change

_____ Encourage drainage of tracheobronchial passages

_____ Tissues that localize and contain organisms to be destroyed by the humoral defense mechanisms

_____ The ability of the tracheobronchial tree to elongate and dilate on inspiration and shorten and narrow on expiration

_____ Remove invading organisms; drain the terminal bronchi

_____ Explosive force that propels foreign material out of the lower tract

_____ Epithelium that secretes a sticky mucus to which airborne organisms adhere

_____ Phagocytes, enzymes, and immunoglobulins secreted by the bronchial epithelium

_____ Keeps mucus flowing; carries microorganisms and other foreign agents away from the lungs to be coughed or swallowed

4. The following terms are related to physical assessment. Match each term with its description.

a. Auscultation   g. Nasal flaring   m. Parietal pleural pain
b. Palpation   h. Head bobbing   n. Diaphragmatic pleural irritation
c. Tachypnea   i. Noisy breathing   o. Clubbing
d. Hyperpnea   j. Grunting   p. Cough
e. Hypopnea   k. Skin color change   q. Percussion
f. Retractions   l. Chest pain

_____ An assessment technique that, along with palpation, provides information regarding areas of pain and tissue density

_____ Mottling, pallor, cyanosis; significant in the infant; suggests cardiopulmonary disease (except circulatory stasis or cyanosis from a cool environment)

_____ Respirations that are too deep

_____ Respirations that are too shallow

_____ May be a complaint of older children; may be caused by disease of any of the chest structures

_____ A sign of dyspnea in the infant who is sleeping or exhausted

_____ May be referred to the base of the neck posteriorly and anteriorly or to the abdomen

_____ An assessment technique that, along with percussion, provides information regarding areas of pain

_____ May be associated with disorders other than respiratory disease; serves as a protective mechanism; indicates irritation

_____ Sinking in of soft tissues relative to the cartilaginous and bony thorax; noted in some pulmonary disorders

_____ Physical assessment technique; helpful in identifying specific abnormalities and assessing response to treatment; used to determine airway patency

_____ Rapid ventilations; observed with anxiety, elevated temperature, severe anemia, and metabolic acidosis

_____ Significant finding in an infant; helps reduce resistance and maintain airway patency

_____ Proliferation of tissue at the terminal phalanges; associated with chronic hypoxia; does not reflect disease progression

_____ Frequently associated with hypertrophied adenoidal tissue, choanal obstruction, polyps, or foreign body in the nasal passages

_____ Usually localized over the affected area and aggravated by respiratory movement

_____ Frequently a sign of chest pain; suggests acute pneumonia, pleural involvement, pulmonary edema, or respiratory distress syndrome; increases end-respiratory pressure and prolongs gas exchange

5. The following terms are related to diagnostic procedures. Match each term with its description.

a. Pulse oximetry
b. Functional hemoglobin
c. Oxyhemoglobin
d. Deoxyhemoglobin
e. Transcutaneous monitoring
f. Arterial blood gas sampling
g. Allen test

_____ Performed to assess adequacy of collateral circulation

_____ Hemoglobin saturated with oxygen

_____ A noninvasive method of determining Sao_2

_____ A noninvasive method of continuously monitoring partial pressure of oxygen in arterial blood; may also be used to measure carbon dioxide

_____ Performed on blood from an artery or capillary

_____ Hemoglobin capable of carrying oxygen

_____ Hemoglobin that is not saturated with oxygen

6. The following terms are related to respiratory therapy. Match each term with its description.

a. Hypoxemia
b. Oxygen hood
c. Nasal cannula
d. Oxygen mask
e. Oxygen tent
f. Atelectasis
g. Oxygen-induced carbon dioxide narcosis
h. Hand-held nebulizer
i. Metered-dose inhaler
j. Spacer device
k. Rotahaler or Turbuhaler
l. Percussion
m. Vibration
n. Squeezing
o. Deep breathing
p. Breathing and postural exercises
q. Bag-valve-mask
r. High-frequency ventilation
s. Extracorporeal membrane oxygenation (ECMO)
t. Endotracheal airway
u. Speaking valves

_____ The method of oxygen administration used for older infants and children; consists of two small tubes inserted into the nares; sometimes called *prongs*

_____ A method of oxygen administration that may be used for children beyond early infancy; advantage—does not require any device to come into direct contact with the face; disadvantage—difficult to control concentration of oxygen within the device

_____ Reduced blood oxygenation

_____ A hazard of oxygen therapy; may occur in persons with chronic pulmonary disease; seldom encountered in children except those with cystic fibrosis

_____ A self-contained, hand-held device that allows for intermittent delivery of a specified amount of medication

_____ Occurs as a result of the washing out of nitrogen from the alveoli by the high concentrations of oxygen; more likely to occur in persons with low tidal volume and retention of secretions

_____ A method of aerosolizing a medication; consists of a mask that the child holds over the nose and mouth

_____ Examples: Passy-Muir, Kistner, and Tucker; not appropriate for use in seriously ill children, children using a tracheostomy cuff, or children with copious secretions

_____ Holding chamber to coordinate breathing and aerosol delivery

_____ A maneuver that is useful while the child is in the drainage position; increases the depth of the expiratory effort by brief, firm pressure from the practitioner's hands compressing the side of the chest

_____ Hand-operated self-inflating ventilation bag with a mask and a nonreturnable valve to prevent rebreathing

_____ Artificial airway that is most often used in association with artificial ventilation (e.g., nasotracheal, orotracheal, tracheostomy)

_____ Used to help move secretions toward the head during exhalation

_____ A new type of metered-dose inhaler that does not require a spacer device

_____ Technique encouraged when the child is relaxed and in the desired position of drainage; uses diaphragmatic breathing; may stimulate a cough; may be facilitated by incentive spirometers, blow bottles, and games that involve blowing

_____ A form of cardiopulmonary bypass; provides both pulmonary and cardiac support

_____ Techniques that are useful with older motivated children with kyphoscoliosis, cystic fibrosis, asthma, or bronchiectasis

_____ Provides information regarding tissue density; the most common technique used in association with postural drainage; accomplished by the practitioner gently striking the chest wall with a cupped hand

_____ The method of oxygen administration that is best tolerated by infants

_____ A generic term for devices that use a rapid cycling rate and deliver small tidal volumes with each cycle

_____ A method of oxygen administration that is not usually well tolerated by children

7. The following terms are related to respiratory emergency. Match each term with its description.

a. Hypercapnia
b. Respiratory insufficiency
c. Respiratory failure
d. Respiratory arrest
e. Apnea
f. Central apnea
g. Obstructive apnea

h. Mixed apnea
i. Obstructive lung disease
j. Restrictive lung disease
k. Primary inefficient gas transfer
l. Respiratory center depression
m. Pulmonary diffusion defect
n. Head tilt

o. Chin lift
p. Jaw thrust
q. Back blows
r. Chest thrusts
s. Heimlich maneuver

_____ Absence of airflow (or absence of breathing that lasts for more than 20 seconds)

_____ Occurs in two conditions: (1) when there is increased work of breathing with near-normal gas exchange function, and (2) when hypoxemia and acidosis develop secondary to carbon dioxide retention

_____ Absence of air flow that occurs when no respiratory efforts are present

_____ Condition in which components of central and obstructive apnea are present

_____ The cessation of respiration

_____ Disease involving increased resistance to airflow

_____ Inadequate carbon dioxide removal

_____ Disease involving impaired lung expansion

_____ May be caused by cerebral trauma, intracranial tumors, central nervous system infection, tetanus

_____ The inability of the respiratory apparatus to maintain adequate oxygenation of the blood

_____ Includes pulmonary edema, fibrosis, embolism

_____ Used to relieve foreign body obstruction in infants; accomplished by placing hands on the sternum

_____ Absence of air flow that occurs when respiratory efforts are present

_____ Used to relieve foreign body obstruction in infants; involves hand placement over the spine between the shoulder blades

_____ Accomplished by placing fingers of the hand under the bony portion of the lower jaw to lift

_____ Involves a series of nondiaphragmatic abdominal thrusts; recommended for children over 1 year of age

_____ Accomplished by placing one hand on the victim's forehead and applying firm, backward pressure with the palm

_____ Insufficient alveolar ventilation due to dysfunction of the respiratory control mechanism or a diffusion defect

_____ Accomplished by grasping the angle of the victim's lower jaw and lifting with both hands

8. Of the following respiratory system structures, the one that does not distribute air is the:
   a. bronchiole.
   b. alveolus.
   c. bronchus.
   d. trachea.

9. The general shape of the chest at birth is:
   a. relatively round.
   b. flattened from side to side.
   c. flattened from front to back.
   d. the same shape as an adult's.

10. The infant relies primarily on:
    a. mouth breathing.
    b. intercostal muscles for breathing.
    c. diaphragmatic abdominal breathing.
    d. all of the above.

11. Because of the position of the diaphragm in the newborn:
    a. there is additional abdominal distention from gas and fluid in the stomach.
    b. the diaphragm does not contract as forcefully as that of an older infant or child.
    c. diaphragmatic fatigue is uncommon.
    d. lung volume is increased.

12. Which of the following statements is true in regard to the anatomy of an infant's nasopharyngeal area?
    a. The glottis is located deeper in infants than in older children.
    b. The laryngeal reflexes are weaker in infants than in older children.
    c. The epiglottis is longer and projects more posteriorly in infants than in adults.
    d. The infant and young child are both less susceptible than adults to edema formation in the nasopharyngeal regions.

13. List four anatomic factors that significantly affect the development of respiratory disorders in infants.

14. The condition that is most likely to reduce the number of alveoli in the newborn is:
    a. maternal heroin use.
    b. increased prolactin.
    c. hyperthyroidism.
    d. kyphoscoliosis.

15. As the child grows, chest wall compliance:
    a. increases.
    b. decreases.

16. As the child grows, elastic recoil of the lungs:
    a. increases.
    b. decreases.

17. Relaxation of the bronchial smooth muscles occurs in response to:
    a. parasympathetic stimulation.
    b. inhalation of irritating substances.
    c. sympathetic stimulation.
    d. histamine release.

18. Room air (ambient air) consists of:
    a. 7% oxygen.
    b. 21% oxygen.
    c. 50% oxygen.
    d. 79% oxygen.

19. A child with anemia tends to be fatigued and breathes more rapidly, because the majority of oxygen is carried through the blood as:
    a. a solute dissolved in the plasma and the water of the red blood cell.
    b. bicarbonate and hydrogen ions.
    c. carbonic acid.
    d. oxyhemoglobin.

20. *Retraction* is defined as:
    a. the sinking in of soft tissues during the respiratory cycle.
    b. proliferation of the tissue near the terminal phalanges.
    c. an increase in the end-expiratory pressure.
    d. contraction of the sternocleidomastoid muscles.

21. In a child, cough may be absent in the early stages of:
    a. cystic fibrosis.
    b. measles.
    c. pneumonia.
    d. croup.

22. Define the term *capacity* in relation to lung volume and pulmonary function.

23. Match each pulmonary function parameter with its description and its significance. Each parameter is used twice.

   a. Forced vital capacity (FVC), or peak flow
   b. Tidal volume (TV or V_T)
   c. Functional residual volume (FRV); functional residual capacity (FRC)

   Description

   _____ Volume of air remaining in lungs after passive expiration

   _____ Maximum amount of air that can be expired after maximum inspiration

   _____ Amount of air inhaled and exhaled during any respiratory cycle

   Significance

   _____ Allows for aeration of alveoli; increased in hyperinflated lungs of obstructive lung disease

   _____ Information needed to determine rate and depth of artificial ventilation; multiplied by respiratory rate to provide minute volume

   _____ Reduced in obesity and obstructive airway disease

24. Match each diagnostic test with its description.

   a. Arterial blood gas
   b. Oximetry
   c. Transcutaneous monitoring
   d. Radiography
   e. Magnetic resonance imaging
   f. Computed tomography

   _____ Photometric measurement of oxygen saturation (Sao_2)

   _____ A sequence of pictures, each representing a cross section or cut through lung tissue at a different depths

   _____ A sensitive indicator to monitor oxygen, carbon dioxide, and pH

   _____ Clearly identifies soft tissues with a two- or three-dimensional image

   _____ Produces images of internal structures of the chest, including air-filled lungs, vascular markings, heart, and great vessels

   _____ Provides a noninvasive, continuous, and reliable measurement of arterial carbon dioxide

25. When an infant's digits are connected to a pulse oximeter, the part of the sensor that is placed on the top of the nail is called the:
   a. photodetector.
   b. microprocessor.
   c. light-emitting diode (LED).
   d. electrode.

26. The nurse conducts a precautionary assessment of the collateral circulation when arterial puncture is performed on the child. This is called the:
   a. cover test.
   b. Allen test.
   c. Miller test.
   d. Weber test.

27. Of the following arterial blood gas results, which value would indicate acidosis in an 8-year-old child?
    a. pH of 7.32
    b. pH of 7.47
    c. P_{CO_2} of 44 mm Hg
    d. Oxygen of 75 mm Hg

28. Oxygen delivered to infants is best tolerated when it is administered by:
    a. an oxygen mask.
    b. a plastic hood with humidified oxygen.
    c. delivery of oxygen directly into the incubator.
    d. nasal cannula or prongs.

29. The oxygen mist tent is a satisfactory means of oxygen administration for children past early infancy because it:
    a. comes into direct contact with the face.
    b. controls and maintains the oxygen above 50%.
    c. does not come into direct contact with the face.
    d. keeps the child warm and dry.

30. When caring for the child receiving oxygen via a mist tent, the nurse should:
    a. encourage the child to have a stuffed animal in the tent.
    b. open the tent as little as possible.
    c. open the tent at the bottom of the bed to allow as little oxygen to escape as possible.
    d. keep the child cool because the tent becomes very warm.

31. In children, oxygen-induced carbon dioxide narcosis is encountered most frequently with:
    a. prematurity.
    b. asthma.
    c. cystic fibrosis.
    d. congenital heart disease.

32. For a child under the age of 5 who needs intermittent delivery of an aerosolized medication, the nurse should consider using a:
    a. hand-held nebulizer.
    b. metered-dose inhaler with a spacer device.
    c. humidified mist tent with low-flow oxygen.
    d. metered-dose inhaler without a spacer device.

33. Postural drainage should be performed:
    a. before meals but after other respiratory therapy.
    b. after meals but before other respiratory therapy.
    c. before meals and before other respiratory therapy.
    d. after meals and after other respiratory therapy.

34. When performing postural drainage, the nurse uses special modifications of the usual techniques for:
    a. infants.
    b. children with head injuries.
    c. children in traction.
    d. all of the above.

35. Which of the following patients is likely to benefit from chest physiotherapy that includes forced expiration combined with postural drainage?
    a. Patients with pneumonia
    b. Uncomplicated surgical patients
    c. Patients with increased sputum production
    d. All of the above

36. Chest percussion is being performed correctly if:
    a. it makes a slapping sound.
    b. it is painful.
    c. a soft circular mask is used.
    d. it is performed over the rib cage and diaphragm.

37. The best method to stimulate deep breathing in a child is to:
    a. encourage the child to cover the mouth and suppress his or her cough.
    b. encourage the child to cough repeatedly.
    c. use games that extend expiratory time and pressure.
    d. leave some balloons at the bedside for the child to blow up.

38. To avoid barotrauma when using the bag-valve-mask device, the nurse should:
    a. use the type without a reservoir.
    b. use the type with a pop-off valve.
    c. use a low oxygen concentration.
    d. hyperextend the infant's neck.

39. In a younger child who weighs 30 kg (66 lb), the urinary output value that most indicates a problem is:
    a. 100 ml from 2 to 3 AM.
    b. 100 ml from 2 to 6 AM.
    c. 200 ml from 2 to 4 AM.
    d. 200 ml from 2 to 5 AM.

40. The most severe complication that can occur during the intubation procedure is:
    a. infection.
    b. sore throat.
    c. laryngeal stenosis.
    d. hypoxia.

41. Of the following vacuum pressures, the most acceptable pressure to use to suction the tracheostomy of a child is:
    a. 30 mm Hg.
    b. 50 mm Hg.
    c. 70 mm Hg.
    d. 120 mm Hg.

42. When suctioning a child's airway, the nurse should always:
    a. use intermittent suction.
    b. inject saline into the tube.
    c. insert the catheter until it meets resistance.
    d. use continuous suction.

43. Suctioning obstructs the airway; therefore the suction catheter should remain in the child's airway no longer than:
    a. 3 seconds.
    b. 5 seconds.
    c. 8 seconds.
    d. 10 seconds.

44. For a tracheostomy dressing, it would be incorrect to use:
    a. DuoDERM CGF.
    b. Allevyn dressing.
    c. a wet 4 × 4 gauze pad cut into the needed shape.
    d. Hollister Restore.

45. After the initial postoperative change, the tracheostomy tube is usually changed:
    a. weekly by the surgeon.
    b. weekly by the nurse or family.
    c. monthly by the surgeon.
    d. monthly by the nurse or family.

46. Describe three factors in the home environment that need to be considered when discharging a child with a tracheostomy.

47. A tracheostomy with a speaking valve:
    a. decreases secretions.
    b. decreases the child's sense of taste and smell.
    c. limits gas exchange.
    d. has no effect on the ability to swallow.

48. List at least 10 conditions that predispose a child to respiratory failure.

49. The pediatric nurse should know that the early subtle indication of hypoxia is:
    a. peripheral cyanosis.
    b. central cyanosis.
    c. hypotension.
    d. mood changes and restlessness.

50. Of the following strategies, the one that is least likely to decrease the oxygen demand of the child with respiratory distress is:
    a. maintain child's body temperature within normal limits.
    b. place the child in the supine position.
    c. control pain.
    d. maintain a warm room temperature.

51. Cardiac arrest in the pediatric population is most often a result of:
    a. atherosclerosis.
    b. congenital heart disease.
    c. prolonged hypoxia.
    d. undiagnosed cardiac conditions.

52. The first action the nurse should take when discovering a child in an emergency outside the hospital is to:
    a. transport the child to an acute care facility.
    b. determine whether the child is unconscious.
    c. administer rescue breathing.
    d. transport the child by car for help.

53. The nurse should place the bag-valve-mask device over both the mouth and the nose for individuals whose age is:
    a. birth to 1 year.
    b. 1 to 3 years.
    c. birth to 3 years.
    d. birth to 2 years.

54. The brachial pulse is the preferred site to use to assess circulation in the:
    a. infant.
    b. school-age child.
    c. adolescent.
    d. adult.

55. In a child who is conscious and choking, the nurse should attempt to relieve the obstruction if the victim:
    a. is making sounds.
    b. has an effective cough.
    c. has stridor.
    d. all of the above.

56. Match each drug with its use during pediatric emergency resuscitation.

    a. Sodium bicarbonate   f. Lidocaine
    b. Calcium chloride   g. Epinephrine
    c. Amiodarone   h. Atropine
    d. Adenosine   i. Naloxone
    e. Dopamine

    _____ Reverses respiratory arrest that is due to excessive opiate administration

    _____ Increases cardiac output and heart rate by blocking vagal stimulation in the heart

    _____ The first choice for ventricular tachycardia that is refractory to defibrillation

    _____ Used for hypermagnesemia; needed for normal cardiac contractility

    _____ Causes vasoconstriction and increases cardiac output

    _____ Used for ventricular dysrhythmias

    _____ Acts on α- and β-adrenergic receptor sites, causing contraction, especially at the site of the heart, vascular, and other smooth muscle

    _____ Administered rapidly; causes a temporary block through the atrioventricular node

    _____ Used to buffer the pH

57. The Heimlich maneuver is recommended for children over the age of:
    a. 4 years.
    b. 3 years.
    c. 2 years.
    d. 1 year.

CRITICAL THINKING—CASE STUDIES

Simon, a 14-month-old boy, is admitted to the pediatric unit with a respiratory tract infection.

58. If Simon has a cough that is characteristic of croup syndromes, the nurse would expect to hear:
    a. paroxysmal cough with an inspiratory "whoop."
    b. a brassy cough.
    c. a very severe cough.
    d. a quiet cough.

59. If the child has no cough at all, the nurse would most likely suspect:
    a. cystic fibrosis.
    b. pertussis.
    c. pneumonia.
    d. measles.

60. Simon is placed under a mist tent at 40% oxygen. Chest physiotherapy and intravenous antibiotics are started. The nurse is monitoring his oxygen saturation with pulse oximetry. The pulse oximeter alarm sounds, and the saturation registers at 76%. The nurse should begin the assessment with an evaluation for changes in:
    a. behavior.
    b. skin color.
    c. placement of the oximeter sensor.
    d. hemoglobin.

61. If Simon were diagnosed as having pneumonia, which of the following adjunctive techniques would be of no value?
    a. Intravenous antibiotics
    b. The mist tent at 40% oxygen
    c. Pulse oximetry
    d. Chest physiotherapy

The Child with Respiratory Dysfunction

1. The following terms are related to respiratory tract infection. Match each term with its description.

a. Upper respiratory tract
b. Lower respiratory tract
c. Strep throat
d. Acute rheumatic fever
e. Acute glomerulonephritis
f. Adenoids
g. Waldeyer tonsillar ring
h. Palatine tonsils
i. Pharyngeal tonsils

j. Lingual tonsils
k. Tubal tonsils
l. Tonsillectomy
m. Adenoidectomy
n. Epstein-Barr
o. Heterophil antibody test
p. Spot test (Monospot)
q. Antigenic shift
r. Antigenic drift

_____ One of the more serious sequelae of strep throat; an inflammatory disease of the heart, joints, and central nervous system

_____ Adenoids; located above the palatine tonsils on the posterior wall of the nasopharynx

_____ One of the more serious sequelae of strep throat; an acute kidney infection

_____ Removal of the adenoids; recommended for those children in whom hypertrophied adenoids obstruct nasal breathing

_____ The mass of lymphoid tissue that encircles the nasal and oral pharynx

_____ Consists of the alveoli, bronchi, and bronchioles (the reactive portion on the airway with smooth muscle and the ability to constrict)

_____ Faucial tonsils; located on either side of the oropharynx, behind and below the pillars of the fauces; usually visible during oral examination; removed during tonsillectomy

_____ A slide test of high specificity for the diagnosis of infectious mononucleosis

_____ Consists primarily of the nose and pharynx; upper airway

_____ Removal of the palatine tonsils; indicated for massive hypertrophy that results in difficulty breathing or eating

_____ Also known as the *pharyngeal tonsils*

_____ Major changes in viruses that occur at intervals of years (usually 5 to 10)

_____ A virus; the principal cause of infectious mononucleosis

_____ Group A β-hemolytic streptococcus (GABHS) infection of the upper airway

_____ Located at the base of the tongue

_____ Minor variations in viruses that occur almost annually

_____ Determines the extent to which the patient's serum will agglutinate sheep red blood cells; used to diagnose infectious mononucleosis (titer of 1:160 required for diagnosis); rapid, sensitive, inexpensive, and easy to perform

_____ Found near the posterior nasopharyngeal opening of the eustachian tubes; not a part of the Waldeyer tonsillar ring

2. The following terms are related to otitis media. Match each term with its description.

a. Otitis media
b. Acute otitis media (AOM)
c. Otitis media with effusion (OME)
d. Swimmer's ear
e. Hearing loss
f. Tympanic membrane retraction
g. Tympanosclerosis
h. Eardrum perforation
i. Adhesive otitis media

j. Chronic suppurative otitis media
k. Labyrinthitis
l. Mastoiditis
m. Meningitis
n. Cholesteatoma
o. Pneumatic otoscopy
p. Tympanometry

_____ An inflammation of the middle ear and mastoid; characterized by perforation and discharge (otorrhea) lasting up to 6 weeks

_____ Assesses the mobility of the tympanic membrane, using air transmission

_____ Middle ear inflammation with rapid and short onset of signs and symptoms lasting approximately 3 weeks

_____ Infection of the inner ear

_____ One of the least common but potentially most dangerous sequelae of OME; the formation of a keratinized epithelial cell lining that forms scales within the middle ear space; erodes all of the structures it encounters, especially bone

_____ An inflammation of the middle ear without reference to etiology or pathogenesis

_____ Eardrum scarring; the deposition of hyaline material into the fibrous layer of the tympanic membrane; associated with repeated inflammatory AOM or with repeated tympanoplasty tube placement

_____ Infection of the mastoid sinus

_____ One of the consequences of prolonged middle ear disorder; usually conductive and not severe

_____ A thickening of the mucous membrane by proliferation of fibrous tissue that can cause fixation of the ossicles with resultant hearing loss; sometimes called "glue ear"

_____ A suppurative intracranial complication from the extension of a middle ear or mastoid infection

_____ A common complication of AOM; often accompanies chronic disease; a complication of tympanoplasty tube placement

_____ Retraction pocket; occurs when continued negative middle ear pressure draws the tympanic membrane inward; may result in impaired sound transmission

_____ The test to assess mobility of the tympanic membrane using sound transmission

_____ Inflammation of the middle ear in which a collection of fluid is present in the middle ear space

_____ Otitis externa; inflammation that occurs when the external ear environment is altered during swimming, bathing, or conditions of increased humidity

3. The following terms are related to croup syndromes and other respiratory tract infections. Match each term with its description.

a. Croup
b. Racemic epinephrine
c. Tracheobronchitis
d. Respiratory syncytial virus (RSV)
e. Ribavirin
f. Palivizumab
g. Meningism
h. Tubercle
i. Miliary tuberculosis (TB)
j. TB infection
k. TB disease

l. Purified protein derivative (PPD)
m. Tuberculin test
n. Positive reaction TB skin test
o. Negative reaction TB skin test
p. Gastric washings
q. Reactive portion of the lungs
r. Pneumonitis
s. Lobar pneumonia
t. Bronchopneumonia
u. Interstitial pneumonia
v. Emphysema

_____ Result that usually means the child has never been infected with the organism

_____ An acute viral infection with maximum effect at the bronchiolar level

_____ Used to make the definitive diagnosis of TB; one means of obtaining material for respiratory smears or culture

_____ The type of pneumonia in which the inflammatory process is confined within the alveolar walls and the peribronchial and interlobular tissues

_____ Nebulized epinephrine; used in children with stridor at rest, retractions, acute epiglottitis, or difficulty breathing

_____ Meningeal symptoms

_____ A symptom complex characterized by hoarseness, a resonant cough described as "barking" or "brassy," inspiratory stridor, and respiratory distress from swelling in the region of the larynx

_____ Includes the bronchi and bronchioles in children because cartilaginous support of the large airways is not fully developed until adolescence

_____ Formed by epithelial cells surrounding and encapsulating multiplying bacilli in an attempt to wall off the invading organisms

_____ The type of pneumonia that begins in the terminal bronchioles, which become clogged with mucopurulent exudates to form consolidated patches in the nearby lobule

_____ An antiviral agent; the only specific therapy approved for hospitalized children with RSV

_____ Progressive overinflation of the lung caused by obstruction of the small airway passages, which prevents air from leaving the lungs

_____ Standard dose is 5 tuberculin units in 0.1 ml of solution, injected intradermally

_____ Widespread dissemination of the tubercle bacillus to near and distant sites

_____ A positive result that indicates a person has been infected; does not confirm the presence of active disease

_____ The type of pneumonia in which all or a large segment of one or more pulmonary lobes is involved; known as "bilateral" or "double pneumonia" when both lungs are affected

_____ RSV monoclonal antibody; the only product available in the United States for prevention of RSV; administered monthly intramuscularly; used to prevent RSV in high-risk infants

_____ Inflammation of the large airways, which is frequently associated with an upper respiratory tract infection; primarily caused by viral agents

_____ Localized acute inflammation of the lung without the toxemia associated with lobar pneumonia

_____ Manifested by a positive skin test; asymptomatic

_____ The single most important test to determine whether a child has been infected with the tubercle bacillus

_____ Diagnosed by positive chest radiograph, positive sputum culture, and presence of signs of the disease

4. The following terms are related to noninfectious irritants. Match each term with its description.

a. Aspiration pneumonia
b. Carbon monoxide
c. Carboxyhemoglobin (COHb)

d. Hyperbaric oxygen
e. Cotinine

_____ Forms when carbon monoxide enters the bloodstream and binds with hemoglobin

_____ A colorless, odorless gas with an affinity for hemoglobin 200 to 250 times greater than that of oxygen

_____ A by-product of nicotine that is considered a valid biochemical marker for environmental smoke exposure; urinary levels increased in children living with smokers

_____ Therapy that lowers carboxyhemoglobin levels rapidly; may be required for severe carbon monoxide poisoning (COHb level >25% in children)

_____ Occurs when food, secretions, inert material, volatile compounds, or liquids enter the lung and cause inflammation and a chemical pneumonitis

5. The following terms are related to long-term respiratory dysfunction. Match each term with its description.

a. Seasonal allergic rhinitis
b. House dust mites
c. Cockroach
d. Long-term control medications
e. Quick-relief medications
f. Nebulized hypertonic saline
g. Exercise-induced bronchospasm
h. Written action plan
i. Peak expiratory flow meters
j. Spacer
k. Cystic fibrosis transmembrane regulator (CFTR)
l. Meconium ileus
m. Distal intestinal obstruction syndrome
n. Prolapse of the rectum
o. Chest physiotherapy

p. Flutter mucus clearance device
q. Mechanical vest
r. Dornase alfa
s. Lung transplantation
t. Specific tissue binding
u. Peak expiratory flow rate (PEFR)
v. Personal best value
w Turbuhaler
x. Salmeterol
y. Status asthmaticus
z. Steatorrhea
aa. Azotorrhea
bb. Quantitative sweat chloride test

_____ Used daily to prevent infection and to maintain pulmonary hygiene in children with cystic fibrosis

_____ Shown to be effective in treating RSV in a few small studies; 3% saline

_____ Used at home by the child with asthma to monitor personal best values

_____ Hay fever

_____ Holding chamber; device that attaches to a metered-dose inhaler and holds medication long enough for the patient to inhale slowly

_____ An important allergen in children with asthma; most common allergen in inner-city environments

_____ The protein product that is located on the long arm of chromosome 7; indicator of cystic fibrosis

_____ Rescue medications; used to treat acute symptoms and exacerbations of asthma

_____ Allergen identified most often in children allergic to inhalants

_____ Should be given to all children with asthma to use in the event of an exacerbation

_____ The earliest postnatal manifestation of cystic fibrosis; seen in 7% to 10% of newborns with the disease; occurs when thick, putty-like tenacious mucilaginous meconium blocks the lumen of the small intestine, usually at or near the ileocecal valve, giving rise to signs of intestinal obstruction

_____ Provides a high-frequency chest wall oscillation to help loosen secretions

_____ Small, hand-held plastic pipe with a stainless steel ball on the inside that facilitates removal of mucus

_____ Acute, reversible, usually self-terminating airway obstruction that develops during or after vigorous activity; reaches its peak 5 to 10 minutes after stopping the activity and usually ceases in another 20 to 30 minutes

_____ The most common gastrointestinal complication associated with cystic fibrosis; occurs most often in infancy and early childhood and is related to large bulky stools and lack of supportive fat pads around the rectum

_____ Preventive medications; used to achieve and maintain control of inflammation in asthma

_____ A final therapeutic option for a few patients with end-stage cystic fibrosis

_____ A partial or complete intestinal obstruction that occurs in some children with cystic fibrosis

_____ Recombinant human deoxyribonuclease; an aerosolized medication that decreases the viscosity of mucus; available in brand name as Pulmozyme

_____ A chlorofluorocarbon-propelled metered-dose inhaler that delivers powdered medication; eliminates the need to coordinate activation of the device with the breath

_____ Excessive protein in the stool

_____ The process whereby the antigen mediates a reaction; the antibody attaches to cells' surfaces, where it reacts with the specific antigen to which the cells have developed a bonding capacity

_____ Serevent; a long-acting bronchodilator that is used twice a day; added to antiinflammatory therapy for prevention of long-term symptoms

_____ An assessment parameter used to monitor pulmonary function; measures the maximum flow of air forcefully exhaled in
1 second; measured in liters per minute

_____ Excessive fat in the stool

_____ Established by measuring values during a 2- to 3-week period when asthma is stable; compared with current PEFR to make care management decisions

_____ A medical emergency in which the child continues to display respiratory distress despite vigorous therapeutic measures such as sympathomimetics

_____ Pilocarpine iontophoresis; a test that involves stimulating the production of sweat and measuring the sweat electrolytes; used to determine presence of cystic fibrosis; should only be carried out by personnel skilled in performing the procedure

6. The largest percentage of respiratory tract infections in children are caused by:
   a. pneumococci.
   b. viruses.
   c. streptococci.
   d. *Haemophilus influenzae.*

7. The most likely reason that the respiratory tract infection rate increases drastically in the age range from 3 to 6 months is that the:
   a. infant's exposure to pathogens is greatly increased during this time.
   b. viral agents that are mild in older children are severe in infants.
   c. maternal antibodies have disappeared and the infant's own antibody production is immature.
   d. diameter of the airways is smaller in the infant than in the older child.

8. A febrile seizure is least likely to be associated with:
   a. fever in a 2-year-old child.
   b. a family history of febrile seizures.
   c. fever in an 8-year-old child.
   d. all of the above.

9. When giving tips for how to increase humidity in the home of a child with a respiratory tract infection, the nurse should emphasize that the primary concern is to ensure that the child has:
   a. a steam vaporizer.
   b. a warm humidification source.
   c. a safe humidification source.
   d. a cool humidification source.

10. Bobby is a child with a respiratory disorder who needs bed rest but who is not cooperating. The nurse's best choice is to:
    a. be sure Bobby's mother takes the advice seriously.
    b. allow Bobby to play quietly on the floor.
    c. insist that Bobby play quietly in bed.
    d. allow Bobby to cry until he stays in bed.

11. For an older child who can tolerate decongestants and who is having difficulty breathing through his stuffy nose, the nurse should recommend:
    a. dextromethorphan nose drops.
    b. phenylephrine nose drops.
    c. dextromethorphan cough squares.
    d. steroid nose drops.

12. Children with nasopharyngitis may be treated with:
    a. decongestants.
    b. antihistamines.
    c. expectorants.
    d. all of the above.

13. The best technique to use to prevent spread of nasopharyngitis is:
    a. prompt immunization.
    b. to avoid contact with infected persons.
    c. mist vaporization.
    d. to ensure adequate fluid intake.

14. Group A β-hemolytic streptococci infection is usually a:
    a. serious infection of the upper airway.
    b. common cause of pharyngitis in children over the age of 15 years.
    c. brief illness that leaves the child at risk for serious sequelae.
    d. disease of the heart, lungs, joints, and central nervous system.

15. The American Academy of Pediatrics recommends that health care providers base their diagnosis of group A β-hemolytic streptococcus on:
    a. antibody responses.
    b. antistreptolysin O responses.
    c. complete blood count.
    d. throat culture.

16. A strategy for the prevention of streptococcal disease would be for the nurse to recommend that:
    a. children with streptococcal infection not return to school until after 48 hours of antibiotic therapy.
    b. children with streptococcal infection discard their toothbrush and replace it with a new one after 24 hours of antibiotic therapy.
    c. children with streptococcal infection not return to school until after 36 hours of antibiotic therapy.
    d. children with streptococcal infection discard their toothbrush and replace it with a new one as soon as the streptococcus is identified.

17. Offensive mouth odor, persistent dry cough, and a voice with a muffled nasal quality are commonly the result of:
    a. pneumonia.
    b. otitis externa.
    c. tonsillitis.
    d. otitis media.

18. An adenoidectomy would be contraindicated in a child:
    a. with recurrent otitis media.
    b. with malignancy.
    c. with thrombocytopenia.
    d. under the age of 3 years.

19. In the postoperative period following a tonsillectomy, the child should be:
    a. placed in Trendelenburg position.
    b. encouraged to cough and deep breathe.
    c. suctioned vigorously to clear the airway.
    d. observed for signs of hemorrhage.

20. Pain medication for the child in the postoperative period following a tonsillectomy should be administered:
    a. orally at regular intervals.
    b. orally as needed.
    c. rectally or intravenously at regular intervals.
    d. rectally or intravenously as needed.

21. Of the following foods, the most appropriate to offer first to an alert child in the postoperative period following a tonsillectomy would be:
    a. ice cream.
    b. red gelatin.
    c. flavored ice pops.
    d. all of the above.

22. An early indication of hemorrhage in a child who has had a tonsillectomy is:
    a. frequent swallowing.
    b. decreasing blood pressure.
    c. restlessness.
    d. all of the above.

23. In about half of all cases of infectious mononucleosis, there will be:
    a. skin rash.
    b. otitis media.
    c. splenomegaly.
    d. failure to thrive.

24. Diagnosis of infectious mononucleosis is established when the:
    a. red blood cell count is depressed.
    b. leukocyte count is depressed.
    c. heterophil agglutination test is positive.
    d. heterophil agglutination test is negative.

25. Infectious mononucleosis is usually a:
    a. disease complicated by pneumonitis and anemia.
    b. self-limiting disease.
    c. disabling disease.
    d. difficult and prolonged disease.

26. Clinical manifestations of influenza usually include all of the following except:
    a. nausea and vomiting.
    b. fever and chills.
    c. sore throat and dry mucous membranes.
    d. photophobia and myalgia.

27. The infant is predisposed to developing otitis media because the eustachian tubes:
    a. lie in a relatively horizontal plane.
    b. have a limited amount of lymphoid tissue.
    c. are long and narrow.
    d. are underdeveloped.

28. List at least five complications of otitis media.

29. The clinical manifestations of otitis media include:
    a. purulent discharge in the external auditory canal.
    b. clear discharge in the external auditory canal.
    c. enlarged axillary lymph nodes.
    d. enlarged cervical lymph nodes.

30. An abnormal otoscopic examination would reveal:
    a. visible landmarks.
    b. a light reflex.
    c. orange tympanic membrane.
    d. mobile tympanic membrane.

31. Of the following antibiotics, the one that would most likely be prescribed for uncomplicated otitis media would be:
    a. tetracycline.
    b. amoxicillin.
    c. gentamicin.
    d. methicillin.

32. To help alleviate the discomfort and fever of otitis media, the nurse may administer:
    a. acetaminophen or ibuprofen.
    b. antihistamines and decongestants.
    c. analgesic ear drops.
    d. all of the above.

33. Recurrent otitis media after a total of 4 to 6 months of bilateral effusion with bilateral hearing deficit would most likely be managed therapeutically by:
    a. tonsillectomy.
    b. steroids.
    c. polyvalent pneumococcal polysaccharide vaccine.
    d. tympanostomy tubes.

34. Children with tympanostomy tubes should:
    a. swim only in freshwater lakes without earplugs.
    b. keep bath water out of the ear.
    c. notify the physician immediately if a grommet appears.
    d. never allow any water to enter their ears.

35. Which of the following techniques would be contraindicated for the nurse to recommend to parents to prevent recurrent otitis externa?
    a. Administer a combination of vinegar and alcohol after swimming.
    b. Allow the child to swim every day for 2 to 4 hours.
    c. Dry the ear canal after swimming with a cotton swab.
    d. Use a hair dryer on low heat at 1 to 2 feet for 30 seconds several times a day.

36. Most children with croup syndromes:
    a. require hospitalization.
    b. will need to be intubated.
    c. can be cared for at home.
    d. are over 6 years old.

37. Of the following croup syndromes, the one that is potentially life threatening is:
    a. spasmodic croup.
    b. laryngotracheobronchitis.
    c. acute spasmodic laryngitis.
    d. epiglottitis.

38. The nurse should suspect epiglottitis if the child has:
    a. cough, sore throat, and agitation.
    b. cough, drooling, and retractions.
    c. drooling, agitation, and absence of cough.
    d. hoarseness, retractions, and absence of cough.

39. In the child who is suspected of having epiglottitis, the nurse should:
    a. have intubation equipment available.
    b. prepare to immunize the child for *H. influenzae*.
    c. obtain a throat culture.
    d. All of the above

40. Since the advent of immunization for *H. influenzae,* there has been a decrease in the incidence of:
    a. laryngotracheobronchitis.
    b. epiglottitis.
    c. Reye syndrome.
    d. croup syndrome.

41. Of the following children, the one who is most likely to be hospitalized for treatment of croup is:
    a. a 2-year-old child whose croupy cough worsens at night.
    b. a 5-year-old child whose croupy cough worsens at night.
    c. a 2-year-old child using the accessory muscles to breath.
    d. a child with inspiratory stridor during the physical examination.

42. The primary therapeutic regimen for croup usually includes:
    a. vigilant assessment, racemic epinephrine, and corticosteroids.
    b. vigilant assessment, racemic epinephrine, and antibiotics.
    c. intubation, racemic epinephrine, and corticosteroids.
    d. intubation, racemic epinephrine, and antibiotics.

43. The condition that is most likely to require intubation is:
    a. acute spasmodic laryngitis.
    b. bacterial tracheitis.
    c. acute laryngotracheobronchitis.
    d. acute laryngitis.

44. RSV is:
    a. an uncommon virus that usually causes severe bronchiolitis.
    b. an uncommon virus that usually does not require hospitalization.
    c. a common virus that usually causes severe bronchiolitis.
    d. a common virus that usually does not require hospitalization.

45. In the infant who is admitted with possible RSV, the nurse would expect the laboratory to perform:
    a. the ELISA antibody test on nasal secretions.
    b. a viral culture of the stool.
    c. a bacterial culture of nasal secretions.
    d. an anaerobic culture of the blood.

46. Nursing care for patients with severe acute respiratory syndrome predominantly involves:
    a. antibiotics.
    b. antivirals.
    c. supportive care.
    d. steroids.

47. Match the age of the child with the most common cause of pneumonia in that age-group.
    a. *Haemophilus influenzae*
    b. *Streptococcus pneumoniae*
    c. *Mycoplasma pneumoniae*

    _____ Over 5 years of age

    _____ 3 months to 5 years old

    _____ Under 3 months

48. Closed chest drainage is most likely to be used with the type of pneumonia that is caused by:
    a. *H. influenzae.*
    b. *M. pneumoniae.*
    c. *S. pneumoniae.*
    d. *Staphylococcus pneumoniae.*

49. Describe four nursing measures to care for the child with pneumonia.

50. In an 8-month-old infant admitted with pertussis, the nurse should particularly assess the:
    a. living conditions of the infant.
    b. labor and delivery history of the mother.
    c. immunization status of the infant.
    d. alcohol and drug intake of the mother.

51. The best test to screen for tuberculosis is the:
    a. chest x-ray.
    b. purified protein derivative (PPD) test.
    c. sputum culture.
    d. multipuncture tests (MPT), such as the tine test.

52. The recommended treatment for the child who has clinically active tuberculosis includes:
    a. isoniazid.
    b. rifampin.
    c. pyrazinamide.
    d. all of the above.

53. Which of the following Mantoux test results would be considered positive?
    a. Induration 5 mm in a 3-year-old child with human immunodeficiency virus (HIV) infection
    b. Induration 2 mm in a 5-year-old child without tuberculosis contacts
    c. Induration 7 mm in an 8-year-old child without any risk factors
    d. All of the above

54. The usual site of bronchial obstruction is the:
    a. left bronchus because it is shorter and straighter.
    b. left bronchus because it is longer and angled.
    c. right bronchus because it is shorter and straighter.
    d. right bronchus because it is longer and angled.

55. The definitive diagnosis of airway foreign bodies in the trachea and larynx requires:
    a. radiographic examination.
    b. fluoroscopic examination.
    c. bronchoscopic examination.
    d. ultrasonographic examination.

56. Parents may be taught to treat aspiration of a foreign body in an infant under 12 months old by using:
    a. back blows and chest thrusts.
    b. back blows only.
    c. the Heimlich maneuver only.
    d. a blind finger sweep.

57. The child who has ingested lighter fluid usually receives:
    a. the same treatment as a child who has hepatitis.
    b. medication to induce vomiting.
    c. the same treatment as a child who has pneumonia.
    d. activated charcoal.

58. List five strategies that may be used to manage acute respiratory distress syndrome in children.

59. Deaths from fires are most often a result of:
    a. full-thickness burns over 50% of the body.
    b. full-thickness burns to the chest and neck.
    c. noxious substances from incomplete combustion.
    d. injuries sustained in escape attempts.

60. Treatment of smoke toxicity with a carboxyhemoglobin level of 10% would most likely consist of:
    a. humidified oxygen at 70%.
    b. humidified oxygen at 100%.
    c. intubation.
    d. use of a hyperbaric oxygen chamber.

61. The biochemical marker for environmental smoke exposure is called _____.

62. List at least five physical findings commonly seen in the child with allergic rhinitis.

63. Of the following children, the one who is most likely suffering from allergy rather than a cold would be the:
    a. 2-year-old with fever and runny nose.
    b. adolescent with itchy eyes and constant sneezing without fever.
    c. 2-year-old with sporadic sneezing and a runny nose.
    d. adolescent with sporadic sneezing and a runny nose.

64. The severity of asthma in a child with daily asthmatic symptoms would be classified as:
    a. mild intermittent.
    b. mild persistent.
    c. moderate persistent.
    d. severe persistent.

CRITICAL THINKING—CASE STUDY

Jason Wilson, 8 years old, is admitted to the pediatric unit with a diagnosis of reactive airway disease. This is his first hospitalization for this disorder. Both of Jason's parents smoke cigarettes, but they try to smoke outdoors. Jason usually does well, although his asthma tends to increase in severity during the winter months. Recently he has had several colds and his asthma has flared up each time. This time, however, he is very uncomfortable, with wheezes in all lung fields.

65. Of the following questions, the one that would be most important for the nurse to ask Jason's mother would be:
    a. "What brings you to the hospital?"
    b. "What is your ethnic background?"
    c. "Do you have any history of asthma in your family?"
    d. "Were your pregnancy and delivery uneventful?"

66. Mrs. Wilson wants the nurse to explain exactly what reactive airway disease is. She says she has been told many times, but it is always when Jason is in so much distress that she is not certain she hears it correctly. The nurse responds that:
    a. asthma is caused by a certain inflammatory mediator.
    b. the one mechanism responsible for the obstructive symptoms of asthma is excess mucous secretion.
    c. the one mechanism responsible for the obstructive symptoms of asthma is spasm of the smooth muscle of the bronchi.
    d. most theories do not explain all types and causes of asthma.

67. In general, Jason does not have difficulty with any food or emotional triggers for asthma. An asthmatic episode for Jason starts with itching all over the upper part of his back. He is usually irritable and restless. He complains of headache, chest tightness, and fatigue. He usually coughs, sweats, and sits in the tripod position with his shoulders hunched over. Today he has no fever, and he is sitting upright. His skin is not sweaty. Based on this information, the nurse would decide that Jason is:
    a. severely ill.
    b. moderately ill.
    c. mildly ill.
    d. not ill at all.

68. Jason's younger sister, Tanya, is an infant. Tanya's disease is much worse than Jason's. Mrs. Wilson states that Tanya often has movements of her chest muscles that make it appear that she is working very hard to breathe; however, her respiratory rate does not change. When this happens, Tanya is not exhaling a long breath like Jason. These differences between Jason and Tanya are confusing to Mrs. Wilson, and she asks the nurse for advice about what to do when this happens to Tanya. The nurse's response is based on the knowledge that:
    a. dyspnea is much more difficult to evaluate in an infant than in a young child.
    b. the bodies of infants and young children respond to the asthmatic episode the same way.
    c. boys tend to have more severe symptoms of asthma than girls do.
    d. dyspnea is much more difficult to evaluate in a young child than in an infant.

69. The nurse examines Jason and finds that he has hyperresonance on percussion. His breath sounds are coarse and loud with sonorous crackles throughout the lung fields. Expiration is prolonged. There is generalized inspiratory and expiratory wheezing. Based on these findings, the nurse suspects that there is:
    a. minimal obstruction.
    b. significant obstruction.
    c. imminent ventilatory failure.
    d. an extrathoracic obstruction.

70. The nurse determines that Jason's peak expiratory flow rate is in the yellow zone. This test result indicates that Jason's asthma control is about:
    a. 80% of his personal best and that his routine treatment plan can be followed.
    b. 50% of his personal best and that he needs an increase in his usual therapy.
    c. 50% of his personal best and that he needs immediate bronchodilators.
    d. less than 50% of his personal best and that he need immediate bronchodilators.

71. Jason's test results are back from the laboratory. The white blood cell count is $11,200/mm^3$. The eosinophils are $728/mm^3$. The chest x-ray film shows hyperexpansion of the airways. The nurse knows that these findings:
    a. support the diagnosis of pneumonia without an episode of asthma.
    b. support the diagnosis of asthma complicated by pneumonia.
    c. do not support the diagnosis of an acute episode of asthma or pneumonia.
    d. support the diagnosis of an acute episode of asthma without pneumonia.

72. The physician orders albuterol via inhaler for Jason. Mrs. Wilson is concerned
    because she says that Jason usually receives theophylline intravenously. The nurse's
    response is based on the fact that:
    a. Jason's asthma episode is probably not as severe as usual.
    b. Jason's physician must be using information that is out of date.
    c. theophylline is a third-line drug that is a weak bronchodilator and not considered as effective as nebulized
       β-agonists.
    d. theophylline is a third-line drug because it has been shown to adversely affect school performance.

73. When preparing for discharge, the nurse would most likely plan to teach the Wilson family to:
    a. keep the humidity at home above 50%.
    b. vacuum the carpets at least twice weekly.
    c. use pesticides to control cockroaches.
    d. launder sheets and blankets regularly in cold water.

74. Jason uses aerosolized steroids at home; therefore he should be taught to rinse his mouth thoroughly with water:
    a. before each treatment to increase absorption.
    b. after each treatment to minimize the risk for oral candidiasis.
    c. before each treatment to minimize the adverse effects of the drug.
    d. after each treatment to increase absorption.

75. Based on the nurse's assessment, a care plan is developed. Of the following nursing diagnoses, the one that would
    least likely appear on Jason's care plan is:
    a. Activity Intolerance related to imbalance between oxygen supply and demand.
    b. Ineffective Airway Clearance related to allergenic response and inflammation in bronchial tree.
    c. High Risk for Infection related to the presence of infective organisms.
    d. Altered Family Process related to a chronic illness.

76. One principle that should be a part of Jason's home self-management program is that:
    a. patients must learn not to abuse their medications so that they will not become addicted.
    b. it is easy to treat an asthmatic episode as long as the child knows the symptoms.
    c. although uncommon, asthma is treatable.
    d. children with asthma are usually able to participate in the same activities
       as nonasthmatic children.

Andrea is an 8-year-old with cystic fibrosis. She is in the fifth percentile for both height and weight.
This failure to thrive persists even though she has a voracious appetite. She has been managed at home most
recently for about 6 months without the need for hospitalization. She is admitted today with blood-tinged sputum.
The sputum culture obtained 2 days ago is positive for *Pseudomonas* organisms. The nurse hears crackles in both lungs,
and Andrea has significant clubbing of her fingers with a capillary refill time of greater than 5 seconds.

77. Based on this information, the nurse suspects that Andrea's:
    a. condition is improving and she will soon return to home care.
    b. condition is progressively worsening.
    c. condition is worse, but intravenous antibiotic therapy will correct the problem.
    d. family has been noncompliant, resulting in this setback.

78. The admission orders included an order for gentamicin at a dosage that the nurse calculated to be higher than usual
    for a child of Andrea's size. Which of the following is an acceptable reason for the high dosage?
    a. The physician used Andrea's age rather than her size to determine the dosage.
    b. The pharmacy has made an error.
    c. Children with cystic fibrosis metabolize antibiotics rapidly.
    d. Children with cystic fibrosis metabolize antibiotics slowly.

79. Which of the following strategies would most likely be contraindicated for Andrea?
    a. Forced expiration
    b. Aerobic exercise
    c. Chest physiotherapy
    d. High-flow oxygen therapy

80. The blood-tinged sputum progresses to an amount greater than 300 ml/day. The nurse recognizes that increased tendency to bleed may be a result of:
    a. iron deficiency anemia.
    b. vitamin K deficiency.
    c. thrombocytopenia.
    d. vitamin D deficiency.

81. At the present time, family support for Andrea will most likely include strategies to help her family cope with all of the following issues except:
    a. pregnancy and genetic counseling.
    b. relief from the continual routine with respite care.
    c. dealing with a chronic illness and anticipatory grieving.
    d. abnormal psychologic adjustment and dysfunctional family patterns.

82. Andrea takes seven pancreatic enzyme capsules about 30 minutes before each meal. She usually has two or three bowel movements per day. The nurse's action in regard to the pancreatic enzymes is based on the knowledge that the dosage:
    a. is adequate.
    b. should always be fewer than five capsules.
    c. should be seven to ten capsules.
    d. is adequate, but she should take it between meals.

33 The Child with Gastrointestinal Dysfunction

1. Which of the following is not a function of the gastrointestinal (GI) system?
   a. Process and absorb nutrients necessary to support growth and development
   b. Maintain thermoregulatory functions
   c. Perform excretory functions
   d. Maintain fluid and electrolyte balance

2. Identify the following as true or false.

   _____ At birth the term infant has the ability to move food particles from the front of the mouth to the back of the mouth.

   _____ The infant has no voluntary control of swallowing for the first 3 months.

   _____ The chewing function is facilitated by eruption of the primary teeth.

   _____ The primary purpose of saliva in the newborn is to moisten the mouth and throat.

   _____ The infant's stomach is smaller in capacity but faster to empty than the child's stomach.

   _____ The infant's stomach at birth has an elongated shape.

3. Fill in the blanks in the following statements.

   a. Three processes, _____, _____, and _____, are necessary to convert nutrients into forms that can be used by the body.

   b. Chemical digestion involves five general types of GI secretions: _____,

   _____, _____ _____, _____, _____,

   and _____.

   c. The _____ _____ is the principal absorption site in the GI system.

4. What are the five most important basic nursing assessments included in a thorough GI assessment?

5. The nurse is preparing Dottie, age 7, for an upper GI endoscopy. Which of the following does the nurse recognize as not being an appropriate preparation for this test?
   a. Bowel cleansing with magnesium citrate or GoLYTELY
   b. Keeping Dottie NPO (nothing by mouth) for 8 hours before the procedure
   c. Giving Dottie sedation before the procedure is begun
   d. Explaining to Dottie in advance about the procedure by use of pictures or play with dolls and demonstration

6. Jenny, an 8-year-old, has been brought to the clinic with continuing pain in the epigastric region of the abdomen. The medical provider has ordered *Helicobacter pylori* testing. Which of the following tests does the nurse recognize as being the most accurate method to determine active infection?
   a. Serology test
   b. C urea breath test
   c. Esophagus manometry
   d. Occult blood guaiac test

7. Match each term with its description.

a. Pica
b. Failure to thrive
c. Regurgitation
d. Projectile vomiting
e. Encopresis
f. Hematemesis

g. Hematochezia
h. Melena
i. Dysphagia
j. Occult blood guaiac test
k. Stool for O&P (ova and parasites)

l. Constipation
m. Sandifer syndrome
n. Phlegmon
o. Obstipation
p. Steatorrhea

_____ An acute suppurative inflammation of subcutaneous connective tissue that spreads

_____ Fatty, foul, frothy, bulky stools

_____ Detects presence of blood in the stool

_____ Vomiting of bright red blood as a result of bleeding in the upper GI tract or from swallowed blood from the upper respiratory tract

_____ Passage of bright red blood from the rectum

_____ Passage of dark-colored "tarry" stools

_____ Characterized by repetitive stretching and arching of the head and neck in an attempt to prevent acid refluxate from reaching the upper portion of the esophagus

_____ Eating disorder in which there is compulsive eating of both food and nonfood substances

_____ A decrease in bowel movement frequency or trouble defecating for more than 2 weeks

_____ Having long intervals between bowel movements

_____ Accompanied by vigorous peristaltic waves

_____ Outflow of incontinent stool, causing soiling

_____ Deceleration from normal pattern of growth or growth below the 5th percentile

_____ Difficulty swallowing

_____ Aids in the diagnosis of parasitic infections

_____ A backward flowing such as the return of gastric contents into the mouth

8. In which of the following children coming to the health clinic should pica be considered?
   a. Seven-year-old with nausea and vomiting for the past 3 days
   b. Four-year-old with history of celiac disease being seen with anemia and abdominal pain
   c. Two-year-old who is still drinking from a bottle and is seen with anemia
   d. Four-month-old who is crying, is irritable, and has reddish stools

9. Lance, a 2-year-old, has been brought to the clinic because his parents are afraid he swallowed a small button battery from his father's watch, which with he was playing. Which of the following is the most appropriate nursing action at this time?
   a. Reassure the parents that Lance has probably not swallowed the battery because he has no symptoms, he is playing in the examination room, and his lung fields are clear.
   b. Explain to the parents that Lance will probably be allowed to normally pass the battery through the GI system because Lance has been able to eat and drink normally since the event.
   c. Start immediate teaching of Lance's parents on how to assess Lance's environment for hazardous objects and how to assess Lance's toys and other items he might play with for safety.
   d. Explain to Lance's parents that x-ray examination will be conducted, and the battery will most probably need to be removed to prevent local damage if lodged in the esophagus.

10. John, age 16, asks the nurse why he has to have an endoscopic examination to determine whether he has *H. pylori* infection. "Why can't they just do the blood test?" Formulate a correct response to this question.

11. Constipation in infancy:
    a. may be due to normal developmental changes.
    b. may be related to dietary practices.
    c. is found more often in breast-feed infants.
    d. may be due to environmental stressors.

12. After fecal impaction is removed, maintenance therapy for constipation may include laxative use. Why is polyethylene glycol considered safe to use for pediatric patients?
    a. Decreases fluid in the colon
    b. Increases fluid in the colon
    c. Increases peristaltic stimulation
    d. Increases osmotic pressure and acidification of the colon contents

13. The nurse is counseling the mother of 12-month-old Brian on methods to prevent constipation. Which of the following methods would be contraindicated for Brian?
    a. Add bran to Brian's cereal.
    b. Increase Brian's intake of water.
    c. Add prunes to Brian's diet.
    d. Add popcorn to Brian's diet.

14. Sally, age 5, has been diagnosed with chronic constipation. Management includes:
    a. decreasing the water and increasing the milk in Sally's diet.
    b. an organized approach of at least 6 to 12 months of treatment to be effective.
    c. daily use of rectal stimulation to promote stool passage.
    d. having Sally sit on the toilet each day until she has a bowel movement.

15. Which of the following is a congenital anomaly that results in mechanical obstruction from inadequate motility of part of the intestine?
    a. Intussusception
    b. Short-bowel syndrome
    c. Crohn disease
    d. Hirschsprung disease

16. To confirm the diagnosis of Hirschsprung disease, the nurse prepares the child for:
    a. barium enema.
    b. upper GI series.
    c. rectal biopsy.
    d. esophagoscopy.

17. What clinical manifestations would the nurse expect to see in the child diagnosed with Hirschsprung disease?
    a. History of bloody diarrhea, fever, and vomiting
    b. Irritability, severe abdominal cramps, fecal soiling
    c. Decreased hemoglobin, increased serum lipids, and positive stool for O&P
    d. History of constipation; abdominal distention; and passage of ribbon-like, foul-smelling stools

18. Explain the defects present in Hirschsprung disease (congenital aganglionic megacolon).

19. The nurse would expect preoperative care for the pediatric patient with Hirschsprung disease to include:
    i. emptying the bowel with repeated saline enemas in the newborn.
    ii. measuring vital signs and blood pressure for signs of shock.
    iii. keeping accurate measurement of abdominal circumference.
    iv. monitoring fluid and electrolyte replacements.
    v. providing daily soap suds enemas.
    vi. explaining to the parents and child that the colostomy is permanent and encouraging them to assume care before discharge.

    a. i, ii, iii, and iv
    b. ii, iii, and iv
    c. i, ii, iii, iv, and vi
    d. i, ii, iv, and v

20. The transfer of gastric contents into the esophagus is termed:
    a. esophageal atresia.
    b. Meckel diverticulum.
    c. gastritis.
    d. gastroesophageal reflux (GER).

21. In preschool children, GER may manifest with:
    a. symptoms of heartburn and reswallowing.
    b. intermittent vomiting.
    c. respiratory conditions such as bronchospasm and pneumonia.
    d. failure to thrive, bleeding, and dysphagia.

22. Which of the following information given to the parents about administration of a proton pump inhibitor for the treatment of GER is correct?
    a. The medication is administered on a full stomach.
    b. The medication is administered 30 minutes before breakfast.
    c. The medication will be immediately effective in suppressing acid formation.
    d. Side effects of the drug include increased fatigue, dry mouth, and bloating.

23. The nurse instructs the parents of a 4-month-old with GER to:
    a. stop breast-feeding, because breast milk is too thin and easily leads to reflux.
    b. place the infant in the prone position after feeding only if the infant is awake and well supervised.
    c. increase the infant's intake of fruit and citrus juices.
    d. try to increase feeding volume right before bedtime because this is the time when the stomach is better able to retain foods.

24. The child with irritable bowel syndrome is most likely to present with:
    a. history of alternating diarrhea and constipation, recurrent abdominal pain, and bloating.
    b. alternating patterns of constipation and bloody diarrhea with little flatulence.
    c. history of parasitic infections, poor nutrition, and low abdominal pain.
    d. history of colic, laxative abuse, and growth retardation.

25. What are the classic first symptoms of appendicitis?

26. Which of the following would alert the nurse to possible peritonitis from a ruptured appendix in a child suspected of having appendicitis?
    a. Colicky abdominal pain with guarding of the abdomen
    b. Periumbilical pain that progresses to the lower right quadrant of the abdomen with an elevated white blood cell count
    c. Low-grade fever of 38° C (100.6° F) with the child demonstrating difficulty walking and assuming a side-lying position with the knees flexed toward the chest
    d. Temperature of 38.8° C (102° F), rigid guarding of the abdomen, and sudden relief from abdominal pain

27. a. What is the name given to the most intense site of pain in appendicitis?

    b. Where is this site located?

    c. What is the term used to describe pain elicited by deep percussion and sudden release, indicating the presence of peritoneal irritation?

28. The clinical manifestations expected with Meckel diverticulum include:
    a. fever, vomiting, and constipation.
    b. weight loss, hypotension, and obstruction.
    c. painless rectal bleeding, abdominal pain, or intestinal obstruction.
    d. abdominal pain, bloody diarrhea, and foul-smelling stool.

29. A common feature of inflammatory bowel diseases (IBD) in pediatric patients is:
    a. growth failure.
    b. chronic constipation.
    c. obstruction.
    d. burning epigastric pain.

30. Describe the pathophysiologic differences between Crohn disease (CD) and ulcerative colitis (UC).

31. Which of the following is used to visualize the surface of the GI tract to diagnose the extent of inflammation and narrowing in IBD?
    a. Computed tomography
    b. Magnetic resonance imaging
    c. Endoscopy
    d. Ultrasound

32. IBD can be treated with immunomodulators such as 6-mercaptopurine and azathioprine. When the patient is receiving these drugs, which of the following adverse effects can occur?
    a. Anemia
    b. Malignancy
    c. Peripheral neuropathy
    d. Decreased serum calcium levels, leading to osteoporosis

33. The pediatric nurse knows that the child diagnosed with IBD needs nutritional support that includes:
    a. avoiding all foods high in fat.
    b. supplementation with multivitamins, iron, and folic acid.
    c. meal planning for three large meals daily.
    d. using bran as a source for high fiber.

34. The most reliable way to detect peptic ulcer disease in children is:
    a. fiberoptic endoscopy.
    b. an upper GI series.
    c. C urea breath test.
    d. complete blood count with differential, erythrocyte sedimentation rate, and stool analysis.

35. Billy, age 14, has an ulcer involving the mucosa of the stomach that has resulted from prolonged use of nonsteroidal antiinflammatory agents. The best term to describe Billy's ulcer is:
    a. secondary duodenal ulcer.
    b. primary duodenal ulcer.
    c. secondary gastric ulcer.
    d. primary gastric ulcer.

36. Which of the following is not thought to contribute to peptic ulcer disease?
    a. *H. pylori*
    b. Alcohol and smoking
    c. Caffeine-containing beverages and spicy foods
    d. Psychologic factors such as stressful life events

37. Triple-drug therapy is the recommended treatment regimen for *H. pylori*. Identify three examples of drug combinations used in triple therapy.

38. Common therapeutic management of peptic ulcer disease includes histamine receptor antagonists. Which of the following medications is an example of this drug class?
    a. Bismuth subsalicylate
    b. Famotidine (Pepcid)
    c. Omeprazole (Prilosec)
    d. Sulfasalazine

39. Which of the following is the term used to describe impaired motility of the GI tract?
    a. Malrotation
    b. Obstipation
    c. Abdominal distention
    d. Paralytic ileus

40. Justin, age 1 month, is brought to the clinic by his mother. The nurse suspects pyloric stenosis. Which of the following symptoms would support this theory?
    a. Diarrhea
    b. Projectile vomiting
    c. Fever and dehydration
    d. Abdominal distention

41. Preoperatively, the nursing plan for suspected pyloric obstruction should include:
     i. observation for dehydration.
     ii. keeping body temperature below 37.7° C (100° F).
     iii. parental support and reassurance.
     iv. observation for coughing and gagging after feeding.
     v. observation of quality of stool.

     a. i, ii, iii, iv, and v
     b. i, iii, and iv
     c. iii, iv, and v
     d. i, iii, and v

42. Postoperative feedings for the infant who has undergone a pyloromyotomy include:
     a. keeping NPO for the first 24 hours, then introducing normal formula.
     b. glucose and electrolyte feedings beginning 4 to 6 hours after surgery and continuing for the first 72 hours.
     c. small, frequent feedings of glucose and electrolytes within 24 hours after surgery.
     d. thickened formula feeding within 24 hours after surgery.

43. An invagination of one portion of the intestine into another is called:
     a. intussusception.
     b. pyloric stenosis.
     c. tracheoesophageal fistula.
     d. Hirschsprung disease.

44. Al, age 5 months, is suspected of having intussusception. What clinical manifestations would he most likely have?
     a. Crampy abdominal pain, inconsolable crying, a drawing up of the knees to the chest, and passage of red currant jelly–like stools
     b. Fever; diarrhea; vomiting; lowered white blood cell count; and tender, distended abdomen
     c. Weight gain, constipation, refusal to eat, and rebound tenderness
     d. Abdominal distention, periodic pain, hypotension, and lethargy

45. Which of the following usually indicates that the intussusception has reduced itself?
     a. Passage of a normal brown stool
     b. Increase in appetite
     c. Hyperactive bowel sounds
     d. Normal complete blood count

46. Al's intussusception is reduced without surgery. The nurse should expect care for Al after the reduction to include:
     a. administration of antibiotics.
     b. enema administration to remove remaining stool.
     c. observation of stools.
     d. rectal temperatures every 4 hours.

47. Abnormal rotation of the intestine is called _____. When the intestine completely twists around itself,

     it is termed _____.

48. Symptoms in celiac disease include stools that are:
     a. fatty, frothy, bulky, and foul smelling.
     b. currant jelly–appearing.
     c. small, frothy, and dark green.
     d. white with an ammonia-like smell.

49. The most important therapeutic management for the child with celiac disease is:
     a. eliminating corn, rice, and millet from the diet.
     b. adding iron, folic acid, and fat-soluble vitamins to the diet.
     c. eliminating wheat, rye, barley, and oats from the diet.
     d. educating the child's parents about the short-term effects of the disease and the necessity of reading all food labels for content until the disease is in remission.

50. The prognosis for children with short-bowel syndrome has improved as a result of:
    a. dietary supplement of vitamin B$_{12}$.
    b. improvement in surgical procedures to correct the defect.
    c. improved home care availability.
    d. total parenteral nutrition and enteral feeding.

51. Jerry, a 4-year-old, is brought to the emergency department by his parents, who say he vomited a large amount of bright red blood. Jerry is pale, is cool to the touch, and has increased respiratory rate and heart rate. The nurse expects priority care at this time to include:
    a. administration of intravenous fluids, usually normal saline or lactated Ringer solution.
    b. stool testing for blood by hemoccult.
    c. insertion of a nasogastric tube for ice-water lavage.
    d. preparation for tracheostomy.

52. Match each type of viral hepatitis with its description. (Types may be used more than once.)

    a. Hepatitis A (HAV)   d. Hepatitis D (HDV)
    b. Hepatitis B (HBV)   e. Hepatitis E (HEV)
    c. Hepatitis C (HCV)   f. Hepatitis G (HGV)

    _____ Spread directly or indirectly by fecal-oral route with a routine vaccination available

    _____ Virus with incubation period of 15 to 50 days

    _____ Non-A, non-B with transmission through the fecal-oral route or with contaminated water

    _____ Spread directly and indirectly by the fecal-oral route

    _____ Occurs in children already infected with HBV

    _____ Often becomes a chronic condition and can cause cirrhosis and hepatocellular carcinoma; the leading reason for liver transplant in the United States

    _____ Incubation period 45 to 160 days; average 120 days

    _____ Universal vaccination recommended for all newborns

    _____ Blood-borne virus that affects high-risk groups, including individuals infected with HCV; transmitted also by organ transplantation; unknown incubation period

53. Sandy, age 2, is brought to the clinic by her mother because a toddler who attends Sandy's daycare center has been diagnosed with hepatitis A. Sandy's mother is concerned that Sandy might develop the disease. Which of the following serum laboratory tests would indicate to the nurse that Sandy has immunity to hepatitis A?
    a. Anti-HAV IgG
    b. Anti-HAV IgM
    c. HAsAg
    d. HAcAg

54. Which of the following would indicate the patient has been immunized with HBV vaccine?
    a. Anti-HBs
    b. Anti-HBs and anti-HBc
    c. HBsAg
    d. Anti-HBc

55. Sandy's testing reflects that she has not had hepatitis A. Because her exposure to hepatitis A occurred within the past 2 weeks, the nurse would expect the physician to order prophylactic administration for:
    a. hepatitis B immune globulin (HBIG).
    b. HBV vaccine.
    c. standard immune globulin (IG).
    d. HAV vaccine.

56. What are the four major goals of management for viral hepatitis?

57. Which of the following would not be expected in the child diagnosed with cirrhosis?
    a. Hepatosplenomegaly
    b. Elevated liver function tests
    c. Decreased ammonia levels
    d. Ascites

58. Brian, 16 years old, has been diagnosed with cirrhosis. The health care practitioner has ordered daily administration of lactulose. What is the rationale for the use of this drug?
    a. Decreases ascites
    b. Decreases bleeding from the esophageal varices
    c. Decreases the formation of ammonia
    d. Improves absorption of fat-soluble vitamins

CRITICAL THINKING—CASE STUDY

Danny, age 17, is a junior in high school. He comes to the clinic with complaints of right lower abdominal pain and slight fever.

59. What questions should be included in the history of present illness if appendicitis is suspected?

60. Which of the following should Danny be advised to avoid until he is seen by the physician?
    a. All activity
    b. All laxatives
    c. Ice to the abdomen
    d. All of the above

61. Danny is admitted to the hospital with a diagnosis of acute appendicitis. Which of the following independent nursing actions should the nurse institute?
    a. Allow clear liquids only.
    b. Start intravenous fluids with antibiotics.
    c. Insert a nasogastric tube and connect to suction.
    d. Monitor closely for progression of symptoms.

62. What laboratory blood evaluation and results would the nurse expect to see in a patient with acute appendicitis?

63. Danny is now 2 hours postoperative. During surgery, his appendix was found to have ruptured before surgery. A priority nursing diagnosis at this time would be:
    a. High risk for spread of infection related to rupture.
    b. Pain related to inflamed appendix.
    c. Altered growth and development related to hospital care.
    d. Anxiety related to knowledge deficit regarding disease.

64. Which of the following is the most critical outcome for Danny after surgery?
    a. Danny's peritonitis has resolved as evidenced by no fever, lack of elevated white blood cell count, and a wound that is clean and healing.
    b. Danny's pain is relieved as evidenced by no verbalization of pain and the fact that Danny is resting quietly.
    c. Danny and his family demonstrate understanding of hospitalization.
    d. Danny is able to express feelings and concerns.

Jose, age 3 years, is brought to the clinic by his mother because he has not had a bowel movement in 3 days. His parents are migrant workers and have just returned home from working in a northern state picking crops. As you enter the examining room, Jose appears active and happy. He is running around in the room and playing with toys.

65. What history would you obtain from the mother related to the chief complaint?

66. It has been determined by physical examination that Jose has no evidence of a pathologic condition that is resulting in his constipation.
    a. What would your major nursing tasks with this family include in relation to Jose's constipation?

    b. What information would you provide to Jose's mother related to his constipation?

34 The Child with Cardiovascular Dysfunction

1. The following terms are related to cardiac structure and function. Match each term with its description.

a. Congenital heart defects
b. Acquired cardiac disorders
c. Mediastinum
d. Myocardium
e. Endocardium
f. Pericardium

g. Pericardial space
h. Pericardial fluid
i. Atria
j. Ventricles
k. Valves
l. Tricuspid valve

m. Mitral valve
n. Atrioventricular (AV) valves
o. Chordae tendineae
p. Semilunar valves

_____ Structures located in the pulmonary artery (pulmonic valve) and the aorta (aortic valve) that prevent backflow of blood

_____ A few drops of serous fluid normally found between the two layers of membrane that cover the heart

_____ Located between left atrium and the left ventricle; prevents flow from the right ventricle back into the left ventricle

_____ The two bottom chambers of the interior of the heart

_____ A double-walled membrane that forms a covering for the heart

_____ The muscular tissue that forms the main mass of the heart

_____ Disease processes or abnormalities that occur after birth; can be seen in the normal heart or in the presence of congenital heart defects

_____ Prevent backflow in the heart

_____ Anatomic abnormalities present at birth that result in abnormal cardiac function

_____ Located between the right atrium and the right ventricle; prevents flow from the right ventricle back into the right atrium

_____ A thin layer of endothelial tissue that lines the inner surface of the myocardium

_____ The two upper chambers of the interior of the heart

_____ The space between the two pleural cavities

_____ Term used to describe both the mitral valve and the tricuspid valve together

_____ Cordlike structures that attach AV valves to the heart muscle

_____ The slight space between the two layers of membrane that cover the heart

2. Match each of the following embryologic development terms with its description.

a. Endocardial cushions
b. Common atrium/ventricle
c. Bulbus cordis
d. Sinus venosus
e. Truncus arteriosus

f. Atrial septum
g. Foramen ovale
h. Ventricular septum
i. Muscular septum
j. Membranous septum

k. Ductus venosus
l. Ductus arteriosus
m. Coronary arteries
n. Coronary veins

_____ Develops into the inferior and superior vena cava

_____ The vessel that allows blood to travel directly to the inferior vena cava before birth

_____ Embryologic internal bulges that eventually merge to divide the heart chambers

_____ The structure that permits blood to be shunted to the descending aorta from the pulmonary artery before birth

_____ Eventually helps to form the outflow tracts of the ventricles

_____ Develops out of an intricate growth of the endocardial cushions, conal cushions, and conotruncal septum

_____ Collect blood and return it directly to the right atrium or through the coronary sinus that drains into the right atrium

_____ Divides into the pulmonary artery and aorta and gives rise to the aortic arch

_____ Structures that begin to be formed at about the fifth week of gestation; ultimately give rise to the heart chambers

_____ Develops from the joining of the muscular and membranous ventricular septa during the fourth to eighth week of embryologic growth

_____ A temporary flap opening that is formed from the overlapping of the septum primum and the septum secundum before they fuse

_____ Develops when the right and left ventricular chambers fuse

_____ Supply the heart muscle with its blood supply; arise above the aortic valve

_____ Formed by the growth of septum primum and septum secundum at about the fourth week of fetal growth

3. The following terms are related to the conduction system and physiology. Match each term with its description.

a. Cardiac cycle	g. Afterload	m. Bradycardia
b. Systole	h. Systemic vascular resistance	n. Tachypnea
c. Diastole	i. Pulmonary vascular resistance	o. Sinoatrial node
d. Cardiac output	j. Contractility	p. AV node
e. Stroke volume	k. Starling's law	q. Bundle of His
f. Preload	l. Tachycardia	r. Purkinje fibers

_____ The efficiency of myocardial fiber shortening; the ability of the cardiac muscle to act as an efficient pump

_____ The amount of blood ejected by the heart in any one contraction

_____ Part of the cardiac conduction system; the heart's usual pacemaker; located within the right atrium near the opening of the superior vena cava

_____ Slow heart rate

_____ Composed of sequential contraction and relaxation of both the atria and the ventricles

_____ Fast heart rate

_____ The volume of blood ejected by the heart in 1 minute

_____ Part of the cardiac conduction system; extends from the AV node along each side of the interventricular septum and divides into right and left bundle branches

_____ Refers to the resistance against which the ventricles must pump when ejecting blood; blood pressure gives some indication of this resistance

_____ Contraction of both the atria and ventricles

_____ The resistance of the pulmonary circulation

_____ Relaxation of both the atria and the ventricles

_____ The volume of blood returning to the heart; the circulation blood volume

_____ Part of the cardiac conduction system; located within the right atrium at the low part of the septum

_____ The principle that demonstrates that an increase in ventricular end-diastolic volume somewhat increases stroke volume

_____ Part of the cardiac conduction system; these strands of conduction tissue extend from the AV bundle into the walls of the ventricles

_____ Resistance of the systemic circulation

_____ Fast respiratory rate

4. Match each wave form term with its description.

a. P wave
b. P-R interval
c. QRS complex

d. T wave
e. Q-T interval
f. ST segment

_____ Represents ventricular repolarization

_____ Represents the spread of the impulse over the atria (atrial depolarization); sinus node's electrical activity not represented in the electrocardiogram (ECG)

_____ Represents ventricular depolarization and repolarization; interval varies with heart rate—faster heart rates decrease the interval, interval is normally shorter in children than in adults

_____ Represents the time that elapses from the beginning of atrial depolarization to the beginning of ventricular depolarization

_____ Represents the time that the ventricles are in absolute refractory period—the period between ventricular depolarization and repolarizaton

_____ Represents ventricular depolarization; actually composed of three separate waves that result from the currents generated when the ventricles depolarize before their contraction

5. Match each test of cardiac function term with its description.

a. Chest radiograph
b. Electrocardiography (ECG, EKG)
c. Holter monitor
d. Echocardiography
e. Transthoracic echocardiography
f. M-mode echocardiography
g. Two-dimensional echocardiography
h. Doppler echocardiography
i. Fetal echocardiography

j. Transesophageal echocardiography
k. Cardiac catheterization
l. Hemodynamics
m. Angiography
n. Biopsy
o. Electrophysiology
p. Exercise stress test
q. Right-sided cardiac catheterization

r. Left-sided cardiac catheterization
s. Interventional cardiac catheterization
t. Diagnostic electrophysiologic catheterization
u. Interventional electrophysiologic catheterization
v. Cardiac magnetic resonance imaging

_____ Uses catheters with tiny electrodes that record the heart's electrical impulses directly from the conduction system to evaluate and treat dysrhythmias

_____ Newest noninvasive imaging technique; used in evaluation of vascular anatomy outside of heart (e.g., coarctation of the aorta, vascular rings) and in estimates of ventricular mass and volume; uses are expanding

_____ Venous; diagnostic catheterization of the venous side in which the catheter is introduced from a vein into the right atrium

_____ Type of echocardiography that uses real-time, cross-sectional views of heart; used to identify cardiac structures and cardiac anatomy

_____ An alternative to surgery in some congenital heart defects, such as isolated valvular pulmonic stenosis and patent ductus arteriosus

_____ Type of echocardiography that obtains a one-dimensional graphic view; used to estimate ventricular size and function

_____ Measures pressure and oxygen saturation in heart chambers

_____ Graphic measure of the electrical activity of the heart

_____ Type of echocardiography that images the fetal heart in utero

_____ Use of contrast material to illuminate heart structures and blood-flow patterns

_____ Use of high-frequency sound waves obtained by a transducer to produce an image of cardiac structures

_____ Type of echocardiography that uses a transducer placed in the esophagus behind the heart to obtain images of the posterior heart structures in patients with poor images from the chest approach

_____ Employs a special catheter with electrodes to record electrical activity from within heart; used to diagnose rhythm disturbances

_____ An alternative to surgery for some congenital heart defects

_____ Use of special catheter to remove tiny samples of heart muscle for microscopic evaluation; used for assessing infection, inflammation, or muscle dysfunction disorders; also used to evaluate for rejection after heart transplant

_____ Provides information about heart size and pulmonary blood flow

_____ Type of echocardiography done with transducer on chest

_____ Type of echocardiography that identifies blood-flow patterns and pressure gradients across structures

_____ Arterial; diagnostic catheterization of the arterial side in which the catheter is threaded retrograde into the aorta or from a right-sided approach to the left atrium by means of a septal puncture or through an existing septal opening

_____ 24-hour continuous ECG recording used to assess dysrhythmias

_____ Imaging study using radiopaque catheters placed in a peripheral blood vessel and advanced into the heart to measure pressures and oxygen levels in heart chambers and to visualize heart structures and blood-flow patterns

_____ Monitoring of heart rate, blood pressure, ECG, and oxygen consumption at rest and during progressive exercise on a treadmill or bicycle

6. Match each congenital heart disease term with its description.

a. Left-to-right shunt
b. Acyanotic-cyanotic defects
c. Hemodynamic characteristics
d. Cor pulmonale

e. Right-sided failure
f. Left-sided failure
g. Cardiac reserve

_____ Dysfunction that results in increased end-diastolic pressure with lung congestion and pulmonary edema

_____ Term for heart failure resulting from obstructive lung diseases such as cystic fibrosis or bronchopulmonary dysplasia

_____ Traditional categories of congenital heart defects that divide defects based on a physical characteristic; problematic because of the complexity of the many defects and the variability of their clinical manifestations

_____ Dysfunction that results in systemic venous hypertension that in turn causes hepatomegaly and edema

_____ The directional flow from an area of higher pressure to one of lower pressure in congenital heart disease

_____ The compensatory mechanisms that initially try to meet the body's demand for increased cardiac output, including hypertrophy and dilation of the cardiac muscle and stimulation of the sympathetic nervous system

_____ A useful classification system for congenital heart defects that uses movements involved in circulation of blood

7. The following terms are related to the clinical manifestations of congenital heart disease. Match each term with its description.

a. Gallop rhythm
b. Diaphoresis
c. Poor perfusion
d. Mild cyanosis
e. Dyspnea
f. Costal retractions
g. Pulmonary edema
h. Orthopnea
i. Wheezing

j. Cough
k. Hoarseness
l. Gasping, grunting respirations
m. Developmental delays
n. Hepatomegaly
o. Edema
p. Weight gain
q. Ascites, pleural effusions
r. Distended veins

_____ Dyspnea in the recumbent position

_____ Manifested by cold extremities, weak pulses, slow capillary refill, low blood pressure, and mottled skin

_____ A late sign of heart failure

_____ Extra heart sounds S_3 and S_4 resulting from ventricular dilation and excess preload

_____ Occurs as the pliable chest wall in the infant is drawn inward during attempts to ventilate the noncompliant lungs

_____ Results from poor weight gain and activity intolerance

_____ Occurs when the pulmonary capillary pressure exceeds the plasma osmotic pressure and fluid is forced into the interstitial space

_____ Caused by mucosal swelling and irritation of the bronchial mucosa

_____ Result from a consistently elevated central venous pressure; venous return is slow; difficult to detect in the short, fat neck of infants; usually observed only in older children

_____ Occurs from pooling of blood in the portal circulation and transudation of fluid into the hepatic tissues

_____ Results from impaired gas exchange and is relieved with oxygen administration

_____ Caused by edema of the bronchial mucosa from obstruction to airflow

_____ Forms from sodium and water retention that causes systemic vascular pressure to rise

_____ Caused by pressure from edema on the laryngeal nerve

_____ Caused by decrease in the distensibility of the lungs; initially may be evident only on exertion; in infants may be accompanied by flaring nares

_____ The earliest sign of edema

_____ Often seen during exertion when myocardial function is impaired; in children, especially noted on the head

_____ Later signs of gross fluid accumulation that is usually generalized and difficult to detect in infants

8. The following terms are related to the therapeutic management of heart failure. Match each term with its description.

a. Digoxin
b. Angiotensin-converting enzyme (ACE) inhibitors
c. Lisinopril, captopril, enalapril
d. Furosemide

e. Chlorothiazide
f. Spironolactone
g. Carvedilol

_____ Coreg; a beta blocker; blocks α- and β-adrenergic receptors, causing decreased heart rate, decreased blood pressure, and vasodilation; used selectively in children; improves symptoms and left ventricular function

_____ Aldactone; blocks action of aldosterone to produce diuresis; allows retention of potassium

_____ Diuril; acts directly on distal tubules and possibly proximal tubules to decrease sodium, water, potassium, chloride, and bicarbonate absorption; decreases urinary diluting capacity; may need to supplement potassium

_____ Cause vasodilation that decreases pulmonary and systemic vascular resistance, decreased blood pressure, reduced afterload, and decreased right and left atrial pressures

_____ Lasix; blocks reabsorption of sodium and water to produce diuresis

_____ Lanoxin; used because of its rapid onset and decreased risk for toxicity; increases the force of contraction (positive inotropic effect), decreases the heart rate (negative chronotropic effect), slows the conduction of impulses through the AV node (negative dromotropic effect), and indirectly enhances diuresis

_____ ACE inhibitors that are frequently used in pediatrics

9. Match each term with its description.

a. Hypoxemia
b. Hypoxia
c. Cyanosis
d. Right-to-left shunting
e. Eisenmenger syndrome
f. Polycythemia

g. Clubbing
h. Modified Blalock-Taussig shunt
i. Tet spells, hypercyanotic spells
j. Cerebrovascular accidents (CVAs)
k. Bacterial endocarditis
l. Palliative shunt

_____ Uses a Gore-Tex or Impra tube graft to create a communication between the subclavian artery and the pulmonary artery to increase blood flow to the lungs; the preferred palliative treatment for severely hypoxemic newborns

_____ May occur in any child whose heart defect includes obstruction to pulmonary blood flow and communication between the ventricles; acute cyanotic episode with hyperpnea; characteristically seen in children with unrepaired tetralogy of Fallot

_____ An increased number of red blood cells

_____ A reduction in tissue oxygenation that results from low Sao_2

_____ A palliative surgical procedure that serves the same purpose as the ductus arteriosus; increases blood flow to the lungs through a systemic-to–pulmonary artery connection

_____ Results from severe obstruction to pulmonary blood flow; desaturated venous blood enters the systemic circulation without passing through the lungs and cyanosis is present; most commonly caused by tetralogy of Fallot

_____ Strokes; occur in about 2% of the children with hypoxia

_____ An arterial oxygen tension (or pressure, Pao_2) that is less than normal and can be identified by decreased arterial oxygen saturation (Sao_2) or decreased Pao_2

_____ Thickening and flattening of the tips of the fingers and toes; thought to occur because of chronic tissue hypoxemia and polycythemia

_____ Increased risk for this disorder in children who are cyanotic, especially those who have systemic-to-pulmonary shunts

_____ A syndrome in which a left-to-right shunt becomes a right-to-left shunt because of a progressive increase in pulmonary vascular resistance

_____ A blue discoloration in the mucous membranes, skin, and nail beds of the child with reduced oxygen saturation; results from the presence of deoxygenated hemoglobin

10. The following terms are related to acquired disorders. Match each term with its description.

a. Rheumatic fever
b. Aschoff bodies
c. Carditis
d. Polyarthritis
e. Erythema marginatum
f. Subcutaneous nodules
g. Chorea, Sydenham chorea
h. Antistreptolysin O (ASLO) titer

i. Ectasia
j. Stage 1 hypertension
k. Primary hypertension
l. Secondary hypertension
m. Stage 2 hypertension
n. Hyperlipidemia
o. Hypercholesterolemia
p. Atherosclerosis
q. Coronary artery disease

r. Cholesterol
s. Triglycerides
t. Chylomicrons
u. Very low–density lipoproteins
v. Low-density lipoprotein
w. High-density lipoproteins
x. Population approach
y. Individualized approach

_____ Fatty plaques on the arteries

_____ Measures the concentration of antibodies formed in the blood against a product that is present in streptococcal infection in children

_____ Primary cause of morbidity and mortality in the adult population

_____ Formed in rheumatic heart disease; inflammatory, hemorrhagic, bullous lesions; causes swelling, fragmentation, and alterations in the connective tissue

_____ Dilation

_____ Major cardiac manifestation of rheumatic fever; involves the endocardium, pericardium, and myocardium

_____ A fatlike steroid alcohol; part of the lipoprotein complex in plasma that is essential for cellular metabolism

_____ Essential hypertension; no identifiable cause

_____ Caused by edema, inflammation, and effusions in joint tissue; reversible; migratory; favors large joints such as knees, elbows, hips, shoulders, and wrists; usually accompanies the acute febrile period in rheumatic fever

_____ Contain low concentrations of triglycerides, high levels of cholesterol, and moderate levels of protein; high levels are a strong risk factor in cardiovascular disease

_____ Small, nontender swellings that persist indefinitely after the onset of rheumatic fever and gradually resolve with no resulting damage

_____ A poorly understood autoimmune reaction to group A β-hemolytic streptococcal pharyngitis; self-limiting disease that involves the joints, skin, brain, serous surface, and heart; cardiac valve damage is the most serious consequence

_____ Contains very low concentrations of triglycerides, relatively little cholesterol, and high levels of protein; thought to protect against cardiovascular disease

_____ A general term for excessive lipids

_____ Also called "St. Vitus dance"; characterized by sudden, aimless, irregular movements of the extremities; involuntary facial grimaces, speech disturbances, emotional lability, and muscle weakness that can be profound in rheumatic fever; exaggerated by anxiety and attempts at deliberate fine motor activity and relieved by rest, especially sleep

_____ Natural fats synthesized from carbohydrates

_____ Blood pressures that fall persistently between the 95th and 99th percentile plus 5 mm Hg for age, sex, and height

_____ A distinct erythematous macule with a clear center and wavy, well-demarcated border; transitory nonpruritic rash found most often on the trunk and proximal portion of the extremities in rheumatic fever

_____ Produced in the intestine in response to the intake of dietary fat; principal transporter of dietary fat

_____ Hypertension that has an identifiable cause; significant hypertension; a blood pressure that is consistently between the 95th and 99th percentile for age and sex

_____ Blood pressure persistently at or above the 99th percentile for age and sex

_____ An approach to controlling hypercholesterolemia that is based on selective screening

_____ Refers to excessive cholesterol in the blood

_____ Contains high concentrations of triglycerides, moderate concentrations of cholesterol, and little protein

_____ Aims to lower the average levels of blood cholesterol among all U.S. children through population-wide changes in nutrient intake and eating patterns

11. The following terms are related to the correction of defects. Match each term with its description.

a. Median sternotomy   d. Intracardiac monitoring   g. Cardiac tamponade
b. Thoracotomy incision   e. Low cardiac output syndrome   h. Seizure
c. Intraarterial monitoring   f. Dysrhythmias   i. Neurologic complications

_____ May occur in the postperative cardiac surgery pediatric patient from hypothermia or inability to maintain systemic circulation

_____ The most common neurologic complication of open-heart surgery; most often occurring in infants

_____ Compression of the heart by blood and other effusion (clots) in the pericardial sac

_____ The most commonly used technique for opening the chest to correct cardiac defects in children; follows the sternum down the center of the chest

_____ Can result from electrolyte imbalance, especially hypokalemia, and surgical intervention to the septum or myocardium

_____ Almost always used after open-heart surgery to measure blood pressure; more reliable than indirect blood pressure readings and provides continuous rather than intermittent monitoring

_____ Uncommon after open-heart surgery, but can be devastating; require ongoing assessments for early intervention—equality of strength and reflexes in both extremities for evidence of paralysis; pupil size, equality, reaction to light, and accommodation; the child's orientation to the environment

_____ Provides data on cardiac function and output; allows assessment of pressures inside the cardiac chambers, giving information about blood volume, cardiac output, ventricular function, pulmonary artery pressures, and responses to drug therapy

_____ The most uncomfortable technique for opening the chest to correct cardiac defects in children; cuts through muscle tissue; allows access to the side of the chest through an incision from under the arm around the back to the scapula

12. The following terms are related to cardiac dysrhythmias. Match each term with its description.

a. Sinus bradycardia
b. Sinus tachycardia
c. Supraventicular tachycardia
d. AV blocks
e. Electrophysiologic cardiac catheterization
f. Transesophageal recording
g. Vagal maneuvers
h. Transesophageal atrial overdrive pacing

i. Synchronized cardioversion
j. Permanent pacemaker
k. Pulse generator
l. Lead
m. Epicardial lead
n. Orthotopic heart transplantation
o. Heterotopic heart transplantation

_____ Applying ice to the face, massaging the carotid artery on one side of the neck only, or having the child perform a Valsalva maneuver; used to treat supraventricular tachycardia

_____ Leaving the recipient's own heart in place and implanting a new heart to act as an additional pump or "piggyback" heart; rarely used in children

_____ The most common dysrhythmia found in children; a rapid, regular heart rate of 200 to 300 beats/min

_____ Most often related to edema around the conduction system and resolved without treatment

_____ Used often for children with postsurgical AV block; takes over or assists in the heart's conduction function

_____ Composed of a battery and the electronic circuitry

_____ Allows for identification of the conduction disturbance and immediate investigation of drugs that may control the dysrhythmia; selective induction of the dysrhythmia and treatment under observation

_____ Accomplished through placement of a protected lead into the esophagus behind the left atrium of the heart; lead is then attached to a stimulator capable of pacing at a very rapid rate to interrupt the tachydysrhythmia

_____ An insulated, flexible wire that conducts electrical impulses

_____ An electrode catheter passed into the esophagus and, when in position at a point proximal to the heart, used to stimulate and record dysrhythmias

_____ May result from the influence of the autonomic nervous system or in response to hypoxia and hypotension

_____ The timed delivery of a preset amount of energy through the chest wall in an attempt to reestablish an organized rhythm

_____ A wire that is directly attached to the heart and conducts impulses

_____ Removing the recipient's own heart and implanting a new heart from a donor

_____ Usually secondary to fever, anxiety, pain, anemia, dehydration, or any factor that requires increased cardiac output

13. The embryologic development of the heart results in a heartbeat by the:
    a. fourth week.
    b. fifth week.
    c. sixth week.
    d. eighth week.

14. During embryologic development of the lower heart, the muscular septum develops from:
    a. fusion of the chambers of the common ventricle.
    b. growth of endocardial cushions.
    c. growth of the conal cushions.
    d. fusion of the conotruncal septum.

15. The process of the formation of the heart's atrial septum results in a temporary flap called the:
    a. truncus arteriosus.
    b. foramen ovale.
    c. sinus venosus.
    d. ductus venosus.

16. In fetal circulation the umbilical vein divides and sends blood directly to the inferior vena cava by way of the ductus venosus. This division occurs at the:
    a. heart.
    b. lungs.
    c. liver.
    d. placenta.

17. In fetal circulation the majority of the most oxygenated blood is pumped through the:
    a. foramen ovale.
    b. lungs.
    c. liver.
    d. coronary sinus.

18. When obtaining a history from the parents of an infant suspected to have altered cardiac function, the nurse would expect to hear:
    a. specific concerns related to palpitations the infant is having.
    b. feeding difficulty, sweating with feedings, and poor weight gain.
    c. specific concerns about the infant's shortness of breath.
    d. all of the above.

19. A clue in the mother's history that is important in the diagnosis of congenital heart disease is:
    a. rheumatoid arthritis.
    b. rheumatic fever.
    c. streptococcal infection.
    d. rubella.

20. Coarctation of the aorta should be suspected when:
    a. the blood pressure in the arms is different from the blood pressure in the legs.
    b. the blood pressure in the right arm is different from the blood pressure in the left arm.
    c. apical pulse is greater than the radial pulse.
    d. point of maximum impulse is shifted to the left.

21. Of the following descriptions, the heart sound that would be considered normal in a young child is:
    a. splitting of S_1.
    b. splitting of S_2.
    c. splitting of S_3.
    d. splitting of S_4.

22. The standard pediatric ECG has:
    a. 6 leads.
    b. 12 leads.
    c. 15 leads.
    d. 18 leads.

23. The test that requires intravenous sedation and has been used increasingly in recent years to confirm the diagnosis of a congenital heart defect without a cardiac catheterization is the:
    a. ECG.
    b. echocardiogram.
    c. transesophageal echocardiogram.
    d. two-dimensional echocardiogram.

24. In children, the usual approach to the left ventricle of the heart in a cardiac catheterization is through the:
    a. left side of the heart.
    b. right side of the heart.

25. List at least five of the most significant signs of complications after a cardiac catheterization in an infant or young child.

26. If bleeding occurs at the insertion site after a cardiac catheterization, the nurse should apply:
    a. warmth to the unaffected extremity.
    b. pressure 1 inch below the insertion site.
    c. warmth to the affected extremity.
    d. pressure 1 inch above the insertion site.

27. When children develop heart failure from a congenital heart defect, the failure is usually:
    a. right-sided only.
    b. left-sided only.
    c. cor pulmonale.
    d. both right- and left-sided.

28. Which of the following heart rates would be considered tachycardia in an infant?
    a. A resting heart rate of 120 beats/min
    b. A crying heart rate of 200 beats/min
    c. A resting heart rate of 170 beats/min
    d. A crying heart rate of 180 beats/min

29. Pulmonary congestion in an infant may be identified by:
    a. inability to feed.
    b. mild cyanosis.
    c. costal retractions.
    d. all of the above.

30. Developmental delays in the infant with heart failure are most pronounced in the:
    a. fine motor areas.
    b. gross motor areas.
    c. social skill areas.
    d. cognitive areas.

31. Evaluation of the infant for edema is different from that of the older child in that:
    a. weight is not reliable as an early sign.
    b. pedal edema is most pronounced in the newborn.
    c. edema is usually generalized and difficult to detect.
    d. distended neck veins are the most reliable sign.

32. In the child taking digoxin, ECG signs that the drug is having the intended effect are:
    a. prolonged P-R interval and slowed ventricular rate.
    b. shortened P-R interval and slowed ventricular rate.
    c. prolonged P-R interval and faster ventricular rate.
    d. shortened P-R interval and faster ventricular rate.

33. The three ACE inhibitors most commonly used for children with heart failure are:
    a. digoxin, furosemide, and captopril.
    b. enalapril, captopril, and lisinopril.
    c. enalapril, captopril, and furosemide.
    d. spironolactone, furosemide, and captopril.

34. The electrolyte that is usually depleted with most diuretic therapy and is most likely to cause dysrhythmias is:
    a. sodium.
    b. chloride.
    c. potassium.
    d. magnesium.

35. The nutritional needs of the infant with heart failure are usually:
    a. the same as an adult's.
    b. less than a healthy infant's.
    c. the same as a healthy infant's.
    d. greater than a healthy infant's.

36. The calories are usually increased for an infant with heart failure by:
    a. increasing the number of feedings.
    b. introducing solids into the diet.
    c. increasing the density of the formula.
    d. gastrostomy feeding.

37. Chronic hypoxemia is manifested clinically by:
    a. fatigue.
    b. polycythemia.
    c. clubbing.
    d. All of the above

38. Prostaglandin is administered to the newborn with a congenital heart defect to:
    a. close the patent ductus arteriosus.
    b. keep the ductus arteriosus open.
    c. keep the foramen ovale open.
    d. close the foramen ovale.

39. The presence of poor ventricular function and atrial arrhythmias increases the risk for:
    a. infection.
    b. CVA.
    c. fever.
    d. air embolism.

40. Air embolism may form in the venous system, traveling directly to the brain by way of the arterial system, in the child with:
    a. a right-to-left shunt.
    b. a left-to-right shunt.
    c. dehydration and hypoxemia.
    d. hypernatremia and hypokalemia.

41. Match the type of defect with the specific disorder. (Defects may be used more than once.)

    a. Defects with decreased pulmonary blood flow
    b. Mixed defects

    c. Defects with increased pulmonary blood flow
    d. Obstructive defects

    _____ Patent ductus arteriosus

    _____ Coarctation of the aorta

    _____ Ventricular septal defect

    _____ Subvalvular aortic stenosis

    _____ Hypoplastic left heart syndrome

    _____ AV canal defect

    _____ Pulmonic stenosis

    _____ Tetralogy of Fallot

    _____ Aortic stenosis

    _____ Tricuspid atresia

    _____ Valvular aortic stenosis

    _____ Truncus arteriosus

    _____ Atrial septal defect

    _____ Transposition of the great vessels

    _____ Total anomalous pulmonary venous connection

42. Which of the following defects has the best prognosis?
    a. Tetralogy of Fallot
    b. Ventricular septal defect
    c. Atrial septal defect
    d. Hypoplastic left heart syndrome

43. Which of the following defects has the worst prognosis?
    a. Tetralogy of Fallot
    b. Atrial ventricular canal defect
    c. Transposition of the great vessels
    d. Hypoplastic left heart syndrome

44. The clinical consequences of congenital heart disease fall into two categories which are:
    a. decreased cardiac output and low blood pressure.
    b. heart failure and murmurs.
    c. increased blood pressure and pulse.
    d. murmurs and decreased pulse.

45. Surgical intervention is always necessary in the first year of life when an infant is born with:
    a. atrial septal defect.
    b. ventricular septal defect.
    c. transposition of the great vessels.
    d. patent ductus arteriosus.

46. The best approach for the nurse to use in advising parents about how to discipline the child with a congenital defect is to:
    a. provide the parents with anticipatory guidance.
    b. teach the parents to overcompensate.
    c. help the parents focus on the child's defect.
    d. teach the parents to use benevolent overreaction.

47. For parents using the Internet to obtain information about their child's cardiac diagnosis, it is important for the nurse to remind them that:
    a. information is difficult to access.
    b. most information found will not be helpful.
    c. not all websites offer accurate information.
    d. all of the above.

48. Parents of the child with a congenital heart defect should know the signs of heart failure, which include:
    a. poor feeding.
    b. sudden weight gain.
    c. increased efforts to breathe.
    d. all of the above.

49. List at least three major categories that should be included in a teaching plan for parents of a child with a congenital heart disorder.

50. A visit to the intensive care unit (ICU) before open-heart surgery for a young child should take place:
    a. 1 week before the surgery.
    b. at a busy time with a lot to see and hear.
    c. the day before surgery.
    d. several weeks before the surgery.

51. Children who will undergo cardiac surgery should be informed about:
    a. the location of the intravenous lines.
    b. the pain at the intravenous insertion sites.
    c. the need to lie still at all times after surgery.
    d. all of the above.

52. Which of the following patterns is indicative of infection in the postoperative period following cardiac surgery?
    a. Temperature of 38.6° C (101.5° F) 72 hours after surgery
    b. Temperature of 37.7° C (100° F) 36 hours after surgery
    c. Hypothermia in the early postoperative period
    d. All of the above

53. After cardiac surgery in a child, the central venous pressure (CVP) line may be used to:
    a. administer fluids.
    b. obtain vital information.
    c. act as a central line outside the ICU.
    d. do all of the above.

54. While suctioning an infant after cardiac surgery, the nurse should:
    a. hyperoxygenate before suctioning.
    b. suction for no more than 5 seconds.
    c. provide supplemental oxygen.
    d. perform all of the above.

55. List five observations the nurse should be making while suctioning an infant after cardiac surgery.

56. Which of the following is not a common reason for chest tube drainage in the child after cardiac surgery?
    a. Removal of secretions
    b. Removal of air
    c. Prevention of pneumothorax
    d. Removal of an empyema

57. Which of the following strategies is not acceptable to include in the care of the child before removing chest tube(s) after cardiac surgery?
    a. Explain that the removal is uncomfortable but not painful.
    b. Administer intravenous fentanyl.
    c. Administer intravenous morphine sulfate.
    d. Use a topical anesthetic on the site.

58. The most painful part of cardiac surgery for the child is usually the:
    a. thoracotomy incision site.
    b. graft site on the leg.
    c. sternotomy incision site.
    d. intravenous insertion sites.

59. An infant who weighs 7 kg (15.4 lb) has just returned to the ICU after cardiac surgery. The chest tube has drained 30 ml in the past hour. In this situation, what is the first action for the nurse to take?
    a. Notify the surgeon.
    b. Identify any other signs of hemorrhage.
    c. Suction the patient.
    d. Identify any other signs of renal failure.

60. An infant who weighs 7 kg (15.4 lb) has just returned to the ICU after cardiac surgery. The urinary output has been 20 ml in the past hour. In this situation, what is the first action for the nurse to take?
    a. Notify the surgeon.
    b. Identify any other signs of hypervolemia.
    c. Suction the patient.
    d. Identify any other signs of renal failure.

61. After cardiac surgery, fluid intake calculations for a child would include:
    a. intravenous fluids.
    b. arterial and CVP line flushes.
    c. fluid used to dilute medications.
    d. all of the above.

62. After cardiac surgery, fluid output calculations in a child would include:
    a. nasogastric secretions.
    b. blood drawn for analysis.
    c. chest tube drainage.
    d. all of the above.

63. Fluids are especially important to monitor after cardiac surgery, because during surgery:
    a. the cardiopulmonary pump uses a large volume of extra fluid.
    b. the patient's blood is diluted by the use of the pump.
    c. there is total body edema.
    d. all of the above may occur.

64. One of the strategies the nurse can use to progressively increase a child's activity in the postoperative period after cardiac surgery is:
    a. to expect some degree of dyspnea.
    b. to ambulate on the first day.
    c. to ambulate after analgesic medication.
    d. all of the above.

65. List at least five complications of cardiac surgery in children.

66. Techniques to provide emotional support to the child and family after cardiac surgery include:
    a. realizing that some procedures are too difficult for the child to perform.
    b. encouraging the child to keep being brave.
    c. reassuring the parents that a child's anger or rejection of them is normal.
    d. all of the above.

67. Which of the following patients with bacterial endocarditis (BE) is at highest risk for death?
    a. A 15-year-old with BE caused by a bacterium that is susceptible to ampicillin
    b. A 2-month-old infant with BE caused by a fungus
    c. A 5-year-old child with BE following a mitral valve replacement
    d. A 9-year-old with BE and aortic stenosis

68. One of the most important factors in preventing BE in high-risk patients is:
    a. administration of prophylactic antibiotic therapy.
    b. surgical repair of the defect.
    c. administration of prostaglandin to correct patent ductus arteriosus.
    d. administration of antibiotics after dental work.

69. One of the most common findings on physical examination of the child with acute rheumatic heart disease is:
    a. a systolic murmur.
    b. pleural friction rub.
    c. an ejection click.
    d. a split S_2.

70. The test that provides the most reliable evidence of recent streptococcal infection is the:
    a. throat culture.
    b. Mantoux test.
    c. elevation of liver enzymes.
    d. ASLO test.

71. Children who have been treated for rheumatic fever:
    a. do not need additional prophylaxis against BE.
    b. are immune to rheumatic fever for the rest of their lives.
    c. will have transitory manifestations of chorea for the rest of their lives.
    d. may need antibiotic therapy for years.

72. The peak age for the incidence of Kawasaki disease is in the:
    a. infant age-group.
    b. toddler age-group.
    c. school-age group.
    d. adolescent age-group.

73. Which of the following dosages of aspirin would be considered adequate for the initial treatment of Kawasaki disease for a child who weighs 20 kg (44 lb)?
    a. 80 mg every 6 hours
    b. 100 mg every 6 hours
    c. 500 mg every 6 hours
    d. 2000 mg every 6 hours

74. Kawasaki disease is treated with:
    a. aspirin and immune globulin.
    b. aspirin and cryoprecipitate.
    c. meperidine hydrochloride and immune globulin.
    d. meperidine hydrochloride and cryoprecipitate.

75. Because of the drug used for long-term therapy, children with Kawasaki disease are at risk for:
    a. chickenpox.
    b. influenza.
    c. Reye syndrome.
    d. myocardial infarction.

76. Most cases of hypertension in children are a result of:
    a. essential hypertension.
    b. secondary hypertension.
    c. primary hypertension.
    d. congenital heart defects.

77. Most children with essential hypertension that is resistant to nonpharmacologic intervention are managed with:
    a. diuretics.
    b. calcium channel blockers.
    c. ACE inhibitors.
    d. any of the above.

78. The nurse's role in relation to hypertension may include:
    a. routine accurate assessment of blood pressure in infants and children.
    b. providing information.
    c. follow-up of the child with hypertension.
    d. all of the above.

79. Elevated cholesterol in childhood:
    a. can predict the long-term risk for heart disease for the individual.
    b. can predict the risk for hypertension in adulthood.
    c. is a major predictor of the adult cholesterol level.
    d. is usually symptomatic.

80. The National Cholesterol Education Program recommends screening for cholesterol in:
    a. all children over 2 years of age.
    b. children over 2 years of age with a family history of elevated cholesterol.
    c. children with congenital heart disease.
    d. all children.

81. The most common kind of cardiomyopathy found in children is:
    a. dilated cardiomyopathy.
    b. hypertrophic cardiomyopathy.
    c. restrictive cardiomyopathy.
    d. secondary cardiomyopathy.

82. The heart transplant procedure where the recipient's own heart is left in place is the:
    a. heterotopic heart transplantation.
    b. orthotopic heart transplantation.

83. Which of the following dysrhythmias would be included on a list of dysrhythmias commonly seen in children?
    a. Ventricular tachycardia
    b. Asystole
    c. Supraventricular tachycardia
    d. All of the above

CRITICAL THINKING—CASE STUDY

Pauline is a 3-year-old child admitted for repair of an atrial septal defect. Her parents have known about the defect since her birth. She has had numerous respiratory tract infections with occasional episodes of heart failure in the past year. Pauline has taken digoxin and furosemide in the past but currently takes only vitamins with iron. Her parents state that they are anxious to have the surgery over with, so that they can treat Pauline like the other children. They have three other children who are all older than Pauline.

84. On admission Pauline is afebrile and playful and has no signs of heart failure. As part of the admission process, the nurse wants to be sure to have a baseline assessment of:
    a. Pauline's sucking and swallowing abilities.
    b. Pauline's reading ability.
    c. Pauline's exercise tolerance level.
    d. all of the above.

85. When developing a nursing care plan for Pauline's admission for the surgical repair of the atrial septal defect, the nurse would most likely have identified a nursing diagnosis of:
    a. Interrupted Family Process.
    b. Impaired Skin Integrity.

86. One of the best ways for the nurse to provide emotional support for Pauline and her family in the stressful postoperative period is to:
    a. facilitate a swift transfer out of the ICU.
    b. expect courage and bravery from Pauline.
    c. limit Pauline's expression of anger toward her parents.
    d. praise Pauline for her efforts to cooperate.

35 The Child with Hematologic or Immunologic Dysfunction

1. Identify the following statements as true or false.

   _____ The major physiologic component of red blood cells (RBCs) is erythropoietin.

   _____ A complete blood count with differential describes the components of blood known as *platelets*.

   _____ A child with a suspected bacterial infection would have a differential count that shows a shift to the left with more mature cells present.

   _____ Erythrocytes supply oxygen and remove carbon dioxide from cells.

   _____ The mature RBC has no nucleus.

   _____ Reticulocytes indicate active RBC production.

   _____ The regulator of erythrocyte production is tissue oxygenation and renal production of erythropoietin.

   _____ The regulatory mechanism for the production of erythrocytes is their circulating numbers.

   _____ The absolute neutrophil count reflects the body's ability to handle bacterial infection.

   _____ Monocytes and lymphocytes are granulocytes.

   _____ In the child with increased numbers of eosinophils, the nurse should suspect allergies or parasitic infection.

   _____ Monocytosis is more evident in acute inflammation.

   _____ The hematocrit is approximately three times the hemoglobin content.

   _____ The mean corpuscular hemoglobin is the average volume of a single RBC.

   _____ Mean corpuscular hemoglobin concentration is the average concentration of hemoglobin in a single cell.

   _____ Bands are immature neutrophils, and they increase in number during bacterial infections.

   _____ The life span of the RBC is 120 days.

   _____ Causes of folate deficiency include inadequate diet, overcooking of vegetables, and malabsorption.

2. The nurse would expect laboratory results for the patient with chronic blood loss to include:
   a. high iron levels.
   b. macrocytic and hyperchromic erythrocytes.
   c. microcytic and hypochromic erythrocytes.
   d. normocytic and normochromic erythrocytes.

3. What are the main causes of anemia?

4. What is the basic physiologic defect caused by anemia?

5. Match the term with its description.

a. Normocytes
b. Macrocytes
c. Microcytes
d. Spherocytes
e. Poikilocytes
f. Drepanocytes
g. Normochromic
h. Hypochromic
i. Leukocytosis

j. Mean corpuscular hemoglobin concentration (MCHC)
k. Mean corpuscular volume (MCV)
l. Petechiae
m. Polycythemia
n. Fetal hemoglobin
o. Mean corpuscular hemoglobin (MCH)
p. Granulocytes
q. Agranulocytes

_____ Indicates the average volume or size of a single RBC

_____ Reduced amount of hemoglobin concentration

_____ Sickle-shaped cells

_____ Indicates the average concentration of hemoglobin in the RBC

_____ Small hemorrhagic areas

_____ Increase in leukocytes

_____ Indicates the average weight of hemoglobin in each RBC

_____ Neutrophils, basophils, eosinophils

_____ Monocytes, lymphocytes

_____ Larger than normal cell size

_____ Smaller than normal cell size

_____ Normal cell size

_____ Sufficient or normal hemoglobin concentration

_____ Two α and two γ chains; has a greater affinity for oxygen

_____ Increase in the number of erythrocytes

_____ Globular-shaped cells

_____ Irregular-shaped cells

6. Identify the cause of leukocytosis.

7. Routine screening of hemoglobin and hematocrit, as recommended by the American Academy of Pediatrics, includes:
   a. Screening should be performed once during infancy (9 to 12 months of age), childhood (1 to 5 years of age), late childhood (5 to 12 years of age), and adolescence (14 to 20 years of age).
   b. All children should be screened once during childhood.
   c. Screening should be performed on all children at high-risk for iron deficiency anemia, preterm infants, infants born of a multiple pregnancy or to iron-deficient woman, and children in low socioeconomic groups.
   d. Screening should not be performed unless history and physical examination suggest anemia.

8. a. In _____ the bone marrow is _____ (producing an increased number of cells).

   b. In _____ _____ the bone marrow is _____ (producing a decreased

   number of cells) or _____ (producing no cells).

9. When the hemoglobin level falls sufficiently to produce clinical manifestations of anemia, the patient experiences:
   a. cyanosis.
   b. tissue hypoxia.
   c. nausea and vomiting.
   d. feelings of anxiety.

10. Which of the following does the nurse expect to include in the care plan of a patient with anemia?
    i. Prepare the child for laboratory tests.
    ii. Observe for complications of therapy.
    iii. Decrease tissue oxygen needs.
    iv. Implement safety precautions.

    a. i and iv
    b. i, ii, iii, and iv
    c. ii and iii
    d. i and ii

11. The nurse is scheduled to administer 100 ml of packed RBCs to 3-year-old Amy. Which of the following is not a correct guideline when administering the blood?
    a. Take vital signs before administration.
    b. Infuse the blood through an appropriate filter.
    c. Administer 50 ml of the blood within the first few minutes to detect for possible reactions before proceeding with the remainder of the infusion.
    d. Start the blood within 30 minutes of its arrival from the blood bank or return it to the blood bank.

12. Lucas, age 7 years, is receiving a transfusion of packed RBCs. After 45 minutes, he begins to have chills, fever, a sensation of tightness in his chest, and headache. The priority action of the nurse is to:
    a. stop the transfusion, maintain a patent intravenous (IV) line with normal saline and new tubing, and administer acetaminophen.
    b. stop the transfusion, maintain a patent IV line with normal saline and new tubing, and notify the practitioner.
    c. slow the transfusion rate until the symptoms subside.
    d. slow the transfusion and send a sample of the patient's blood and urine to the laboratory.

13. At birth the normal full-term newborn has maternal stores of iron sufficient to last for:
    a. the first 5 to 6 months of life.
    b. the first 2 to 3 months of life.
    c. the first 8 months of life.
    d. less than 1 month of life.

14. Which of the following laboratory values is diagnostic of anemia caused by inadequate intake or absorption of iron?
    a. Elevated total iron-binding capacity (TIBC) and reduced serum iron concentration (SIC)
    b. Reduced TIBC and SIC
    c. Elevated TIBC and SIC
    d. Reduced TIBC and elevated SIC

15. Angie, age 11 months, is brought into the clinic by her mother for a routine checkup. On physical examination, the nurse observes that Angie appears chubby; that her skin looks pale, almost porcelain-like; and that Angie has poor muscle development. Based on these observations, which of the following questions is most important for the nurse to include when completing Angie's history?
    a. "Did you have any complications during pregnancy or delivery of Angie?"
    b. "Tell me about what you are currently feeding Angie."
    c. "Has Angie had any recent infections or high fevers?"
    d. "Have you noticed whether Angie is having difficulty with her movements or advancing in her growth and development abilities?"

16. The nurse is instructing a new mother in how to prevent iron deficiency anemia in her new premature infant when she takes her home. The mother intends to breast-feed. Which of the following statements reflects a need for further education of the new mother?
    a. "I will use only breast milk or formula as a source of milk for my baby until she is at least 12 months old."
    b. "My baby will need to have iron supplements introduced when she is 2 months old."
    c. "As my baby is able to tolerate other foods, such as cereal, I should limit her formula intake to about 1 L/day to encourage intake of iron-rich cereals."
    d. "I will need to add iron supplements to my baby's diet when she is 6 months old."

17. When teaching the parents of 4-year-old Tony how to administer the iron supplement ordered for his iron deficiency, which of the following should be included in the teaching plan?
    a. Give the iron twice daily in divided doses with orange juice.
    b. Give the iron twice daily with milk.
    c. Administer the oral liquid iron preparation with the use of a syringe or medicine dropper directly into each side of the mouth in the cheek areas.
    d. Make certain the parents have at least 3 months' supply of the iron preparation on hand so that they will not run out.

18. On a return clinical visit after Tony has been taking the iron supplement, his mother tells the nurse she is concerned because Tony's stools are now greenish black. What would your response be?

19. Hereditary spherocytosis is:
    a. always transmitted as an autosomal recessive disease.
    b. a hemolytic disorder caused by a defect in the proteins that form the RBC membrane.
    c. rarely evident until the infant is 4 to 6 months of age.
    d. usually resolved when additional folic acid supplements are administered.

20. Sally and David Brown are returning with Jason, their 6-week-old infant, for a routine newborn examination. Sally is a carrier for sickle cell anemia; David is not. What is the chance that Jason was born with sickle cell anemia?
    a. 25% chance
    b. 50% chance
    c. 75% chance
    d. 0% chance

21. Infants are often not diagnosed with sickle cell anemia until they are 1 year of age. Why?
    a. Usually there are no symptoms until after age 1 year.
    b. High intake of fluids from formulas prevents sickle cell crises during this age.
    c. Fetal hemoglobin is present during the first year of life.
    d. Increased hemoglobin and hematocrit amounts compensate during this period.

22. The basic defect responsible for the sickling effect of erythrocytes is in the globin fraction of hemoglobin.

    Under conditions of _____, _____, _____, and _____

    _____, the relatively insoluble HgbS changes its molecular structure to filamentous crystals that cause distortion of the cell membrane to a crescent- or sickle-shaped RBC.

23. Persons diagnosed with sickle cell trait:
    a. have 50% or more of the total hemoglobin in HgbS.
    b. cannot pass the trait to their children.
    c. can have painful gross hematuria as a major complication.
    d. never develop symptoms of anemia.

24. Bruce, age 12 years, is admitted to your unit with a diagnosis of sickle cell crisis. Which of the following activities is most likely to have precipitated this episode?
    a. Attending the football game with his friends
    b. Going camping and hiking in the mountains with his friends
    c. Going to the beach and surfing with his friends
    d. Staying indoors and reading for several hours

25. Pat is a 5-year-old being admitted because of diminished RBC production triggered by a viral infection. What type of sickle cell crisis is she most likely experiencing?
    a. Vasoocclusive crisis
    b. Splenic sequestration crisis
    c. Aplastic crisis
    d. Hyperhemolytic crisis

26. Which of the following diagnostic tests can distinguish between children with sickle cell trait and those with sickle cell disease?
    a. Complete blood count with differential
    b. Sickledex
    c. Bleeding time
    d. Hemoglobin electrophoresis

27. Therapeutic management of sickle cell crisis generally includes:
    a. Long-term oxygen use to enable the oxygen to reach the sickled RBCs
    b. Decrease in fluids to increase hemoconcentration
    c. Diet high in iron to decrease anemia
    d. Bed rest to minimize energy expenditure

28. _____ is a useful noninvasive diagnostic test that screens for stroke risk in children with sickle cell disease. It is performed yearly on children ages 2 to 16 years and measures the vascular flow within the large cerebral arteries.
    a. Cat scan of the head
    b. Transcranial Doppler
    c. Ultrasound of the carotid arteries
    d. Magnetic resonance imaging of the head

29. To control pain related to vasoocclusive sickle cell crisis, which of the following can the nurse expect to be included in the care plan?
    a. Administration of long-term oxygen
    b. Application of cold compresses to the area
    c. Administration of meperidine (Demerol) titrated to a therapeutic level
    d. Codeine added to acetaminophen or ibuprofen if neither one of these is effective in relieving the pain alone

30. In planning for a child's discharge after a sickle cell crisis, which of the following is a critical factor to include in the teaching plan?
    a. Ingestion of large quantities of liquids to promote adequate hydration
    b. Rigorous exercise schedule to promote muscle strength
    c. A high-caloric diet to improve nutrition
    d. At least 12 hours of sleep per night to promote adequate rest

31. Which of the following is the homozygous form of β-thalassemia, which results in a severe anemia and is not compatible with life without transfusion support?
    a. Thalassemia minor
    b. Thalassemia intermedia
    c. Thalassemia major
    d. Thalassemia trait

32. Norma, age 2 years, is to begin therapy for β-thalassemia. Which of the following would be appropriate for the nurse to include in the educational session held with the parents?
    i. Norma will need frequent blood transfusions to keep her hemoglobin level above 12 g/dl.
    ii. Large doses of vitamin C will be needed throughout the disease.
    iii. Chelation therapy is delayed until after 6 years of age to promote normal physical development.
    iv. To minimize the effect of iron overload, deferoxamine (Desferal), an iron-chelating agent, will be given intravenously or subcutaneously.
    v. Deferasirox is an oral iron-chelating agent available for patients 2 years and older with chronic iron overload secondary to recurrent blood transfusions.

    a. i, ii, and iv
    b. iii, iv, and v
    c. i, ii, iii, iv, and v
    d. iv and v

33. Which of the following does the nurse recognize as an appropriate nursing objective when caring for the child with β-thalassemia?
    a. Promote compliance with transfusion and chelation therapy.
    b. Foster the family's adjustment to the acute illness.
    c. Teach the family to prevent tissue deoxygenation.
    d. Promote physical therapy and range-of-motion techniques to prevent bone changes.

34. What are the two types of aplastic anemia?

35. a. How is a definite diagnosis of aplastic anemia determined?

    b. Acquired aplastic anemia is first seen with clinical manifestations of _____, _____, and _____ _____ _____.

    c. Identify two main approaches aimed at restoring function to the marrow in aplastic anemia.

36. Danny is scheduled to receive antithymocyte globulin (ATG) for treatment of his aplastic anemia. Based on knowledge about this therapy, which of the following does the nurse recognize as true?
    a. ATG is administered intramuscularly every 3 to 4 weeks.
    b. ATG is administered intravenously in a peripheral vein over a 3-hour period.
    c. All reactions to ATG, including skin rash and fever, occur within the first hour of administration.
    d. ATG suppresses T cell–dependent autoimmune responses but does not cause bone marrow suppression.

37. Match the term with its description.

a. Bleeding time
b. Prothrombin time (PT)
c. Partial thromboplastin time (PTT)
d. Thromboplastin generation test (TGT)
e. Fibrinogen

f. Hemophilia A
g. Hemophilia B
h. Hemostasis
i. Fibrinolysis

_____ Allows for determination of specific factor deficiencies, especially factors VIII and IX

_____ Clot breakdown

_____ Blood clotting factor number I

_____ Function depends on platelet aggregation and vasoconstriction

_____ Measures factors necessary for prothrombin conversion to thrombin and fibrinogen

_____ Measures the activity of thromboplastin; specific for factor deficiencies except factor VII

_____ Factor IX deficiency

_____ Factor VIII deficiency

_____ Process that stops bleeding when a bleed vessel is injured

38. When discussing hemophilia with the parents of a child recently diagnosed with this disease, the nurse tells the parents that:
   a. hemophilia is an X-linked disorder in which the mother is the carrier of the illness but is not affected by it.
   b. hemophilia is a recessive disorder carried by either the mother or the father.
   c. all of the daughters of the parents will be carriers.
   d. each of their sons has a 75% chance of being affected.

39. Which of the following is the most frequent form of internal bleeding in the child with hemophilia?
   a. Hemarthrosis
   b. Epistaxis
   c. Intracranial hemorrhage
   d. Gastrointestinal tract hemorrhage

40. Which of the following is no longer recommended for use in treating factor VIII deficiency because the risk for hepatitis or human immunodeficiency virus (HIV) cannot be safely eliminated?
   a. Factor VIII concentrate
   b. Cryoprecipitate
   c. DDAVP (1-deamino-8-D-arginine vasopressin)
   d. ε-Aminocaproic acid (Amicar, EACA)

41. Donald, age 5 years and previously diagnosed with hemophilia A, is being admitted with bleeding into the joints. Which of the following is contraindicated in his care plan?
   i. Ice packs to the affected area
   ii. Application of a splint or sling to the area
   iii. Administration of corticosteroids
   iv. Administration of aspirin, indomethacin (Indocin), or phenylbutazone (Butazolidin)
   v. Passive range-of-motion exercises
   vi. Active range-of-motion exercises
   vii. Teaching Donald how to administer antihemophilic factor (AHF) to himself

   a. i, iii, and vi
   b. ii, iii, iv, and vi
   c. i, v, and vii
   d. iv, v, and vii

42. Which of the following statements about von Willebrand disease is true?
    a. The characteristic clinical feature is an increased tendency toward bleeding from mucous membranes.
    b. It affects females but not males.
    c. It will be unsafe for the female affected with the disease to have children because of hemorrhage.
    d. It is an inherited autosomal recessive disease.

43. Sammy, age 8 years and diagnosed with von Willebrand disease, is brought to the school nurse with a nosebleed. Which of the following is an appropriate action for the nurse to take?
    a. Call Sammy's parents immediately so that they can arrange for him to have a dose of DDAVP to control the bleeding.
    b. After Sammy is lying down, apply cold packs to the back of the neck and over the bridge of the nose.
    c. Have Sammy sit up, lean forward, and apply continuous pressure to his nose with the thumb and forefinger.
    d. Notify emergency services for transport of Sammy to the hospital emergency room, because all bleeding with von Willebrand disease is a medical emergency.

44. Which of the following is an acquired hemorrhagic disorder characterized by excessive destruction of platelets; normal bone marrow with increase in large, young platelets; and a discoloration caused by petechiae beneath the skin?
    a. Idiopathic thrombocytopenic purpura
    b. Disseminated intravascular coagulation
    c. Acute onset neutropenia
    d. Henoch-Schönlein purpura

45. Which of the following does the nurse recognize as true when administering anti-D antibody for idiopathic thrombocytopenic purpura?
    a. The platelet count will increase immediately after administration.
    b. Eligible patients include those with lupus.
    c. Bone marrow examination to first rule out leukemia is necessary before administration.
    d. The patient should be premedicated with acetaminophen before medication is infused.

46. In severe cases of disseminated intravascular coagulation, treatment may include the administration of heparin. What is the rationale for this therapy?
    a. Inhibit thrombin formation
    b. Decrease platelet count
    c. Increase RBCs
    d. Increase prothrombin

47. Disseminated intravascular coagulation is:
    a. a primary disease characterized by abnormal coagulation.
    b. a secondary disorder characterized by bleeding and clotting, which occur simultaneously.
    c. characterized by an increased tendency to form clots, along with diagnostic findings that include low prothrombin levels and increased fibrinogen levels.
    d. treated with blood transfusion of whole blood and factor VIII concentrate.

48. Which of the following statements about chronic benign neutropenia is true?
    a. Nursing care management includes educating the parents to keep their child away from crowded areas and individuals who are ill.
    b. Diagnosis is usually made when the child is seen with weight loss and fatigue.
    c. The absolute neutrophil count is usually 1500/mm^3 or less at the time of diagnosis.
    d. Children with chronic benign neutropenia do not receive routine childhood immunizations because of the abnormal cellular immunity and antineutrophil antibodies associated with this disorder.

49. What are the four characteristics of Henoch-Schönlein purpura?

50. HIV is likely to be transmitted by:
    a. exposure in utero or through breast milk from an infected mother.
    b. receipt of infected blood products by transfusion before 1985.
    c. adolescent engagement in high-risk behaviors (sex or IV drugs).
    d. All of the above

51. What are the seven most common clinical manifestations of HIV infection in children?

52. Goals of therapy for HIV infection in children are:

53. Identify the following as true or false.

    _____ Combinations of antiretroviral drugs are more likely to delay the emergence of drug resistance in the treatment of HIV than is single-drug therapy.

    _____ *Pneumocystis carinii* pneumonia (PCP) is the most common opportunistic infection of children infected with HIV.

    _____ HIV-infected children who are already receiving PCP prophylaxis antibiotics derive significant additional benefit from the administration of IV immune globulin.

    _____ Children who are diagnosed with acquired immunodeficiency syndrome (AIDS) in the first year of life, particularly as a result of PCP, are more likely to have a shorter life expectancy.

    _____ Developmental delays in children with AIDS include receptive language delays rather than expressive language delays.

54. Immunization needs of the child with HIV infection include:
    a. delay of all immunizations until the child has the HIV infection under control.
    b. withholding of pneumococcal and influenza vaccines.
    c. administration of varicella vaccine at the age of 12 months only if there is no evidence of severe immunocompromise.
    d. provision of MMR vaccine to children receiving IV γ-globulin prophylaxis.

55. Why are the ELISA and Western blot immunoassay tests not used to determine HIV infection in infants born to HIV-infected mothers?

56. Two-year-old Jennifer is HIV infected. Her mother is concerned about placing Jennifer in daycare and is discussing this with the nurse at a routine pediatric follow-up visit. Which of the following is the best information to provide Jennifer's mother?
    a. The risk for HIV transmission is significant in daycare centers. Jennifer should not go to daycare until she is older.
    b. It will be all right for Jennifer to attend the daycare, but Jennifer's mother must tell the daycare that Jennifer is infected.
    c. Jennifer can go to daycare but will not be allowed to participate in sports or physical activity that could lead to injury.
    d. Jennifer should be admitted to the daycare without restrictions and allowed to participate in all activities as her health permits.

57. The Centers for Disease Control and Prevention recommend that all infants born to HIV-infected women should receive prophylaxis during the first year of life. Which of the following is the drug of choice?
    a. Amoxicillin
    b. Trimethoprim-sulfamethoxazole (TMP-SMZ)
    c. IV immune globulin
    d. Dapsone

58. In Wiskott-Aldrich syndrome, the most notable effect of the disease at birth is:
    a. bleeding.
    b. infection.
    c. eczema.
    d. malignancy.

59. Which of the following would be the definitive therapeutic management for the infant diagnosed with severe combined immunodeficiency disease?
    a. Histocompatible hematopoietic stem cell transplantation from a sibling with human leukocyte antigen (HLA)–matched bone marrow
    b. Histocompatible hematopoietic stem cell transplantation from an identical twin with HLA-matched bone marrow
    c. IV immune globulin
    d. Fetal liver and thymus transplants

CRITICAL THINKING—CASE STUDY

Mary, age 9, has sickle cell anemia. She is admitted to the hospital with knee and back pain and is diagnosed as being in vasoocclusive crisis.

60. The nurse, in developing a care plan for Mary, formulates a diagnosis of pain. The nurse understands that Mary's pain is related to:
    a. pooling of large amounts of blood in the liver and spleen.
    b. shorter life span of the RBCs and the fact that the bone marrow cannot produce enough RBCs.
    c. tissue anoxia brought on by sickle cells occluding blood vessels.
    d. RBC destruction related to a viral infection or transfusion reaction.

61. Describe interventions that the nurse can include in the care plan to control pain during this vasoocclusive crisis to prevent undermedicating Mary.

62. The nurse is developing an educational plan about sickle cell anemia for Mary and her parents. To prevent recurrence of a crisis, which of the following is most important to include in the educational session?
    a. Explaining the signs of dehydration
    b. Explaining that frequent rest periods are required when the child is in a low-oxygen atmosphere
    c. Explaining that the child should avoid injury to joints to decrease sickling of blood cells
    d. Explaining the importance of avoiding infection by routine immunization and protection from known sources of infection

63. Evaluation of Mary's progress is best based on the observation that:
    a. Mary's verbalization that she no longer has pain or need for pain medication.
    b. Mary's ability to perform active range-of-motion exercises.
    c. Mary's desire to drink the required level of fluids for hydration.
    d. Mary's verbalization of how to prevent future sickle cell crisis.

64. Cindy is a 12-month-old being treated for HIV infection. Describe nursing interventions to prevent the spread of the disease to others.

65. In preparing a nursing care plan for Cindy, expected goals would be:

36 The Child with Cancer

1. Match each of the following terms with its description.

   a. Germ-line mutations
   b. Oncogenes
   c. Leukemia
   d. Gram-negative bacteria
   e. Apoptosis
   f. Biologic response modifiers (BRMs)
   g. Bone marrow test
   h. Alopecia
   i. Tumor suppressor genes

   _____ Programmed cell death

   _____ Genes that keep tumor growth in check

   _____ Used to determine the presence or absence of tumor or response to therapy in this specific location

   _____ Chromosome abnormalities that are not confined to the tumor alone but are present elsewhere; may be present in all cells

   _____ Hair loss

   _____ Genes that activate tumor growth

   _____ A broad term given to a group of malignant diseases of the bone marrow and lymphatic system

   _____ Agents that modify the relationship between tumor and host by therapeutically changing the host's reaction to tumor cells

   _____ Examples are *Pseudomonas aeruginosa*, *Escherichia coli*, and *Proteus* and *Klebsiella* organisms.

2. The following terms are related to modes of therapy and complications of therapy. Match each term with its description.

   a. Philadelphia chromosome
   b. Neutropenia
   c. Alkylating agents
   d. Antimetabolites
   e. Plant alkaloids
   f. Antitumor antibiotics
   g. Hormones
   h. Lethal damage
   i. Sublethal damage
   j. Total body irradiation
   k. Monoclonal antibody
   l. Mono
   m. Clone
   n. Human leukocyte antigen (HLA) system complex
   o. Haplotype
   p. Graft-versus-host disease (GVHD)
   q. Allogeneic bone marrow transplantation
   r. Umbilical cord blood stem cell transplantation
   s. Autologous bone marrow transplantation
   t. Peripheral stem cell transplant
   u. Acute tumor lysis syndrome
   v. Hyperleukocytosis
   w. Obstruction
   x. Superior vena cava syndrome
   y. Overwhelming infections

   _____ Genes inherited as a single unit

   _____ Natural products that interfere with cell division by reacting with deoxyribonucleic acid (DNA) in such a way as to prevent further replication of DNA and transcription of ribonucleic acid (RNA)

   _____ Autologous transplant; stem cells first stimulated to grow, then collected and filtered from whole blood; whole blood then returned to the patient; performed without problems on very small children

   _____ The system used to select a suitable donor

   _____ One of the three main consequences of the proliferation of cells in the bone marrow of children with leukemia; may result in infection

   _____ Both adrenal and gonadal agents with antineoplastic properties; mechanism of action unclear

   _____ Resemble essential metabolic elements needed for cell growth but are sufficiently altered in molecular structure to inhibit further synthesis of DNA and/or RNA

_____ Refers to the death of the cell

_____ The first chromosome abnormality found in a malignancy; associated with myelogenous leukemia

_____ Damage to injured cells that may subsequently be repaired

_____ Replace a hydrogen atom of a molecule by an alkyl group; irreversible; cause unbalanced growth of unaffected cell constituents so that the cell eventually dies; similar action as irradiation

_____ Associated with the most severe reactions; employed to prepare the immune system for bone marrow transplantation

_____ Arrests cells in metaphase by binding to microtubular protein needed for spindle formation

_____ Antibodies that recognize a single specific antigen; currently used to diagnose subclasses of leukemia cells to understand how the cancer responds

_____ The most common complication in allogeneic transplants; characterized by a hardening of the tissues and drying of the mucous membranes

_____ A new source of hematopoietic stem cells for use in children with cancer; allows for partially matched unrelated transplants to be successful; lowers risk for GVHD-related problems

_____ Life-threatening condition; peripheral white blood cell count greater than $100,000/mm^3$; can lead to capillary obstruction, microinfarction, and organ dysfunction

_____ Also means "one"

_____ Compression of the mediastinal structures, leading to airway compromise and potentially to respiratory failure

_____ Exact duplicate

_____ Caused by space-occupying lesions such as Hodgkin disease and non-Hodgkin lymphoma structures

_____ Involves matching a histocompatible donor with the recipient

_____ May constitute an emergency situation; can result in complications such as disseminated intravascular coagulation, hemorrhage, thrombocytopenia, and leukocytosis

_____ Uses the patient's own marrow that was collected from disease-free tissue, frozen, and sometimes treated to remove malignant cells; has been used to treat neuroblastoma, Hodgkin disease, non-Hodgkin lymphoma, rhabdomyosarcoma, Ewing sarcoma, and Wilms tumor

_____ Life-threatening condition caused by the rapid release of intracellular metabolites during the initial treatment of malignancies such as Burkitt and T-cell lymphomas and acute leukemia; leads to hyperuricemia, hypocalcemia, hyperphosphatemia, and hyperkalemia

3. The following terms are related to the signs and symptoms of cancer. Match each term with its description.

a. Pain
b. Fever
c. Skin assessment
d. Anemia

e. Abdominal mass
f. Swollen lymph glands
g. White reflection

_____ Classic sign of retinoblastoma; cat's eye reflex or leukocoria

_____ Common finding in children; if enlarged and firm for more than a week, may indicate a serious disease

_____ Typical finding in children with Wilms tumor and neuroblastoma

_____ Caused by the replacement of normal cells with malignant cells in the bone marrow

_____ May show signs of low platelet count, ecchymosis, petechiae

_____ A frequent occurrence caused by numerous illnesses other than cancer; with cancer, usually caused by infection secondary to the malignant process

_____ May be an early or late initial sign of cancer

4. The following terms are related to the nursing care of children with cancer. Match each term with its description.

a. Absolute neutrophil count
b. Colony-stimulating factors
c. Granulocyte colony-stimulating factor

d. Postirradiation somnolence
e. Mood changes
f. Cushingoid appearance

_____ Filgrastim; pegfilgrastim; directs granulocyte development and can decrease the duration of neutropenia following immunosuppressive therapy

_____ One of the effects of long-term steroid treatment that can be extremely distressing to older children; child's face becomes rounded and puffy

_____ May be experienced shortly after beginning steroid therapy; range from feelings of well-being and euphoria to depression and irritability

_____ If lower than 500/mm^3, risk for infection and major complications

_____ A neurologic syndrome that may develop 5 to 8 weeks after central nervous system irradiation; characterized by somnolence with or without fever, anorexia, and nausea and vomiting; may be an early indicator of long-term neurologic sequelae after cranial irradiation

_____ A family of glycoprotein hormones that regulate the reproduction, maturation, and function of blood cells; used as a supportive measure to prevent the side effects caused by low blood counts

5. Match each term with its description.

a. Cryotherapy
b. Induction
c. Intensification
d. Central nervous system prophylactic therapy
e. Maintenance phase
f. Ann Arbor Staging Classification
g. Leukocoria

h. Sternberg-Reed cell
i. Involved field radiation
j. Extended field radiation
k. Total nodal irradiation
l. Burkitt lymphoma
m. Brain tumors
n. Neuroblastoma
o. Infratentorial
p. Supratentorial

q. Astrocytes
r. Astrocytomas
s. Stereotactic surgery
t. Lasers
u. Brain mapping
v. Phantom limb pain
w. Somatic mutations
x. Photocoagulation
y. Plaque brachytherapy

_____ Vaporize tumor tissue

_____ Consolidation therapy; the phase of leukemia treatment that decreases the tumor burden

_____ The phase of leukemia therapy that serves to preserve the remission of the disease

_____ Determines the precise location of critical brain areas that are avoided during surgery

_____ Cat's eye reflex; a whitish glow in the pupil that is a sign of retinoblastoma and is often first visualized by the parent

_____ Freezing the tumor; destroys the microcirculation to the tumor and the cells themselves through microcrystal formation

_____ The phase of leukemia therapy that prevents leukemic cells from invading the central nervous system; administered to all children with leukemia

_____ The phase of leukemia treatment that achieves a complete remission or disappearance of leukemic cells

_____ Treatment for which children with stage I Hodgkin disease are candidates

_____ A staging system to classify Hodgkin disease

_____ Entire axial lymph node system irradiated; usually combined with chemotherapy

_____ A type of cancer that is rare in the United States but endemic in parts of Africa; a rapidly growing neoplasm that is most commonly seen as a mass in the jaw, abdomen, or orbit

_____ A giant cell with a dark-staining nucleolus; considered diagnostic of Hodgkin but may occur in mononucleosis

_____ May be benign or malignant, although because of the location, the designation of any tumor as "benign" should be made cautiously

_____ Involved areas and adjacent nodes irradiated

_____ The most common malignant tumors of infancy; the most common extracranial solid tumor of childhood

_____ May develop after amputation; characterized by sensations such as tingling, itching, and, more frequently, pain felt in the amputated limb; amitriptyline may decrease the pain

_____ Below the tentorium cerebelli

_____ Those retinoblastomas occurring in the general body cells as opposed to the germ cells or gametes; sporadic, nonhereditary events; result in unilateral retinoblastoma tumors

_____ Within the anterior two thirds of the brain, mainly the cerebrum

_____ Use of a laser beam to destroy retinal blood vessels that supply nutrition to the tumor

_____ Cells that form most of the supportive tissue for the neurons

_____ Surgical implantation of an iodine-125 applicator on the sclera until the maximum radiation dose has been delivered to the tumor

_____ The most common glial tumor

_____ Involves the use of computed tomography and magnetic resonance imaging in conjunction with other special computer techniques to reconstruct the tumor in three dimensions

6. The cancer that occurs with the most frequency in children is:
   a. lymphoma.
   b. neuroblastoma.
   c. leukemia.
   d. melanoma.

7. Which of the following carcinogenic agents has been definitely implicated in the development of childhood cancer?
   a. Low doses of radiation
   b. Excessive sun exposure
   c. Exposure to cigarette smoke
   d. Intramuscular vitamin K at birth

8. Of the following assessment findings, the one that would most likely be seen in a child with leukemia is:
   a. weakness of the eye muscle.
   b. bruising, nosebleeds, paleness, and fatigue.
   c. wheezing and shortness of breath.
   d. abdominal swelling.

9. When a clinical trial is used to evaluate an aspect of childhood cancer care, the parents can expect the treatment the child receives to always be:
   a. better than the current treatment usually used.
   b. an evaluation of an investigational drug.
   c. intermittent intravenous infusion of drugs.
   d. at least as good as the best possible treatment currently known.

10. The use of clinical trials and protocols for cancer treatment has resulted in an increased use of:
    a. intermittent intravenous therapy.
    b. continuous intravenous therapy.
    c. lower doses of single-drug therapy.
    d. prolonged duration of maintenance therapy.

11. The severe cellular damage that is caused by chemotherapy drugs infiltrating into surrounding tissue occurs when the chemotherapeutic agent is a(n):
    a. hormone.
    b. steroid.
    c. vesicant.
    d. antimetabolite.

12. Match each type of chemotherapeutic agent with the side effect or nursing consideration that most pertains to that type of drug.

   a. Alkylating agents　　　　　　　　　　　d. Hormones
   b. Antimetabolites　　　　　　　　　　　　e. Enzymes
   c. Plant alkaloids

   _____ Neurotoxicity

   _____ Renal toxicity or hemorrhagic cystitis

   _____ Usually no short-term acute toxicity

   _____ Mucosal ulceration, stomatitis

   _____ Allergic reactions

13. A candidate for bone marrow transplantation is the child who:
   a. is unlikely to be cured by other means.
   b. has acute leukemia.
   c. has chronic leukemia.
   d. has a compatible donor in his or her family.

14. Name four types of early side effects of radiotherapy, and describe one nursing intervention for each type.

15. A major benefit of using umbilical cord blood for stem cell transplantation is:
   a. stem cells are found in low frequency in newborns.
   b. umbilical cord blood is relatively immunodeficient.
   c. there is a lower risk for acute tumor lysis syndrome.
   d. all of the above.

16. List five cardinal symptoms of cancer in children.

17. The family of glycoprotein hormones that regulate the function of blood cells is called _____

   _____ _____.

18. Children who have profound anemia during induction therapy should:
   a. strictly limit their activities.
   b. regulate their own activity with adult supervision.
   c. receive transfusions until the hemoglobin level approaches 10 g/dl.
   d. receive chemotherapy until the hemoglobin level reaches 10 g/dl.

19. The nursing intervention that would be most helpful for the child who has stomatitis from cancer chemotherapy would be:
   a. an anesthetic preparation without alcohol.
   b. viscous lidocaine (Xylocaine).
   c. lemon glycerin swabs.
   d. a mild sedative.

20. Describe three strategies the nurse can use to prevent sterile hemorrhagic cystitis.

21. Parents sometimes view the child's moon face from steroids as an appearance of:
    a. an anorexic, undernourished child.
    b. a malnourished child with a swollen abdomen.
    c. an overweight but undernourished child.
    d. a well-nourished, healthy child.

22. The child who receives a bone marrow transplant will require:
    a. meticulous personal hygiene.
    b. multiple peripheral sites for intravenous therapy.
    c. less chemotherapy before the transplant.
    d. a room with laminar air flow.

23. After bone marrow aspiration is performed on a child, the nurse should:
    a. apply an adhesive bandage.
    b. place the child in the Trendelenburg position.
    c. ask the child to remain in the supine position.
    d. apply a pressure bandage.

24. Dental care for a child whose platelet count is $32,000/mm^3$ and granulocyte count is $450/mm^3$ should include daily:
    a. toothbrushing with flossing.
    b. toothbrushing without flossing.
    c. flossing without toothbrushing.
    d. wiping with moistened sponges.

25. Delaying vaccinations is usually recommended in the immunosuppressed child because the immune response is likely to be suboptimal; however, it is considered safe to administer:
    a. any vaccines.
    b. any live attenuated vaccines.
    c. any inactivated vaccines.
    d. the varicella vaccine.

26. Leukemia is characterized by:
    a. a high leukocyte count.
    b. destruction of normal cells by abnormal cells.
    c. low numbers of blast cells.
    d. overproduction of blast cells.

27. Identify the three main consequences of bone marrow dysfunction.

28. The most important prognostic factors in determining long-term survival for children with acute lymphoblastic leukemia include:
    a. leukocyte count and leukemia cell burden.
    b. age and gender.
    c. immunologic subtype, FAB morphology, and cytogenetics.
    d. all of the above.

29. Children who receive reinduction therapy for a relapse in their acute lymphocytic leukemia are likely to:
    a. recover rapidly.
    b. receive vincristine and prednisone.
    c. receive a bone marrow transplant.
    d. relapse 5 years after a complete remission.

30. Which of the following children with acute lymphoid leukemia has the best prognosis?
    a. A 1-year-old girl with a leukocyte count of 30,000/mm^3
    b. A 6-year-old boy with a leukocyte count of 120,000/mm^3
    c. A 6-year-old boy with a leukocyte count of 30,000/mm^3
    d. A 1-year-old girl with a leukocyte count of 120,000/mm^3

31. To attempt to prevent central nervous system invasion of malignant cells, children with leukemia usually receive prophylactic:
    a. cranial-spinal irradiation.
    b. intravenous steroid therapy.
    c. intrathecal chemotherapy.
    d. intravenous methotrexate and cytarabine.

32. The fact that 95% of children with acute lymphoid leukemia will achieve an initial remission should be interpreted as:
    a. the percentage of children who will live 5 years or longer.
    b. an estimate that applies to children treated with the most successful protocols since diagnosis.
    c. the number to use only for the low-risk group of children.
    d. the estimate that may be used to determine the probability of a cure.

33. Hodgkin disease increases in incidence in children between the ages of:
    a. 1 and 5 years.
    b. 5 and 10 years.
    c. 11 and 14 years.
    d. 15 and 19 years.

34. Using present treatment protocols, prognosis for Hodgkin disease may be estimated with:
    a. the Ann Arbor Staging Classification.
    b. histologic staging.
    c. degree of tumor burden.
    d. initial leukocyte count.

35. A child with Hodgkin disease who has lesions in both the left and the right supraclavicular area, the mediastinum, and the lungs would be classified as:
    a. stage I.
    b. stage II.
    c. stage III.
    d. stage IV.

36. The Sternberg-Reed cell is a significant finding, because it:
    a. is absent in all diseases other than Hodgkin disease.
    b. is absent in all diseases other than the lymphomas.
    c. eliminates the need for laparotomy to determine the stage of the disease.
    d. is absent in all lymphomas other than Hodgkin disease.

37. A particular area of concern for the adolescent receiving radiotherapy is:
    a. frequent vomiting.
    b. altered sexual function.
    c. the high risk for sterility.
    d. precocious puberty.

38. Burkitt lymphoma is a type of:
    a. Hodgkin disease.
    b. non-Hodgkin lymphoma.
    c. acute myelocytic leukemia.
    d. neuroblastoma.

39. The early signs and symptoms of brain tumor in the infant:
    a. are similar to those of a young child's.
    b. may be undetectable while the sutures are open.
    c. will be demonstrated as vomiting after feedings.
    d. will be demonstrated as headache and vomiting.

40. Match each major brain tumor of childhood with its corresponding characteristics.

    a. Medulloblastoma   d. Ependymoma
    b. Astrocytoma   e. Brainstem glioma
    c. Craniopharyngioma

    _____ Arise from pons or medulla; 10% of childhood brain tumors; slow growing

    _____ Considered to have benign properties but is life threatening because of its location near vital structures (pituitary gland)

    _____ Arise from lining tissue of the ventricle; supratentorial and infratentorial tumors comprise 13% of all brain tumors in children

    _____ Invade surrounding tissue, but a slow-growing tumor

    _____ Fast growing; arise from the cerebellum; can invade fourth ventricle and subarachnoid space and cerebrospinal fluid; 18% of all brain tumors in children

41. The surgical technique that uses computed tomography and magnetic resonance imaging is called:
    a. sclerotherapy.
    b. microsurgery.
    c. laser surgery.
    d. stereotactic surgery.

42. An assessment finding that is consistent with the presence of a brain tumor is increased:
    a. temporal headaches.
    b. appetite.
    c. pulse rate.
    d. blood pressure.

43. Describe three strategies the nurse can use to help prepare the child for shaving the hair before surgery to remove a brain tumor.

44. If a child vomits in the postoperative period following surgery for a brain tumor, it may predispose the child to:
    a. incisional rupture.
    b. increased intracranial pressure.
    c. aspiration.
    d. all of the above.

45. Of the following assessment findings in the postoperative care of a child who had surgery to remove a brain tumor, the one with the most serious implications is:
    a. a comatose child.
    b. serosanguinous drainage on the dressing.
    c. colorless drainage on the dressing.
    d. decreased muscle strength.

46. Neuroblastoma is often classified as a silent tumor because:
    a. diagnosis is not usually made until after metastasis.
    b. the primary site is intracranial.
    c. the primary site is the bone marrow.
    d. diagnosis is made based on the location of the primary site.

47. The peak age for the appearance of bone tumors is:
    a. 5 years.
    b. 10 years.
    c. 15 years.
    d. 20 years.

48. The most common bone cancer is most likely to occur in a child age:
    a. birth to 4 years.
    b. 4 years to 8 years.
    c. 8 years to 10 years.
    d. 11 years or older.

49. Treatment for Ewing sarcoma usually involves:
    a. radiation alone.
    b. radiation and chemotherapy.
    c. amputation and chemotherapy.
    d. chemotherapy alone.

50. Treatment for Wilms tumor in children is based on clinical stage and histologic pattern and includes:
    a. chemotherapy and radiation.
    b. radiation alone.
    c. surgery, chemotherapy, and radiation.
    d. surgery alone.

51. Rhabdomyosarcoma is a:
    a. malignant bone neoplasm.
    b. nonmalignant soft tissue tumor.
    c. nonmalignant solid tumor.
    d. malignant solid tumor of the soft tissue.

52. With a multimodal approach to treatment for nonmetastatic rhabdomyosarcoma, what percentage of patients are expected to survive?
    a. 15%
    b. 35%
    c. 50%
    d. 80%

53. Hereditary retinoblastomas are almost always considered to be transmitted as:
    a. an autosomal dominant trait.
    b. a somatic mutation.
    c. a chromosomal aberration.
    d. an autosomal recessive trait.

54. Preoperative instructions to prepare parents of a child who is scheduled for eye enucleation should include:
    a. there will be a cavity in the skull where the eye was.
    b. the child's face may be edematous and ecchymotic.
    c. the eyelids will be open and the surgical site will be sunken.
    d. all of the above.

CRITICAL THINKING—CASE STUDY

Cory is a 6-year-old child who is diagnosed with acute lymphoid leukemia. She receives chemotherapy regularly. Her parents are divorced, and she is an only child. She lives with her mother and rarely sees her father. Cory attends first grade when she can. She had little difficulty with school before her diagnosis, but lately she has had trouble keeping up with the activities because she is so tired.

55. Today Cory arrives at the chemotherapy clinic for her regular medication regimen. A complete blood count shows that her white blood count is lower than expected. The best nursing diagnosis for the nurse to use for Cory today based on the above information would be:
    a. Altered Family Process related to the therapy.
    b. High Risk for Hemorrhagic Cystitis related to white cell proliferation.
    c. High Risk for Infection related to depressed body defenses.
    d. Altered Mucous Membranes related to administration of chemotherapy.

56. Cory's mother tells the nurse that she has noticed Cory's appetite is usually poor after the chemotherapy. The mother knows that nutrition is essential, so she is trying everything to get Cory to eat even when she is nauseated after the chemotherapy. Strategies the nurse might suggest include:
    a. gargling with viscous lidocaine to relieve pain.
    b. permitting only nutritious snacks.
    c. establishing regular mealtimes.
    d. offering small snacks frequently.

57. To plan for the body image disturbance related to loss of hair, moon face, and debilitation, which of the following actions by Cory's mother would be considered most beneficial?
    a. Emphasize the benefits of the therapy.
    b. Encourage Cory to select a wig to wear.
    c. Suggest that Cory keep her hair long for as long as possible.
    d. All of the above

58. Which of the following expected outcomes would be appropriate for the nurse to use to measure Cory's mother's progress toward coping with the possibility of her child's death?
    a. Cory's mother frequently talks to the staff about her fear of living without her daughter.
    b. Cory's mother is able to verbalize an understanding of the procedures and tests that have been performed.
    c. Cory's mother is able to provide the care at home that is needed.
    d. Cory's mother complies with the suggestions the nurses make.

37 The Child with Cerebral Dysfunction

1. Match each term with its description.

a. Central nervous system
b. Peripheral nervous system
c. Autonomic nervous system
d. Meninges
e. Dura mater
f. Epidural space
g. Falx cerebri
h. Falx cerebelli
i. Tentorium
j. Tentorial hiatus

k. Arachnoid membrane
l. Subdural area
m. Pia mater
n. Subarachnoid space
o. Arachnoid trabeculae
p. Longitudinal fissure
q. Corpus callosum
r. Basal ganglia
s. Brainstem
t. Autoregulation

_____ Cerebral nuclei; situated deep within each hemisphere and on each side of the midline; serve as vital sorting areas for messages passing to and from the hemispheres

_____ The large gap through which the brainstem passes; the site of herniation in untreated increased intracranial pressure

_____ The part of the nervous system that is composed of the sympathetic and parasympathetic systems, which provide automatic control of vital functions

_____ A potential space that normally contains only enough fluid to prevent adhesion between the arachnoid and the dura mater

_____ A double-layered membrane that serves as the outer meningeal layer and the inner periosteum of the cranial bones

_____ Located between the pia mater and the arachnoid membrane; filled with cerebrospinal fluid (CSF), which acts as a protective cushion for the brain tissue

_____ A segment of the sheet of dura that separates the cerebral hemispheres

_____ Connected to the hemispheres by thick bunches of nerve fibers; all nerve fibers traverse through this structure as they pass from the hemispheres to the cerebellum and the spinal cord; extends from the base of the hemispheres through the foramen magnum, where it is continuous with the spinal cord

_____ A segment of the sheet of dura that separates the cerebellar hemispheres

_____ The part of the nervous system that is composed of the cranial nerves that arise from or travel to the brainstem and the spinal nerves that travel to or from the spinal cord and which may be motor (efferent) or sensory (afferent)

_____ A segment of dura that separates the cerebellum from the occipital lobe of the cerebrum; a tentlike structure

_____ Separates the outer meningeal layer and the inner periosteum of the cranial bones

_____ The middle meningeal layer; a delicate, avascular, weblike structure that loosely surrounds the brain

_____ The innermost covering layer of the brain; a delicate, transparent membrane that, unlike other coverings, adheres closely to the outer surface of the brain, conforming to the folds (gyri) and furrows (sulci)

_____ The unique ability of the cerebral arterial vessels to change their diameter in response to fluctuating cerebral perfusion pressure

_____ Fibrous filaments that provide protection by helping to anchor the brain

_____ The membranes that cover and protect the brain; the dura mater, arachnoid membranes, and pia mater

_____ Separates the upper part of the two large cerebral hemispheres that occupy the anterior and medial fossae of the skull

_____ The part of the nervous system that is composed of two cerebral hemispheres, the brainstem, the cerebellum, and the spinal cord

_____ The largest fiber bundle in the brain; joins the central part of the cerebral hemispheres; interconnects cortical areas of the right and left hemispheres

2. The following terms are related to the evaluation of neurologic status. Match each term with its description.

a. Neurologic physical examination
b. Choreiform movements
c. Level of development
d. Alertness
e. Cognitive power
f. Unconsciousness
g. Coma
h. Comatose state
i. Glasgow Coma Scale
j. Brain death

k. Descriptive and detailed documentation
l. Pulse, respiration, blood pressure
m. Autonomic activity
n. Body temperature
o. Corneal reflex
p. Doll's head maneuver
q. Caloric test
r. Papilledema
s. Flexion posturing
t. Extension posturing

_____ Quick, jerky, grossly uncoordinated movements that may disappear on relaxation

_____ An arousal-waking state that includes the ability to respond to stimuli; an aspect of consciousness

_____ Includes observation of the size and shape of the head, spontaneous activity, postural reflex activity, sensory responses, symmetry of movement

_____ Depressed cerebral function; the inability to respond to sensory stimuli and have subjective experiences

_____ Provide information regarding the adequacy of circulation and the possible underlying cause of altered consciousness

_____ The aspect of consciousness that includes the ability to process stimuli and produce verbal and motor responses

_____ The continuum of diminished alertness as a result of pathologic conditions

_____ Provides essential information about neurologic function; developmental tests used to determine this element of the neurologic assessment

_____ Often elevated in head injury; sometimes extreme and unresponsive to therapeutic measures

_____ Consists of a three-part assessment; created to meet a clinical need of experienced nurses for objective criteria for the consciousness level; the most popular tool that attempts to standardize the description and interpretation of depressed consciousness

_____ A sign of increased intracranial pressure observed in the eyes

_____ The total cessation of brainstem and cortical brain function

_____ A sign of dysfunction at the level of the midbrain; characterized by rigid extension and pronation of the arms and legs

_____ Most intensively disturbed in deep coma and in brainstem lesions

_____ Blinking of the eyelids when the cornea is touched with a wisp of cotton; used to test the integrity of the ophthalmic division of cranial nerve

_____ The fashion in which neurologic examination should be documented; enables detection of subtle changes in neurologic status over time

_____ Child's head rotated quickly to one side and then the other; normally, eyes will move in the direction opposite the head rotation

_____ A state of unconsciousness from which the patient cannot be aroused, even with powerful stimuli

_____ Oculovestibular response; elicited by irrigating the external auditory canal with ice water; causes movement of the eyes toward the side of the stimulation

_____ Seen with severe dysfunction of the cerebral cortex; includes adduction of the arms and shoulders; arms flexed on the chest; wrists flexed; hands fisted; lower extremities extended and adducted

3. The following terms are related to head injury. Match each term with its description.

a. Acceleration/deceleration
b. Deformation
c. Coup
d. Contrecoup
e. Shearing stresses
f. Cytotoxic edema
g. Vasogenic edema
h. Concussion
i. Contusion, laceration
j. Linear fractures

k. Depressed fractures
l. Compound fractures
m. Basilar fracture
n. Growing fracture
o. Acute subdural hematoma
p. Chronic subdural hematoma
q. Postconcussion syndrome
r. Posttraumatic seizures
s. Structural complications

_____ A fracture in which the bone is locally broken, usually into several irregular fragments that are pushed inward, causing pressure on the brain

_____ Bruising at the point of impact

_____ Physical forces that act on the head when the stationary head receives a blow; the circumstances responsible for most head injuries; when the head receives a blow

_____ A common sequela to brain injury with or without loss of consciousness; symptoms typically develop within days of the injury and typically resolve within 3 months; involves headaches, dizziness, fatigue, irritability, anxiety, insomnia, loss of concentration, and memory impairment

_____ Caused by hemorrhage; associated with contusions or lacerations and develops within minutes or hours of injury

_____ Involves the basilar portion of the frontal, ethmoid, sphenoid, temporal, or occipital bones

_____ Actual bruising and tearing of cerebral tissue

_____ An effect of brain movement that is caused by unequal movement or different rates of acceleration at various levels of the brain; may tear small arteries; the area of the brainstem often most seriously affected

_____ Distortion and cavitation that occur as the brain changes shape in response to the force transmitted from impact to the brain

_____ Occur in a number of children who survive a head injury; more common in children than in adults; more likely to occur with severe head injury; usually occur within the first few days after injury

_____ Results from fracture with an underlying tear in the dura that fails to heal properly; parietal bone is the most common location

_____ A result of direct cell injury; caused by intracellular swelling

_____ Bruising at a distance from the point of impact

_____ Nerve cells not primarily injured; caused by increased permeability of capillary endothelial cells, which results in increased intracellular fluid

_____ Occur as a result of head injuries; include hydrocephalus and motor deficits

_____ The most common head injury; a transient and reversible neuronal dysfunction with instantaneous loss of awareness and responsiveness from trauma to the head

_____ Consists of a skin laceration that extends to the site of the bony fracture

_____ Uncommon before age 2 or 3, but constitute the majority of childhood skull fractures; often asymptomatic in older children

_____ Caused by hemorrhage; associated with contusions or lacerations, symptoms are delayed; more commonly seen in children with open fontanels and sutures

4. The following terms are related to intracranial infections. Match each term with its description.

   a. Meningitis
   b. Encephalitis
   c. Human diploid cell rabies vaccine
   d. Bacterial meningitis
   e. Viral meningitis

   f. Tuberculous meningitis
   g. *Streptococcus pneumoniae* meningitis
   h. Meningococcal sepsis
   i. Waterhouse-Friderichsen syndrome
   j. Hydrophobia

   _____ The sudden, severe, and fulminating onset of meningococcemia

   _____ Inflammatory process that affects the brain

   _____ The term used to describe the symptoms of rabies; severe spasm of respiratory muscles resulting in apnea, cyanosis, and anoxia

   _____ An acute inflammation of the meninges and CSF; antimicrobial therapy has a marked effect on course and prognosis; dramatic decrease in incidence with increased use of *Haemophilus influenzae* type B and *S. pneumoniae* vaccines

   _____ Vaccine administered to confer active immunity after a rabid animal bite; administered with immune globulin and followed with injections at 3, 7, 14, and 28 days after the first dose

   _____ Aseptic meningitis

   _____ Has decreased in incidence since the use of vaccine in 2000; remains the most common cause of bacterial meningitis in children between 3 months and 10 years of age

   _____ Inflammatory process that affects the meninges

   _____ Meningococcemia; one of the most dramatic and serious complications associated with meningococcal infection

   _____ Meningitis that is more likely to disseminate in very young or immunosuppressed children; more children predisposed to this form of meningitis with the increase in drug-resistant tuberculosis

5. Match each neurologic diagnostic procedure with its description.

   a. Lumbar puncture (LP)
   b. Subdural tap
   c. Ventricular puncture
   d. Electroencephalography (EEG)
   e. Nuclear brain scan
   f. Endocephalography

   g. Real-time ultrasonography (RTUS)
   h. Radiography
   i. Computed tomography (CT) scan
   j. Magnetic resonance imaging (MRI)
   k. Positron emission tomography (PET)
   l. Digital subtraction angiography (DSA)

   _____ Needle inserted into anterior fontanel or coronal suture

   _____ Identifies shifts in midline structures from their normal positions as a result of intracranial lesions; simple, safe, and rapid procedure; fontanel must be patent

   _____ After contrast dye injected intravenously, computer "subtracts" all tissues without contrast medium, leaving clear image of contrast medium in vessels; safe alternative to angiography

   _____ Similar to CT but uses ultrasound instead of ionizing radiation; especially useful in neonatal central nervous system problems

   _____ Detects and measures blood volume and flow in brain, metabolic activity, biochemical changes within tissue; requires lengthy period of immobility; minimal exposure to radiation occurs; patient often needs sedation

   _____ Needle inserted into lateral ventricle via coronal suture

   _____ Pinpoint x-ray beam directed on horizontal or vertical plane to provide series of images that are fed into a computer and assembled in image displayed on video screen; uses ionizing radiation; rapid

   _____ Radioisotope injected intravenously, then counted and recorded after fixed time intervals; radioisotope accumulates in areas where blood-brain barrier is defective; visualizes CSF pathways

_____ Records changes in electrical potential of brain; used to determine brain death and to indicate the potential for seizures

_____ Skull films taken from different views—lateral, posterolateral, axial; shows fractures

_____ Radiofrequency images produced from elements and converted to visual images by computer; no exposure to radiation; may require sedation

_____ Spinal needle inserted between L3-L4 or L4-L5 vertebral spaces into subarachnoid space; measures spinal fluid pressure; can obtain CSF for laboratory analysis

6. Cerebral blood flow, oxygen consumption, and brain growth are all:
   a. less in adults than in children.
   b. greater in adults than in children.
   c. greater in adults than in infants.
   d. less in infants than in children.

7. Match each seizure term with its description.

   a. Cryptogenic seizures
   b. Acute symptomatic seizures
   c. Epileptogenic focus
   d. Ictal state
   e. Postictal state
   f. Simple partial seizures with motor signs
   g. Aversive seizure
   h. Rolandic (Sylvan) seizure
   i. Jacksonian march
   j. Simple partial seizures with sensory signs
   k. Partial seizures
   l. Generalized seizures
   m. Unclassified epileptic seizures
   n. Psychomotor seizures
   o. Aura

   p. Déjà vu
   q. Impaired consciousness
   r. Automatism
   s. Tonic phase
   t. Clonic phase
   u. Status epilepticus
   v. Drop attacks
   w. Infantile spasms
   x. Salaam seizure
   y. Tonic-clonic seizures
   z. Lennox-Gastaut syndrome
   aa. West syndrome
   bb. Resective surgery
   cc. Callosotomy
   dd. Multiple subpial transection

   _____ Seizures that occur as a result of an insult such as head injury

   _____ Simple motor seizure; consists of orderly, sequential progression of clonic movements that begin in a foot, hand, or face and, as electrical impulses spread from the irritable focus to contiguous regions of the cortex, move body parts activated by these cerebral regions

   _____ Seizures with no clear cause

   _____ Formerly called "focal seizures"; limited to a particular local area of the brain

   _____ A period of the seizure where the eyes roll upward and the patient immediately loses consciousness

   _____ A feeling of familiarity in a strange environment

   _____ All seizures that cannot be classified

   _____ Arise from the area of the brain that controls muscle movement

   _____ Tonic-clonic movements involving the face, salivation, and arrested speech; most common during sleep

   _____ Horizontal fibers of the motor cortex divided to reduce seizures; vertical fibers spared to allow for function

   _____ A group of hyperexcitable cells that initiate the spontaneous electrical discharge that produces a seizure

   _____ The period during the time the seizure is occurring

   _____ The period following a seizure

   _____ Characterized by various sensations, including numbness, tingling, prickling, paresthesia, or pain that originates in one area and spreads to other parts of the body

   _____ Seizures that involve both hemispheres of the brain

   _____ Partial seizures with complex symptoms

_____ A characteristic of the complex partial seizure; repeated activities without purpose and carried out in a dreamy state such as smacking, chewing, drooling, or swallowing

_____ The period in the seizure where there are intense jerking movements as the trunk and extremities undergo rhythmic contraction and relaxation

_____ Atonic seizures; manifested as a sudden, momentary loss of muscle tone

_____ A common motor seizure in children; the eye(s) and head turn away from the side of the focus

_____ A rare disorder that has an onset within the first 6 to 8 months of life; also known as *infantile myoclonus, West syndrome*

_____ Separation of the connections between the two hemispheres of the brain; used to treat some generalized seizures

_____ A characteristic of the complex partial seizure; child may appear dazed and confused and be unable to respond when spoken to or to follow instruction

_____ Also known as *jackknife seizures*; observed as sudden, brief, symmetric muscular contractions by which the head is flexed, the arms extended, and the legs drawn up; observed in infantile spasms

_____ Focal area of seizure activity excised with the expectation that serious deficits will not be produced and that existing deficits will not be increased

_____ A seizure that lasts 30 minutes or longer or a series of seizures at intervals too brief to allow the child to regain consciousness between each seizure; requires emergency intervention

_____ Onset occurs between 1 and 7 years of age; multiple tonic seizures daily are typical

_____ Disorder also known as *massive spasms, salaam seizures, flexion spasms, jackknife seizures, massive myoclonic jerks*, or *infantile myoclonic spasms*; more common in males than in females

_____ Sensation or sensory phenomenon that reflects the complicated connections and integrative functions of that area of the brain

_____ Formerly know as "grand mal seizures"

8. The blood-brain barrier in an infant is:
   a. less permeable than in the adult.
   b. impermeable to protein.
   c. impermeable to glucose.
   d. permeable to large molecules.

9. Which of the following signs is used to evaluate increased intracranial pressure in the infant but not in the older child?
   a. Projectile vomiting
   b. Headache
   c. Nonpulsating fontanel
   d. Pulsating fontanel

10. Which of the following indicators best determines the depth of the comatose state?
    a. Motor activity
    b. Level of consciousness
    c. Reflexes
    d. Vital signs

11. Define the term *persistent vegetative state.*

12. The guidelines for establishing brain death in children:
    a. differ from age to age.
    b. are the same as in the adult.
    c. require an observation period of at least 7 days.
    d. require an observation period of at least 48 hours.

13. Of the following neurologic conditions, the one that is most associated with hypothermia is:
    a. intracranial bleeding.
    b. barbiturate ingestion.
    c. heatstroke.
    d. serious infection.

14. A child in a very deep comatose state would exhibit:
    a. hyperkinetic activity.
    b. purposeless plucking movements.
    c. few spontaneous movements.
    d. combative behavior.

15. After a seizure in a child over 3 years of age, the Babinski reflex often:
    a. remains positive.
    b. remains negative.
    c. fluctuates.
    d. is unable to be tested correctly.

16. A cerebral dysfunction gait that is described as narrow-based gait with a tendency to walk on toes, along with flexion at knees and hips and shuffling, is:
    a. ataxia.
    b. spastic hemiplegic gait.
    c. extrapyramidal gait.
    d. spastic paraplegic gait.

17. If the patient has an increase in intracranial pressure, one test that is contraindicated is the:
    a. LP.
    b. subdural tap.
    c. CT.
    d. DSA.

18. The diagnostic procedure that is usually noninvasive and permits visualization of the neurologic structures using radiofrequency emissions from elements is called:
    a. DSA.
    b. PET.
    c. MRI.
    d. CT.

19. The factor that is likely to have the greatest impact on the outcome and recovery of the unconscious child is the:
    a. gradual reduction in intracranial pressure.
    b. level of nursing care and observation skills.
    c. emotional response of the parents.
    d. level of discomfort the child experiences.

20. The nurse should suspect pain in the comatose child if the child exhibits:
    a. increased flaccidity.
    b. increased oxygen saturation.
    c. decreased blood pressure.
    d. increased agitation.

21. Intracranial pressure monitoring has been found to be useful in pediatric critical care to:
    a. provide quick and effective relief of increased pressure.
    b. evaluate children with Glasgow Coma Scale scores less than 7.
    c. maintain $Paco_2$ at 25 to 30 mm Hg.
    d. prevent herniation.

22. Of the following activities, the one that has been shown to increase intracranial pressure is:
    a. using earplugs to eliminate noise.
    b. range-of-motion exercises.
    c. suctioning.
    d. osmotherapy.

23. The medications that are controversial in the management of increased intracranial pressure are:
    a. barbiturates.
    b. paralyzing agents.
    c. sedatives.
    d. antiepileptics.

24. If a child is permanently unconscious, it would be inappropriate for the nurse to:
    a. permit the parents to bring a child's favorite toy.
    b. provide guidance and clarify information that the physician has already given.
    c. suggest the parents plan for periodic relief from the continual care of their child.
    d. use reflexive muscle contractions as a sign of hope for recovery.

25. Because of the ability of the cranium to expand, which of the following neurologic conditions might very young children tolerate better than an adult?
    a. Cerebral edema
    b. Hypoxic brain damage
    c. Epilepsy
    d. Subdural hemorrhage

26. Head injury that causes the brain to be forced though the tentorial opening is usually referred to as:
    a. tentorial contrecoup.
    b. concussion.
    c. tentorial herniation.
    d. deformation.

27. Of the following symptoms, the one that would not be considered a hallmark of concussion in a child is:
    a. alteration of mental status.
    b. amnesia.
    c. loss of consciousness.
    d. confusion.

28. Epidural hemorrhage is less common in children under 2 years of age than in adults because:
    a. the middle meningeal artery is embedded in the bone surface of the skull until approximately 2 years of age.
    b. fractures are less likely to lacerate the middle meningeal artery in children under 2 years of age.
    c. separation of the dura from bleeding is more likely to occur in children than in adults.
    d. there is an increased tendency for the skull to fracture in children under 2 years of age.

29. Which of the following features is usually associated with supratentorial subdural hematoma?
    a. Arterial hemorrhage is usually present.
    b. Skull fracture is almost always present.
    c. It is more common than epidural hematoma.
    d. It occurs in patients older than 2 years.

30. The goal in the management of a child with a head injury is to:
    a. eliminate ischemic brain damage.
    b. eliminate original primary insult.
    c. care for the secondary brain injuries.
    d. carry out all of the above.

31. Emergency treatment of a child with a head injury would generally not include:
    a. administering analgesics.
    b. checking pupils' reaction to light.
    c. stabilizing the neck and spine.
    d. checking level of consciousness.

32. The clinical manifestation that indicates a progression from minor head injury to severe head injury is:
    a. confusion.
    b. mounting agitation.
    c. an episode of vomiting.
    d. pallor.

33. Compared with adults who have suffered craniocerebral trauma, children usually have a:
    a. lower incidence of psychologic disturbances.
    b. higher mortality rate.
    c. less favorable prognosis.
    d. higher incidence of psychologic disturbances.

34. Family support for the child who has suffered head injury includes all of the following except encouraging the parents to:
    a. hold and cuddle the child.
    b. bring familiar belongings into the child's room.
    c. make a tape recording of familiar voices or sounds.
    d. search for clues that the child is recovering.

35. What should the nurse emphasize when providing anticipatory guidance for parents in regard to children spending time near the water?

36. Physiologic factors that influence the extent of damage from immersion include resistance to asphyxia and anoxia. Which of the following best describes this?
    a. Primitive neurologic response of bradycardia and breath-holding
    b. Triggered by immersion of the body in cold water
    c. Blood shunted away from the vital organs except for the lungs
    d. Response terminated and reflex inspiration occurs as the child comes up for air

37. Of the following factors, the best predictor of outcome in near-drowning victims is:
    a. respiratory rate.
    b. degree of acidosis on admission.
    c. level of consciousness.
    d. length of time the child was submerged.

38. The etiology of bacterial meningitis has changed in recent years because of the:
    a. increased surveillance of tuberculosis.
    b. increased awareness of rubella and polio vaccines.
    c. routine use of *H. influenzae* type B and *S. pneumoniae* vaccines.
    d. routine use of hepatitis B and hepatitis A vaccines.

39. The most common mode of transmission for bacterial meningitis is:
    a. vascular dissemination of a respiratory tract infection.
    b. direct implantation from an invasive procedure.
    c. direct extension from an infection in the mastoid sinuses.
    d. direct extension from an infection in the nasal sinuses.

40. A child who is ill and develops a purpuric or petechial rash may possibly have developed:
    a. aseptic meningitis.
    b. Waterhouse-Friderichsen syndrome.
    c. *Citrobacter diversus* meningitis.
    d. herpes simplex encephalitis.

41. Secondary problems from bacterial meningitis are most likely to occur in the:
    a. child with meningococcal meningitis.
    b. infant under 2 months of age.
    c. infant over 2 months of age.
    d. child with *H. influenzae* type B meningitis.

42. Which of the following types of meningitis is self-limiting and least serious?
    a. Meningococcal meningitis
    b. Tuberculous meningitis
    c. *H. influenzae* meningitis
    d. Nonbacterial (aseptic) meningitis

43. Although an uncommon disease, the type of encephalitis that is responsible for 30% of cases in children is caused by:
    a. herpes simplex.
    b. measles.
    c. mumps.
    d. rubella.

44. In the United States, most human fatalities associated with rabies occur in people who:
    a. are unaware of their exposure.
    b. have not been immunized.
    c. live near raccoons and bats.
    d. provoke an unvaccinated dog.

45. The recommended postexposure treatment for rabies includes:
    a. mass immunization using human rabies immune globulin.
    b. administration of human diploid cell rabies vaccine according to schedule for 3 months after the exposure.
    c. mass immunization using human diploid cell rabies vaccine.
    d. administration of human rabies immune globulin 90 days after the exposure.

46. The decrease in the incidence of Reye syndrome is widely believed to be linked to:
    a. improved definitive diagnosis using liver biopsy as a criterion.
    b. earlier diagnosis and more aggressive therapy.
    c. public education about the potential hazard of using aspirin for the treatment of children with varicella or influenza.
    d. mass immunization programs.

47. Symptoms that are similar to those of Reye syndrome have occurred during viral illnesses when the child was given an:
    a. antiemetic drug.
    b. analgesic drug.
    c. antiepileptic drug.
    d. antiarrhythmic drug.

48. The drug that reduces the chance that the human immunodeficiency virus (HIV)–infected pregnant mother will infect her infant is called:
    a. valproate.
    b. zidovudine.
    c. nitrazepam.
    d. felbamate.

49. Name two factors that contribute to childhood seizures.

50. A child having a complex partial seizure rather than a simple partial seizure is more likely to exhibit:
    a. impaired consciousness.
    b. clonic movements.
    c. a seizure duration of less than 1 minute.
    d. all of the above.

51. One strategy that may provide a clue to the origin of a seizure is:
    a. to attempt to place an airway in the mouth.
    b. to gently open the eyes to observe their movement.
    c. to provide a clear description of the seizure.
    d. all of the above.

52. Which of the following types of seizures is most common in children between the ages of 5 and 12 years?
    a. Salaam seizures
    b. Absence seizures
    c. Atonic seizures
    d. Jackknife seizures

53. The therapy for infantile spasms is likely to include:
    a. adrenocorticotropic hormone or vigabatrin.
    b. valproic acid and vigabatrin.
    c. ethosuximide only.
    d. felbamate only.

54. The drug of choice for the treatment of Lennox-Gastaut syndrome is:
    a. nitrazepam.
    b. clonazepam.
    c. felbamate.
    d. valproate.

55. Therapy for epilepsy should begin with:
    a. short-term drug therapy.
    b. combination drug therapy.
    c. only one drug, if possible.
    d. drugs that correct the brain wave pattern.

56. The intravenous medication that is used to treat seizures and may be given in either saline or glucose is:
    a. fosphenytoin.
    b. phenytoin.
    c. valproic acid.
    d. felbamate.

57. A simple, effective, and safe treatment for home or prehospital management of status epilepticus is:
    a. rectal diazepam.
    b. intravenous valproic acid.
    c. intravenous phenytoin.
    d. rectal fosphenytoin.

58. The highest morbidity for the child with status epilepticus is associated with:
    a. previous developmental delays.
    b. previous neurologic abnormalities.
    c. history of recurrent seizures.
    d. nonfebrile, nonidiopathic seizures.

59. Nursing intervention for a child during a tonic-clonic seizure should include attempts to:
    a. halt the seizure as soon as it begins.
    b. restrain the child.
    c. remain calm and prevent the child from sustaining any harm.
    d. place an oral airway in the child's mouth.

60. Emergency care of the child during a seizure includes:
    a. giving ice chips slowly.
    b. restraining the child.
    c. putting a tongue blade in the child's mouth.
    d. loosening restrictive clothing.

61. To prevent submersion injuries in children with epilepsy, the child should be instructed to:
    a. never go swimming.
    b. take showers.
    c. wear a bicycle helmet.
    d. do all of the above.

62. In most children who have a febrile seizure, the factor that triggers the seizure tends to be:
    a. rapidity of the temperature elevation.
    b. duration of the temperature elevation.
    c. height of the temperature elevation.
    d. any of the above.

63. When a child has a febrile seizure, it is important for the parents to know that the child will:
    a. probably not develop epilepsy.
    b. most likely develop epilepsy.
    c. most likely develop neurologic damage.
    d. usually need tepid sponge baths to control fever.

64. Migraine headaches in children:
    a. have typical symptoms of abdominal pain, as well as episodic pallor in the older child.
    b. occur most often in the morning, awakening the child from sleep.
    c. are more common in boys, after the onset of puberty.
    d. have typical symptoms of nausea, vomiting, and abdominal pain that are relieved by sleep.

65. Treatment for migraine headaches in adolescents over 12 years of age may include:
    a. ergots.
    b. opioids.
    c. sumatriptan.
    d. all of the above.

CRITICAL THINKING—CASE STUDY

Jackson was riding his bike in the street by his house when he was hit by a car. He is 9 years old. He was not wearing a helmet at the time. He has been unconscious since the accident 8 hours ago. His mother and father both work full-time, and there are five other siblings at home ranging in ages from 7 to 19 years old.

66. Based on the preceding information, which of the following nursing diagnoses would have the highest priority?
    a. Risk for Impaired Skin Integrity related to immobility
    b. Self-Care Deficit related to physical immobility
    c. Interrupted Family Process related to potential permanent disability
    d. Risk for Aspiration: Ineffective Airway Clearance related to depressed sensorium

67. To effectively deal with the interrupted family process related to the hospitalization, the nurse should:
    a. provide information about bicycle safety helmets.
    b. encourage expression of feelings.
    c. encourage the family to take care of Jackson's hygiene needs.
    d. provide auditory stimulation for Jackson.

68. To help Jackson receive appropriate sensory stimulation, the nurse should:
    a. hang a black-and-white mobile above his bed.
    b. hang a calendar at the foot of his bed.
    c. encourage the family to bring a tape of his favorite music.
    d. administer pain medications as needed.

69. Jackson's parents visit him every day, but they never come together. The nurse should be concerned about:
    a. marital problems that usually occur during stressful times like this.
    b. whether Jackson's parents are able to receive adequate support from each other with this arrangement.
    c. whether Jackson's siblings are receiving adequate care.
    d. all of the above.

38 The Child with Endocrine Dysfunction

1. The following terms are related to hormones. Match each term with its description.

a. Cell
b. End organ
c. Environment
d. Local hormones
e. General hormones
f. Target tissues
g. Anterior pituitary

h. Tropic hormones
i. Inhibitory hormones
j. Neuroendocrine system
k. Autonomic nervous system
l. Parasympathetic system
m. Sympathetic system
n. Neurotransmitting substances

_____ The master gland

_____ Substances produced in one organ or part of the body and carried through the bloodstream to a distant part, or parts, of the body, where they initiate or regulate physiologic activity of an organ or group of cells (e.g., thyroid)

_____ The component of the endocrine system that sends a chemical message by means of a hormone

_____ Acetylcholine released by cholinergic fibers and norepinephrine released by adrenergic fibers

_____ Substances secreted to produce their effects on specific tisues called _target tissues_

_____ The component of the endocrine system through which the chemical is transported (blood, lymph, extracellular fluid) from the site of synthesis to the site of cellular action

_____ Consists of the sympathetic and parasympathetic systems; controls nonvoluntary functions, specifically of the smooth muscle myocardium and glands

_____ Specific tissues on which hormones produce their effect (e.g., the pituitary hormones stimulating the adrenal glands to secrete adrenocorticotropin)

_____ Secreted by the hypothalamus and transported by way of the pituitary portal system to the anterior pituitary, where they stimulate the secretion of tropic hormones

_____ Target cell; the component of the endocrine system that receives the chemical message

_____ The system that maintains homeostasis through interaction between endocrine glands and the nervous system

_____ Primarily involved in regulating digestive processes

_____ Substances produced and secreted into body fluids that exert a physiologic controlling effect on cells near the point of secretion (e.g., acetylcholine)

_____ Functions to maintain homeostasis during stress

2. The following terms are related to pituitary disorders. Match each term with its description.

a. Idiopathic hypopituitarism
b. Familial short stature
c. Constitutional growth delay
d. Creutzfeldt-Jakob disease
e. Biosynthetic growth hormone
f. Human Growth Foundation
g. Acromegaly

h. Hypothalamic-pituitary-gonadal axis
i. Central precocious puberty
j. Peripheral precocious puberty
k. Desmopressin acetate (DDAVP)
l. Luteinizing hormone–releasing hormone
m. Neurogenic diabetes insipidus
n. Vasopressin

_____ Early puberty resulting from hormones other than hypothalamic and pituitary gonadotropic releasers

_____ Hormone that will alleviate the polyuria and polydipsia associated with neurogenic diabetes insipidus

_____ Refers to individuals (usually boys) with delayed linear growth generally beginning in toddler years; skeletal and sexual maturation is behind that of age-mates

_____ Prepared by recombinant deoxyribonucleic acid (DNA) technology

_____ Regulates pituitary secretions; a synthetic analog is used to manage precocious puberty of central origin

_____ An organization that provides research, education, support, and advocacy for professionals and for families of a child with growth defects

_____ The sequence of events that stimulates the secretion of gonadotropic hormones from the anterior pituitary at the time of puberty

_____ Growth failure; usually related to growth hormone deficiency

_____ Results from premature activation of the hypothalamic-pituitary-gonadal axis, which produces early maturation and development of the gonads with secretion of sex hormones, development of secondary sexual characteristics, and occasional production of mature sperm or ova; more common among girls

_____ A rare and fatal neurodegenerative condition that has been iatrogenically transmitted through human tissue from cadaver-derived growth hormone

_____ A long-acting analog of arginine vasopressin used to treat diabetes insipidus

_____ The condition that is produced when hypersecretion of growth hormone occurs after epiphyseal closure; growth occurs in transverse direction

_____ Hyposecretion of antidiuretic hormone, or vasopressin; produces a state of uncontrolled diuresis

_____ Refers to otherwise healthy children who have ancestors with adult height in the lower percentiles and whose height during childhood is appropriate for genetic background

3. The following terms are related to endocrine disorders. Match each term with its description.

a. Thyroid hormone
b. Calcitonin
c. Thyroid-stimulating hormone
d. Hashimoto disease
e. Exophthalmos
f. Parathyroid hormone
g. Vitamin D therapy
h. Hyperparathyroidism
i. Adrenal cortex
j. Glucocorticoids
k. Mineralocorticoids
l. Sex steroids
m. Corticotropin-releasing factor
n. Adrenocorticotropic hormone
o. Aldosterone
p. Renin
q. Adrenal crisis
r. Waterhouse-Friderichsen syndrome
s. 21-Hydroxylase deficiency
t. 11-Hydroxylase deficiency
u. Ambiguous genitalia

_____ Most pronounced in the female with masculinization of the external genitalia; the term to use for any infant with hypospadias or micropenis and no palpable gonads

_____ The thyroid gland secretes this type of hormone in addition to thyroid hormone (T_3 and T_4); one of the two types of hormones secreted by the thyroid gland

_____ Juvenile autoimmune thyroiditis; lymphocytic thyroiditis; the most common cause of thyroid disease in children and adolescents; accounts for the largest percentage of juvenile hypothyroidism

_____ Produced by the anterior pituitary; controls the secretion of thyroid hormones

_____ Protruding eyeballs; observed in many children with Hashimoto disease; accompanied by a wide-eyed staring expression, increased blinking, lid lag, lack of convergence, and absence of wrinkling of the forehead when looking upward

_____ Treatment used in hypoparathyroidism

_____ Secreted by the parathyroid glands; maintains serum calcium levels

_____ The mineralocorticoid that promotes sodium retention and potassium excretion in the renal tubules

_____ Androgens, estrogens, and progestins

_____ Causes the pituitary gland to produce adrenocorticotropic hormone

_____ Rare in childhood; causes include adenoma, chronic renal disease, renal osteodystrophy, and congenital urinary tract anomalies; hypercalcemia is present

_____ Cortisol and corticosterone

_____ The acute form of adrenocortical insufficiency

_____ Secretes the glucocorticoids, mineralocorticoids, and sex steroids

_____ Aldosterone; one of the three groups of hormone secreted by the adrenal cortex

_____ Stimulates the adrenal glands to synthesize glucocorticoids

_____ Converts angiotensinogen to angiotensin I and then to angiotensin II, stimulating the adrenal cortex to secrete aldosterone, which preserves sodium, retains water, and increases blood pressure

_____ The presentation of generalized hemorrhagic and necrotic manifestations in adrenocortical insufficiency; may be caused by a prolonged, difficult labor and rapidly progressing infections, such as meningococcemia

_____ The most common biochemical defect associated with congenital adrenogenital hyperplasia

_____ A type of hormone secreted by the thyroid gland; consists of the hormones thyroxine (T_4) and triiodothyronine (T_3)

_____ The form of adrenal hyperplasia in which there is an increase in the mineralocorticoid that leads to hypertension

4. The following terms are related to diabetes. Match each term with its description.

a. Type 1 diabetes
b. Immune-mediated diabetes mellitus
c. Idiopathic type 1 diabetes
d. Type 2 diabetes
e. Maturity-onset diabetes of the young
f. Insulin
g. Hyperglycemia
h. Glycosuria
i. Polyuria
j. Polydipsia
k. Glucogenesis

l. Polyphagia
m. Ketonuria
n. Acetone breath
o. Ketonemia
p. Ketoacidosis
q. Ketones
r. Kussmaul respirations
s. Nephropathy, retinopathy, neuropathy
t. Glycosylation
u. Diabetic ketoacidosis

_____ Excessive thirst

_____ The rare form of type 1 diabetes that has no known cause

_____ Elevated blood glucose levels and glucose in the urine

_____ The form of diabetes that results from an autoimmune destruction of beta cells; typically starts in slim children or young adults

_____ Organic acids that readily produce excessive quantities of free hydrogen ions

_____ May be a result of sluggish or insensitive secretory response of insulin from the pancreas or a defect in body tissues that requires unusual amounts of insulin, or the insulin secreted may be rapidly destroyed, inhibited, or inactivated

_____ β-Hydroxybutyric acid, acetoacetic acid, and acetone in the urine

_____ Elimination of ketones through the lungs

_____ The metabolic hormone that supports the metabolism of carbohydrates, fats, and proteins

_____ Osmotic diversion of water, a cardinal sign of diabetes

_____ Associated with monogenetic defects in beta-cell function; characterized by impaired insulin secretion with minimal defects in insulin action; inherited in an autosomal dominant pattern, with the onset of hyperglycemia occurring at an early age (generally before age 25 years)

_____ Process where protein is broken down and converted to glucose by the liver

_____ Dehydration, electrolyte imbalance, and acidosis from diabetes

_____ Characterized by the destruction of the pancreatic beta cells that produce insulin; usually leads to absolute insulin deficiency

_____ The lowering of the serum pH; results from ketone bodies in the blood

_____ Glucose in the urine

_____ Proteins from the blood become deposited in the walls of small vessels; these substances cause narrowing of the vessels and interfere with the microcirculation in the affected areas over time

_____ Increased food intake

_____ Long-term complications of diabetes that involve the microvasculature

_____ β-Hydroxybutyric acid, acetoacetic acid, and acetone in the blood

_____ Hyperventilation characteristic of metabolic acidosis

5. The following terms are related to the therapeutic management of diabetes. Match each term with its description.

a. Regular insulin
b. NPH or Lente insulin
c. Adrenergic symptoms
d. Insulin pump
e. Islet cell or whole pancreas transplant
f. Self-monitoring of blood glucose

g. Insulin reaction
h. Glucagon
i. Somogyi effect
j. Inject-Ease
k. NovoPen

_____ An intermediate-acting drug

_____ An electromechanical device designed to deliver fixed amounts of a diluted solution of regular insulin continuously; more closely imitates the release of insulin

_____ A rapid-acting drug

_____ Has improved diabetes management; diabetes management depends on these values

_____ Used in persons who have serious diabetes complications, particularly those who require renal transplantation with immunosuppressive therapy

_____ Releases stored glycogen from the liver; prescribed for home treatment of hypoglycemia

_____ A syringe-loaded injector for use by children who do not wish to give themselves injections

_____ Often the most feared aspect of diabetes due to possible development of severe brain symptoms

_____ Rebound hyperglycemia

_____ Early signs of hypoglycemia; help to raise the blood glucose level; sweating, trembling

_____ A self-contained, compact device resembling a fountain pen, which eliminates conventional vials and syringes

6. For each of the following hormones, write the name of the target tissue or gland in the blank following the hormone. Then match each hormone and gland with the corresponding effect in the list below.

a. Thyroid-stimulating hormone _____ _____

b. Luteinizing hormone _____ and _____

c. Somatotropic hormone _____

d. Gonadotropin _____

e. Melanocyte-stimulating hormone _____

f. Adrenocorticotropic hormone _____ _____

g. Antidiuretic hormone _____ _____

h. Follicle-stimulating hormone _____ and _____

i. Oxytocin _____ and _____

j. Prolactin _____ and _____

_____ Increases reabsorption of water

_____ Promotes growth of bone and soft tissue

_____ Stimulates the secretion of glucocorticoids

_____ Initiates spermatogenesis

_____ Regulates metabolic rate

_____ Maintains corpus luteum during pregnancy

_____ Promotes pigmentation of the skin

_____ Causes the let-down reflex

_____ Produces sex hormones

_____ Stimulates the secretion of testosterone in the male

7. A hormone that produces its effect on a specific tissue would be classified as a _____ hormone.

8. Overproduction of the anterior pituitary hormones can result in:
   a. hyperthyroidism.
   b. hypercortisolism.
   c. precocious puberty.
   d. all of the above.

9. The most common organic cause of pituitary undersecretion is:
   a. tumor in the adrenocortical region.
   b. autoimmune hypophysitis.
   c. tumor in the pituitary or hypothalamic region.
   d. perinatal trauma.

10. A child with growth hormone deficiency will exhibit the signs of:
    a. retarded height and weight.
    b. abnormal skeletal proportions.
    c. malnutrition.
    d. short stature but proportional height and weight.

11. In a child with hypopituitarism, the growth hormone levels would usually be:
    a. elevated after 20 minutes of strenuous exercise.
    b. elevated 45 to 90 minutes after the onset of sleep.
    c. lower than normal or not measurable at all.
    d. increased in response to insulin.

12. Treatment of choice for the child with idiopathic hypopituitarism may include:
    a. biosynthetic growth hormone.
    b. human growth hormone.
    c. chemotherapy to shrink the tumor.
    d. any of the above.

13. In the child with idiopathic hypopituitarism, growth hormone replacement therapy:
    a. will continue for life.
    b. will not result in achievement of a normal familial height.
    c. requires subcutaneous injection.
    d. requires intramuscular injection.

14. Tests that use neuromodulators to stimulate the release of growth hormone:
    a. are the best method to diagnose growth hormone deficiency.
    b. suppress the release of growth hormone.
    c. may be less sensitive indicators than growth hormone assays.
    d. are recommended whenever growth delays occur.

15. Explain the difference between acromegaly and the pituitary hyperfunction that is not considered to be acromegaly.

16. Parents of the child with precocious puberty need to know that:
    a. dress and activities should be aligned with the child's sexual development.
    b. heterosexual interest will usually be advanced.
    c. the child's mental age is congruent with the chronologic age.
    d. overt manifestations of affection represent sexual advances.

17. Desmopressin acetate may be administered:
    a. by mouth.
    b. intranasally.
    c. topically.
    d. by all of the above routes.

18. The immediate management of syndrome of inappropriate antidiuretic hormone (SIADH) consists of:
    a. increasing fluids.
    b. administering antibiotics.
    c. restricting fluids.
    d. administering vasopressin.

19. One of the most common causes of thyroid disease in children and adolescents is:
    a. Hashimoto disease.
    b. Graves disease.
    c. goiter.
    d. thyrotoxicosis.

20. The initial treatment for the child with hyperthyroidism would most likely be:
    a. subtotal thyroidectomy.
    b. total thyroidectomy.
    c. ablation with radioactive iodide.
    d. administration of antithyroid medication.

21. When a thyroidectomy is planned, the nurse should explain to the child that:
    a. iodine preparations will be mixed with flavored foods and then eaten.
    b. he or she will need to hyperextend the neck postoperatively.
    c. the skin, not the throat, will be cut.
    d. laryngospasm can be a life-threatening complication.

22. The child with longstanding hypoparathyroidism will usually exhibit:
    a. short, stubby fingers.
    b. dimpling of the skin over the knuckles.
    c. skeletal growth retardation.
    d. a short, thick neck.

23. A common cause of secondary hyperparathyroidism is:
    a. maternal hyperparathyroidism.
    b. chronic renal disease.
    c. maternal diabetes mellitus.
    d. adenoma of the parathyroid gland.

24. Hyperfunction of the adrenal medulla results in:
    a. release of epinephrine and norepinephrine from the sympathetic nervous system.
    b. pheochromocytoma.
    c. adrenal crisis.
    d. myxedema.

25. Diagnosis of acute adrenocortical insufficiency is based on:
    a. elevated plasma cortisol levels.
    b. the clinical presentation.
    c. depressed plasma cortisol levels.
    d. depressed aldosterone levels.

26. Parents of a child who has Addison disease should be instructed to:
    a. use extra hydrocortisone only when signs of crisis are present.
    b. discontinue the child's cortisone if side effects develop.
    c. decrease the cortisone dose during times of stress.
    d. administer hydrocortisone intramuscularly.

27. Which of the following tests is particularly useful in diagnosing congenital adrenogenital hyperplasia?
    a. Chromosomal typing
    b. Pelvic ultrasound
    c. Pelvic x-ray
    d. Testosterone levels

28. The temporary treatment for hyperaldosteronism before surgery would usually involve administration of:
    a. spironolactone.
    b. phentolamine.
    c. furosemide.
    d. phenoxybenzamine.

29. Definitive treatment for pheochromocytoma consists of:
    a. surgical removal of the thyroid.
    b. administration of potassium.
    c. surgical removal of the tumor.
    d. administration of beta blockers.

30. Most children with diabetes mellitus tend to exhibit characteristics of:
    a. maturity-onset diabetes of youth.
    b. gestational diabetes.
    c. type 2 diabetes.
    d. type 1 diabetes.

31. The currently accepted etiology of type 1 diabetes mellitus takes into account:
    a. genetic factors.
    b. autoimmune mechanisms.
    c. environmental factors.
    d. all of the above.

32. An early sign of type 2 diabetes mellitus in the adolescent would be:
    a. a vaginal candidal infection.
    b. obesity.
    c. Kussmaul respirations.
    d. all of the above.

33. Of the following blood glucose levels, the value that most certainly indicates a diagnosis of diabetes would be a:
    a. fasting blood glucose of 120 mg/dl.
    b. random blood glucose of 160 mg/dl.
    c. fasting blood glucose of 160 mg/dl.
    d. glucose tolerance test (oral) value of 160 mg/dl for the 2-hour sample.

34. State the goal of insulin replacement therapy.

35. Glycosolated hemoglobin is an acceptable method to use to:
    a. assess for ketoacidosis.
    b. assess the control of diabetes.
    c. assess oxygen saturation of the hemoglobin.
    d. determine blood glucose levels most accurately.

36. Even with good glucose control, a child with type 1 diabetes mellitus may frequently encounter the acute complication of:
    a. retinopathy.
    b. ketoacidosis.
    c. hypoglycemia.
    d. hyperosmolar nonketotic coma.

37. Describe the treatment for a mild hypoglycemic episode in a young child with diabetes mellitus.

38. Which of the following is not one of the principles of managing diabetes during illness?
    a. Blood glucose should be monitored every 3 hours.
    b. Dosage requirements may increase, decrease, or remain the same.
    c. Insulin should always be omitted when excessive vomiting occurs.
    d. Fluids should be encouraged to avoid dehydration.

39. Diabetic ketoacidosis in children with diabetes mellitus:
    a. is the most common chronic complication.
    b. is a result of too much insulin.
    c. is a life-threatening complication.
    d. rarely requires hospitalization.

40. Which of the following cardiac wave patterns is indicative of hypokalemia?
    a. Widening of the Q-T interval with a flattened T wave
    b. Shortening of the Q-T interval with an elevated T wave
    c. Shortening of the Q-T interval with a flattened T wave
    d. Widening of the Q-T interval with an elevated T wave

41. The best approach to effectively teach a child and his or her family the complex concepts of the home management of diabetes mellitus is to:
    a. provide intensive training a day or so after diagnosis.
    b. provide intensive training the first 3 or 4 days after diagnosis.
    c. teach nothing until 2 weeks after diagnosis.
    d. teach essentials at diagnosis, followed by intense information later.

42. The child with diabetes mellitus is taught to weigh and measure food to:
    a. receive the nutrients prescribed.
    b. prevent hypoglycemia.
    c. learn to estimate food portions.
    d. prevent hyperglycemia.

43. In regard to meal planning for the child with diabetes mellitus, parents should be aware that:
    a. fast foods must be eliminated.
    b. foods must be always be weighed and measured.
    c. the exchange list is limited to one type of food.
    d. foods with sorbitol are metabolized into glucose.

44. The most efficient rotation pattern for insulin injections involves giving injections in:
    a. one area of the body 1 inch apart.
    b. different areas of the body each day.

45. In regard to insulin administration:
    a. insulin should never be premixed.
    b. insulin syringes should never be reused.
    c. insulin doses under 2 units may be diluted.
    d. an air bubble in the syringe is insignificant.

46. The child with diabetes mellitus needs to test his or her urine:
    a. for ketones every day.
    b. for ketones at times of illness.
    c. for glucose every day.
    d. for glucose at times of illness.

47. Exercise for the child with diabetes mellitus may:
    a. be restricted to noncontact sports.
    b. require a decreased intake of food.
    c. necessitate an increased insulin dose.
    d. require an increased intake of food.

48. Problems with the child adjusting to the self-management of diabetes are most likely to occur when diabetes is diagnosed in:
    a. infancy.
    b. adolescence.
    c. the toddler years.
    d. the school-age years.

49. Describe the feelings that parents may have when they are raising a child with diabetes mellitus.

CRITICAL THINKING—CASE STUDY

Rebecca Bennett is an 8-year-old who was recently diagnosed with diabetes mellitus. She is hospitalized with diabetic ketoacidosis, and she is beginning to learn about the disease process. Her parents are with her continually. She has an identical twin sister who is staying with her maternal grandparents.

50. Mrs. Bennett is concerned that Rebecca's sister will also develop diabetes. Based on the preceding information, an acceptable response for the nurse to make would be to:
    a. reassure the parents that the disease is not contagious.
    b. discuss the hereditary and viral factors of type 1 diabetes.
    c. discuss the hereditary factors of type 1 diabetes.
    d. discuss the viral factors of type 1 diabetes.

51. Which of the following nursing diagnoses is most likely to become a priority after the first few days of Rebecca's hospitalization?
    a. Fluid Volume Deficit related to uncontrolled diabetes
    b. Fluid Volume Excess related to hormonal disturbances
    c. Deficient Knowledge related to newly diagnosed type 1 diabetes mellitus
    d. Impaired Respiratory Function related to fluid imbalance

52. In preparing the Bennett family for discharge, the nurse should plan to teach:
    a. only Rebecca how to inject insulin.
    b. only Rebecca's parents how to inject insulin.
    c. both Rebecca and her parents how to inject insulin.
    d. the family how to administer oral hypoglycemics.

53. To evaluate Rebecca's progress in relation to her diabetes self-management, the best measure would be Rebecca's:
    a. parents' verbalizations about the disease process.
    b. blood glucose levels.
    c. glycosylated hemoglobin values.
    d. demonstration of her insulin injection technique.

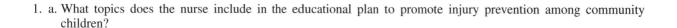

39 The Child with Musculoskeletal or Articular Dysfunction

1. a. What topics does the nurse include in the educational plan to promote injury prevention among community children?

   b. Besides conducting educational programs, what methods can the nurse use to promote injury prevention in children?

2. The nurse is suspicious of child abuse when:
     i. there is a delay in seeking medical assistance for the injury.
     ii. the parent's history of the injury is not congruent with the actual injury.
     iii. x-ray studies demonstrate previous fractures in different stages of healing.
     iv. the child is crying and fearful of separation from the parent.

   a. i, ii, iii, and iv
   b. i, ii, and iii
   c. ii and iii
   d. ii, iii, and iv

3. A nurse discovers 5-year-old Jimmy, a neighbor, lying in the street next to his bicycle. The nurse sends another witness to activate the emergency medical services (EMS) while the nurse begins a primary assessment of Jimmy. Which of the following best describes the primary assessment and its correct sequence?
   a. Body inspection, head-to-toe survey, and airway patency
   b. Airway patency, respiratory effectiveness, circulatory status
   c. Open airway, head-to-toe assessment for injuries, and chest compressions
   d. Weight estimation, symptom analysis, blood pressure measurement

4. The nurse suspects that Jimmy (from question 3) has a spinal cord injury. Describe the immobilization technique.

5. Major consequences of immobility in the pediatric patient include:
   a. bone demineralization leading to osteoporosis.
   b. orthostatic hypertension.
   c. dependent edema in the lower extremities.
   d. decrease in the metabolic rate.

6. What are the three major cardiovascular consequences of immobility?

7. Name four symptoms of neurologic impairment that should be immediately evaluated.

8. Nursing interventions aimed at preventing problems associated with immobility include:
   a. encouraging self-care and allowing patients to do as much for themselves as they are able.
   b. restricting fluids with strict intake and output.
   c. limiting active range-of-motion exercises to once per day.
   d. decreasing sensory stimulation to allow adequate rest.

9. Match each term with its description.
   a. Orthotics

   b. Prosthetics
   c. Parapodium
   d. Ankle-foot orthosis (AFO)
   e. Knee-ankle-foot orthosis (KAFO)
   f. Hip-knee-ankle-foot orthosis (HKAFO)
   g. Reciprocal gait orthosis (RGO)
   h. Thoracolumbosacral orthosis (TLSO)

   i. Boston brace
   j. Jewett-Taylor brace
   k. Axillary swing-through crutches
   l. Forearm crutches
   m. Trough crutches

   _____ Standing frame on a circular base

   _____ The fabrication and fitting of braces

   _____ Provides support for the knee, ankle, and hip; used for flail lower limb and paralysis

   _____ The fabrication and fitting of artificial limbs

   _____ Sometimes used to support the spine and trunk during ambulation to prevent compression after fracture of the spinal column

   _____ Used to prevent buckling of the knee, to support the extremity when there is paralysis or marked weakness of the knee extension or quadriceps muscle

   _____ Custom molded and fits snugly around the truck of the body to exert pressure on the ribs and back to support the spine in a straight position

   _____ An underarm orthosis customized from prefabricated plastic shells, with corrective forces for each patient supplied by lateral pads; prevent progression of curves in the spine

   _____ Allows children with paraplegia to walk on a flat surface; used in children with spinal cord injury, sacral agenesis, and spina bifida

   _____ Used to prevent footdrop due to bed rest, trauma to the foot, or paralysis of muscles that flex the foot

   _____ Usual selection for children who anticipate permanent use; used for paraplegic children who are unable to use braces

   _____ Used most frequently for temporary assistance

   _____ Allows the weight to be assumed by the elbow

10. Which of the following is a complication of immobility that is easily prevented by an appropriate nursing intervention?
    a. Disuse atrophy and loss of muscle mass
    b. Constipation
    c. Hypocalcemia
    d. Pain

11. Which of the following is not included in the teaching plan of a child with a brace or prosthesis?
    a. Frequent assessment of all areas in contact with the brace for signs of skin irritation
    b. Assessment of the stump area before application of the prosthesis
    c. Removal of the prosthesis limited to bedtime unless skin breakage occurs
    d. Use of protective clothing under the brace

12. List five effects that prolonged immobilization or disability of the child may have on the family.

13. Bone healing is characteristically more rapid in children because:
    a. children have less constant muscle contraction associated with the fracture.
    b. children's fractures are less severe than adult's.
    c. children have an active growth plate that helps speed repair with less likelihood of deformity.
    d. children have thickened periosteum and a more generous blood supply.

14. The method of fracture reduction is not determined by:
    a. the child's age.
    b. the manner in which the fracture occurred.
    c. the degree of displacement.
    d. the amount of edema.

15. Match each term with its description.

    a. Diaphysis
    b. Epiphysis
    c. Epiphyseal plate
    d. Complete fracture
    e. Incomplete fracture
    f. Transverse fracture
    g. Simple, or closed, fracture
    h. Open, or compound, fracture
    i. Complicated fracture
    j. Comminuted fracture

    k. Greenstick fracture
    l. Buckle, or torus, fracture
    m. Bend fracture
    n. Osteopenia
    o. Ossification
    p. Periosteum
    q. Oblique
    r. Spiral
    s. Butterfly

    _____ Fracture with an open wound from which the bone has protruded

    _____ Complete fracture with a large central fragment at the site

    _____ Major portion of the long bone

    _____ Fracture in which fracture fragments are separated

    _____ Fracture in which fracture fragments remain attached

    _____ Located at the ends of the long bones

    _____ Also called the *growth plate* because it plays a major role in the longitudinal growth of the developing child

    _____ Fracture that is crosswise, at right angles to the long axis of the bone

    _____ Conversion of cartilage to bony structure

    _____ Membrane covering all bone; contains blood vessels to nourish bone

    _____ Fracture in which small fragments of bone are broken from the fractured shaft and lie in surrounding tissue

    _____ Fracture in which bone fragments cause damage to surrounding organs or tissue

    _____ Fracture that is slanting and circular, twisting around the bone shaft

    _____ Demineralization of the bone

    _____ Appears as a raising or bulging at the site of the fracture

    _____ Occurs more commonly in the ulna and fibula and can produce some deformity

    _____ Occurs when a bone is angulated beyond the limits of bending

    _____ Fracture that has not produced a break in the skin

    _____ Fracture that is slanting but straight, between a horizontal and a perpendicular direction

16. What are the "five *P*s" of ischemia that are included when assessing fractures to rule out vascular injury?

17. Emergency treatment for the child with a fracture includes:
    a. moving the child to allow removal of clothing from the area of injury.
    b. immobilization of the limb, including joints above and below the injury site.
    c. pushing the protruding bone under the skin.
    d. keeping the area of injury in a dependent position.

18. What are the four goals of fracture management?

19. Wolff's law, as applied to treating children with orthopedic problems, states that:
    a. bone will grow in the direction of the stress that is applied to it.
    b. bone will grow in the opposite direction of the stress that is applied to it.
    c. bone healing is directly influenced by the general health of the traumatized person.
    d. the amount of fragment angulation or rotation influences the degree of correction that can be accomplished.

20. An appropriate nursing intervention for the care of a child with an extremity in a new cast is:
    a. keeping the cast covered with a sheet.
    b. using the fingertips when handling the cast to prevent pressure areas.
    c. using heated fans or dryers to circulate air and speed the cast-drying process.
    d. turning the child at least every 2 hours to help dry the cast evenly.

21. To reduce anxiety in the child undergoing cast removal, which of the following nursing interventions would the nurse expect to be least effective?
    a. Demonstrate how the cast cutter works to the child before beginning the procedure.
    b. Use the analogy of having fingernails or hair cut.
    c. Explain that it will take only a few minutes.
    d. Continue to reassure that all is going well and that their behavior is acceptable during the removal process.

22. Julie, age 10, has been placed in a long leg cast for an open fracture. The nurse immediately notifies the physician if assessment findings include:
    a. appearance of blood-stained area the size of a quarter on the cast.
    b. 2+ pedal pulse.
    c. inability to move the toes.
    d. ability of the nurse to insert one finger under the edge of the cast.

23. The three primary purposes of traction for reduction of fractures are:

24. The nurse is caring for 7-year-old Charles after insertion of skeletal traction. Which of the following is contraindicated?
    a. Gently massage over pressure areas to stimulate circulation.
    b. Release the traction when repositioning Charles in bed.
    c. Inspect pin sites for bleeding or infection.
    d. Assess for alterations in neurovascular status.

25. Nursing intervention for the child with an Ilizarov external fixator device includes:
    a. teaching the child to walk with crutches.
    b. observing for the common problem of infection.
    c. allowing full weight bearing once the fixation device has been applied.
    d. allowing full weight bearing after removal of the device.

26. The nurse is assessing Carol, age 8, for complications related to her recent fracture and the application of a flexion cast to her forearm and elbow. Carol is crying with pain, the nurse is unable to locate pulses in the affected extremity, and there is lack of sensitivity to the area as well as some edema. Which of the following would the nurse suspect as most likely to be occurring?
    a. Normal occurrence for the first few hours after application of traction
    b. Volkmann contracture
    c. Nerve compression syndrome
    d. Epiphyseal damage

27. Johnny, a 12-year-old with fracture of the femur, has developed chest pain and shortness of breath. The nurse suspects a pulmonary embolism. The priority nursing action is to:
    a. elevate the affected extremity.
    b. administer oxygen.
    c. administer pain medication.
    d. start an intravenous (IV) infusion of heparin.

28. Match each term with its best description.

    a. Compartment syndrome
    b. Epiphyseal damage
    c. Buck extension
    d. Russell traction
    e. 90-90 traction
    f. Balance suspension traction
    g. Thomas splint
    h. Pearson attachment
    i. Cervical traction
    j. Manual traction
    k. Skin traction
    l. Skeletal traction
    m. Distraction
    n. Osteomyelitis
    o. Internal fixation
    p. Nonunion
    q. Malunion

    _____ Insertion of a wire or pin into the bone

    _____ Requires surgery and includes screw and plate fixation and intramedullary fixation

    _____ Used to realign bone fragments for cast application

    _____ Applied when there is minimal displacement and little muscle spasticity but contraindicated when there is associated skin damage

    _____ Occurs when increased pressure within a group of muscles, surrounded by inelastic tissue, compromises circulation to the muscles and nerves within the space

    _____ Can result in unequal length of the extremities

    _____ Infection of the bone

    _____ Results when bone fragments cannot be maintained in correct alignment for repair due to inadequate reduction, poor immobilization, or a damaged or softened cast

    _____ Increased angulation or deformity at the fracture site

    _____ Uses skin traction on the lower leg and a padded sling under the knee

    _____ A type of skin traction with the leg extended; used primarily for short-term immobilization

    _____ Skeletal traction where the lower leg is put in a boot cast or supported in a sling and a pin is placed in the distal fragment of the femur

    _____ Used with or without skin or skeletal traction; suspends the leg in a flexed position to relax the hip and hamstring muscles

_____ Process of separating opposing bone to regenerate new bone in the created space

_____ Accomplished by insertion of Crutchfield tongs through burr holes

_____ Supports the lower leg

_____ Extends from the groin to midair above the foot

29. Nursing interventions for the child after surgical amputation of a lower extremity include:
    a. applying special elastic bandaging to the stump, using a circular pattern to decrease stump edema.
    b. keeping the stump elevated for at least 72 hours postsurgery.
    c. encouraging the child to lie prone at least three times a day, increasing the time prone to tolerance of an hour at a time.
    d. recognizing that the child is only trying to gain the nurse's attention when the child says there is pain in the missing limb.

30. Jeff has accidentally amputated the distal one third of his thumb. The camp nurse knows that the amputated thumb part should be:
    a. placed directly in ice water and transported to the emergency department with Jeff.
    b. immediately rinsed with water to remove dirt, placed back on the injury site, secured with a sterile gauze dressing, and transported with Jeff to the emergency department.
    c. rinsed in normal saline, wrapped in a sterile dressing, placed in a watertight bag in iced solution without freezing, and transported with Jeff to the emergency department.
    d. placed in a sterile dressing into a cold milk solution and transported with Jeff to the emergency department.

31. When matching children to participate in sports competition, which of the following is the least important consideration?
    a. Age
    b. Height and weight
    c. Physical fitness
    d. Physical skills

32. Match the term with its description.

a. Contusion	e. Sprain
b. Ecchymosis	f. Myositis ossificans
c. Dislocation	g. Stress fracture
d. Strain	h. Phantom limb pain

    _____ Occurs when the force of stress on the ligament is so great that it displaces the normal position of the opposing bone ends or the bone end in relation to its socket

    _____ Occurs as a result of repeated muscle contraction from repetitive weight-bearing sports

    _____ Damage to the soft tissue, subcutaneous structures, and muscle

    _____ Occurs when trauma to a joint is so severe that a ligament is either stretched or partially or completely torn by the force created as a joint is twisted or wrenched

    _____ May persist for years and is an expected experience because the nerve-brain communication is still present

    _____ Occurs from deep contusions to the biceps or quadriceps muscles, resulting in a restriction of the flexibility of the affected limb

    _____ Escape of blood into the tissues

    _____ Microscopic tear to the musculotendinous unit

33. Which of the following statements about "nursemaid's elbow" is correct?
    a. This most common partial dislocation of the radial head of the elbow is usually found in children ages 1 to 3 years.
    b. This condition is caused by a sudden pull at the wrist while the arm is fully extended and the forearm is pronated.
    c. The longer the dislocation is present, the longer it takes the child to recover mobility after treatment.
    d. All of the above

34. Immediate treatment of sprains and strains includes:
    a. rest and cold application.
    b. disregarding the pain and "working out" the sprain or strain.
    c. rest, elevation, and pain medication.
    d. compression of the area and heat application.

35. Major sprains or tears to the ligamentous tissues rarely occur in growing children because the _____ are stronger than bone. The _____ and the _____

    _____ are the weakest parts of the bone and the usual sites of injury.

36. Match the term with its description.

    a. Shin splints
    b. Frictional injury
    c. Tractional injury
    d. Cyclic injury
    e. Plantar fasciitis
    f. Osgood-Schlatter disease
    g. Achilles tendinitis
    h. Johansson syndrome (jumper's knee)
    i. Little League elbow
    j. Little League shoulder

    _____ Caused by repeated forcible traction on the short tendon; pain with plantar flexion against resistance

    _____ Manifests with pain in the elbow, is aggravated by use, and is caused by repetitive strain from throwing

    _____ Pain in arch or heel

    _____ Repetitive loading of impact forces; stress fractures

    _____ Traction apophysitis on inferior pole of patella

    _____ Repeated pull on a ligament or tendon

    _____ Pain and characteristic contracture; loss of internal rotation and increased external rotation; microfracture of proximal humeral growth plate

    _____ Experienced by athletes who run extensively; ligaments torn away from the tibial shaft, causing pain

    _____ Rubbing of one structure against another

    _____ Traction apophysitis of tibial tubercle; overprominence of involved tubercle; occurs in children who do a lot of jumping

37. Ben, a 15-year-old high school student, is at a track event. He has been running multiple events. He was feeling unwell before the event and had been vomiting. Now he is complaining of thirst, headache, fatigue, dizziness, and nausea. He seems to be somewhat disoriented and is sweating. Ben's temperature is normal. Which of the following is the most likely to describe Ben's condition?
    a. Heat cramps
    b. Heatstroke
    c. Heat exhaustion

38. Which of the following statements made to the athlete by the nurse is correct?
    a. It is more important to replace sodium and chloride than water.
    b. Recommended dietary energy intake for adolescents involved in sports is 50% of caloric intake from carbohydrates.
    c. Iron replacement is necessary only for the female athlete.
    d. Energy for prolonged exercise is best obtained from high-carbohydrate foods eaten 2 hours before the event.

39. Sixteen-year-old Ben has been brought to the school nurse's office for heatstroke. He has a temperature of 40° C (104° F) and is awake but disoriented. Which of the following is contraindicated?
    a. Immediate removal of clothing and application of cool water to the skin
    b. Administration of antipyretics
    c. Use of fans directed at Ben
    d. Activation of EMS for transport to hospital

40. Zac, a 16-year-old football star at the local high school, is at the school nurse practitioner's office for acne that is not clearing. During the physical examination the nurse notes that Zac has achieved a marked increase in muscle and strength in a very short time. Which of the following would the nurse suspect caused these changes?
    a. Use of an ergogenic aid, anabolic steroids
    b. More frequent and more strenuous workouts in the gym
    c. Increased protein and vitamins in the diet
    d. Use of methylphenidate (Ritalin) or phenmetrazine (Preludin)

41. Commotio cordis:
    a. occurs after a blunt, nonpenetrating blow to the chest, which produces ventricular fibrillation.
    b. rarely causes death.
    c. occurs in athletes with hypertrophic cardiomyopathy.
    d. occurs in athletes who have a history of sudden death in a relative under the age of 50 years.

42. The condition recognized in the infant with limited neck motion, where the neck is flexed and turned to the affected side as a result of shortening of the sternocleidomastoid muscle, is:
    a. torticollis.
    b. paralysis of the brachial nerve.
    c. Legg-Calvé-Perthes disease.
    d. a self-limiting injury.

43. Bob, age 7, is diagnosed with Legg-Calvé-Perthes disease. Which of the following manifestations is not consistent with this diagnosis?
    a. Intermittent appearance of a limp on the affected side
    b. Hip soreness, ache, or stiffness that can be constant or intermittent
    c. Pain and limp most evident on arising and at the end of a long day of activities
    d. Specific history of injury to the area

44. Slipped femoral capital epiphysis is suspected when:
    a. an adolescent or preadolescent begins to limp and complains of continuous or intermittent pain in the hip.
    b. an examination reveals no restriction on internal rotation or adduction but restriction on external rotation.
    c. referred pain goes into the sacral and lumbar areas.
    d. all of the above occur.

45. An accentuation of the lumbar curvature beyond physiologic limits is termed _____.
    An abnormally increased convex angulation in the curvature of the thoracic spine is termed

    _____. _____ is the forward slipping of one vertebral body onto another, usually L5 and S1.

46. Diagnostic evaluation is important for early recognition of scoliosis. Which of the following is the correct procedure for the school nurse conducting this examination?
    a. View the child, who is standing and walking fully clothed, to look for uneven hanging of clothing.
    b. View all children from the left and right side to look mainly for asymmetry of the hip height.
    c. Completely undress all children before the examination.
    d. View the child, who is wearing underpants, from behind when the child bends forward.

47. The surgical technique for the correction of scoliosis consists of:

48. Marilyn, age 13, has been diagnosed with scoliosis and placed in a thoracolumbosacral orthotic (TLSO) brace. Which of the following information provided by the nurse to Marilyn is correct?
    a. "The brace will cure your curvature."
    b. "The brace is an underarm brace made of plastic that will be molded and shaped to your body to correct the curvature."
    c. "The brace includes a neck ring to extend the neck."
    d. "The brace will only be worn in bed, since it prevents walking because of the severity of the trunk bend."

49. Nursing implementation directed toward nonsurgical management in a teenager with scoliosis primarily includes:
    a. promoting self-esteem and positive body image.
    b. preventing immobility.
    c. promoting adequate nutrition.
    d. preventing infection.

50. Osteomyelitis resulting from a blood-borne bacterium that could have developed from an infected lesion is termed:
    a. acute hematogenous osteomyelitis.
    b. exogenous osteomyelitis.
    c. subacute osteomyelitis.
    d. any of the above.

51. The care plan for the child during the acute phase of osteomyelitis always includes:
    a. performing wound irrigations.
    b. maintaining the IV infusion site.
    c. isolating the child.
    d. incorporating passive range-of-motion exercises for the affected area.

52. Which of the following statements about septic arthritis is true?
    a. The most common causative agent in children under 2 years of age is *Haemophilus influenzae*.
    b. Knees, hips, ankles, hands, and feet are the joints most commonly affected.
    c. Early radiographic findings show soft tissue swelling and erosions of the bone.
    d. IV antibiotic use is based on Gram stain and clinical presentation.

53. The most common sites for tubercular infection of the bones in older children are:
    a. carpals and phalanges and corresponding bones of the feet.
    b. vertebrae.
    c. long bones of the legs.
    d. radius and ulna.

54. Nursing considerations for the patient diagnosed with osteogenesis imperfecta include:
    a. preventing fractures by holding onto the child's ankles when changing diapers.
    b. providing nonjudgmental support while parents are dealing with accusations of child abuse.
    c. providing guidelines to the parents in avoiding all exercise and sports for the child.
    d. educating parents that the use of braces and splints can increase the rate of fracture.

55. Which of the following nursing goals is most appropriate for the child with juvenile idiopathic arthritis?
    a. Child will exhibit signs of reduced joint inflammation and adequate joint function.
    b. Child will exhibit no signs of impaired skin integrity due to rash.
    c. Child will exhibit normal weight and nutritional status.
    d. Child will exhibit no alteration in respiratory patterns or respiratory tract infection.

56. What should the nurse teach the patient and family of the child diagnosed with systemic lupus erythematosus (SLE) regarding each of the following topics?

    a. Methotrexate

    b. Diet

    c. Sun exposure

    d. Birth control medication

57. What are the two goals of therapeutic management for SLE?

58. The principal drugs used in SLE to control inflammation are the _____.

59. What are the two primary nursing goals for the child with SLE?

CRITICAL THINKING—CASE STUDY

Sandy, age 10, has developed joint and leg pain, some joint swelling, fever, malaise, and pleuritis. The physician has ordered laboratory testing to include sedimentation rate, rheumatoid factor, and a complete blood count. Tentative diagnosis has been established as juvenile idiopathic arthritis (JIA).

60. If the diagnosis is correct, which of the following would represent the expected laboratory results?
    a. Leukocytosis
    b. Elevated sedimentation rate
    c. Negative rheumatoid factor
    d. All of the above

61. A group of drugs prescribed for JIA are nonsteroidal antiinflammatory drugs. Education regarding the use of these drugs should include the statement that:
    a. they produce excellent analgesic and antiinflammatory effects but little antipyretic effect.
    b. they are administered in the lowest effective dose and given on alternate days rather than daily.
    c. antiinflammatory effect occurs 3 to 4 weeks after therapy is begun.
    d. because there is a narrow margin between effective and toxic dosage, levels need to be monitored regularly until therapeutic dosage is established.

62. Which of the following is the most appropriate nursing intervention to promote adequate joint function in the child with JIA?
    a. Incorporate therapeutic exercises in play activities.
    b. Provide heat to affected joints by use of tub baths.
    c. Provide written information for all treatments ordered.
    d. Explore and develop activities in which the child can succeed.

63. An expected outcome for the nursing diagnosis of High Risk for Body Image Disturbance related to the disease process of JIA is:
    a. the patient and family members are able to explain the disease process.
    b. the patient is accepted by peers.
    c. the patient will express feelings and concerns.
    d. the child will understand and use effective communication techniques.

64. What laboratory monitoring is required if Sandy is started on methotrexate?

65. What is the nutritional goal for Sandy?

40 The Child with Neuromuscular or Muscular Dysfunction

1. Identify the following as true or false.

   _____ Upper motor neuron lesions produce weakness associated with spasticity, increased deep tendon reflexes, and abnormal superficial reflexes.

   _____ The primary disorder of lower motor neuron dysfunction is cerebral palsy (CP).

   _____ Lower motor neuron lesions interrupt the reflex arc, causing weakness and atrophy of the skeletal muscles involved with associated hypotonia or flaccidity, with final progression to varying degrees of contracture.

   _____ Lower motor neuron involvement is most often asymmetric.

   _____ In most instances the sudden appearance of flaccid paralysis in a previously healthy child can be attributed to an infectious process.

   _____ Hereditary factors and metabolic disease are more often responsible for muscular weakness and atrophy of gradual onset.

   _____ The most useful classification of neuromuscular disorders defines the source of the lesion.

   _____ Deep tendon reflexes are briskly active in upper motor neuron disease and diminished or absent in lower motor neuron disease.

   _____ CP has four primary types of movement disorders: spastic, dyskinetic, ataxic, and mixed.

2. Match each diagnostic tool with its description.

   a. Electromyogram (EMG)   c. Muscle biopsy
   b. Nerve conduction velocity   d. Creatine kinase

   _____ Elevated in skeletal muscle disease; not elevated in neurogenic disease

   _____ Ketamine used to decrease the pain with this procedure

   _____ Measures electric impulse conduction along motor nerves

   _____ Measures electric potential of individual muscle

3. The nurse knows that the etiology of CP is most commonly related to:
   a. existing prenatal brain abnormalities.
   b. maternal asphyxia.
   c. childhood meningitis.
   d. preeclampsia.

4. The nurse is preparing the long-term care plan for a child with CP. Which of the following is included in the plan?
   a. No delay in gross motor development is expected.
   b. The illness is not progressively degenerative.
   c. There will be no persistence of primitive infantile reflexes.
   d. All children will need genetic counseling as they get older before planning for a family.

5. Match each term with its description.

    a. Hemiparesis   g. Parietal lobe syndrome
    b. Quadriparesis   h. Spastic CP
    c. Diplegia   i. Dyskinetic CP
    d. Monoplegia   j. Ataxic CP
    e. Triplegia   k. Mixed-type CP
    f. Paraplegia   l. Opisthotonic posture

    _____ Pure cerebral paraplegia of lower extremities

    _____ Involving three extremities

    _____ Exaggerated arching of the back

    _____ Involves only one extremity

    _____ Similar parts of both sides of the body involved

    _____ Most common form of spastic CP; motor deficit greater in upper extremity; one side of the body affected

    _____ Cortical sensory function impaired and therefore impaired two-point discrimination and position sense

    _____ All four extremities equally affected

    _____ Characterized by abnormal involuntary movement, such as athetosis—slow, wormlike, writhing movements that usually involve the extremities, trunk, neck, facial muscles, and tongue

    _____ Characterized by wide-based gait; rapid, repetitive movements performed poorly; disintegration of movements of the upper extremities when the child reaches for objects

    _____ Combination of spasticity and athetosis

    _____ Characterized by persistent primitive reflexes, positive Babinski reflex, ankle clonus, and exaggerated stretch reflexes

6. Children with CP often have manifestations that include alterations of muscle tone. Which of the following is an example of a finding in a child with altered muscle tone?
    a. Demonstrates increased or decreased resistance to passive movements
    b. Develops hand dominance by the age of 5 months
    c. Has an asymmetric crawl
    d. When placed in prone position, maintains hips higher than trunk, with legs and arms flexed or drawn under the body

7. Associated disabilities and problems related to the child with CP include:
    a. All children with CP have intelligence testing in the abnormal range.
    b. A large number of eye cataracts are associated with CP and require surgical correction.
    c. Seizures are a common occurrence among children with athetosis and diplegia.
    d. Coughing and choking, especially while eating, predispose children with CP to aspiration.

8. The nurse is completing a physical examination on 6-month-old Brian. Which of the following would be an abnormal finding suggestive of CP?
    a. Brian is able to hold onto the nurse's hands while being pulled to a sitting position.
    b. Brian has no Moro reflex.
    c. Brian has no tonic neck reflex.
    d. Brian has an obligatory tonic neck reflex.

9. Recommended diagnostic evaluation for infants at risk for CP includes:
    a. magnetic resonance imaging of the brain.
    b. computed tomographic scan of the brain.
    c. laboratory testing.
    d. metabolic and genetic testing when structural abnormality is identified.

10. The goal of therapeutic management for the child with CP is:
    a. assisting with motor control of voluntary muscle.
    b. maximizing the child's capabilities.
    c. delaying the development of sensory deprivation.
    d. surgically correcting deformities.

11. What factors should be taken into account in planning therapy for a child with CP?

12. Identify the following as true or false.

    _____ Ankle-foot orthoses are molded to fit the feet and worn inside shoes to reduce deformity.

    _____ The use of an infant walker helps the child with CP develop independent mobilization.

    _____ Surgical intervention is used in the child with CP to correct contractures or spastic deformities and provide stability.

    _____ Baclofen and diazepam are effective in improving muscle coordination in children with CP and in decreasing overall spasticity.

    _____ Prime candidates for botulinum toxin type A (Botox) injections are children with spasticity confined to the lower extremities.

    _____ CP patients are screened before pump placement by the infusion of a "test dose" of intrathecal baclofen delivered via a lumbar puncture.

    _____ The application of technical aids makes it possible for older persons with CP to eventually function in their own apartments and can be extended into the workplace.

    _____ Children receiving phenytoin are at risk for developing gum hyperplasia.

    _____ Physical therapy consisting of stretching, passive, active, and resistive movements applied to specific muscle groups is able to achieve spectacular changes in the ultimate outcome of the CP child.

    _____ Children who have CP and sucking and swallowing difficulty should be held in a semireclining posture during feeding to make use of gravity flow.

    _____ Feeding techniques such as forcing the child to use the lips and tongue in eating can facilitate speech.

    _____ Education requirements of all children with CP are determined by the child's needs and potential.

    _____ Sports, physical fitness, and recreation programs are encouraged for children with CP.

    _____ Approximately 30% to 50% of children with CP are cognitively impaired; however, many children with severe spastic quadriplegic CP have normal intelligence.

13. Which of the following would be expected in the infant with hypotonia?
    a. When held in horizontal suspension, the infant responds by slightly raising the head.
    b. When pulled to a sitting position, the infant demonstrates head lag that is quickly corrected to a normal position.
    c. When placed in horizontal suspension position, the infant's head droops over the examiner's supporting hand and the infant's extremities hang loosely.
    d. The infant has a slower weight gain but a good sucking reflex.

14. Infantile spinal muscular atrophy (SMA):
    a. is diagnosed prenatally by genetic analysis of circulating fetal cells in maternal blood or amniotic fluid.
    b. can be cured with surgery performed in utero.
    c. is associated with nutritional failure to thrive, the most serious complication, often leading to the infant's early death.
    d. is associated with children who are intellectually slower.

15. The disease inherited only as an autosomal recessive trait and characterized by progressive weakness and wasting of skeletal muscles caused by degeneration of anterior horn cells is:
    a. infantile SMA (Werdnig-Hoffmann disease).
    b. CP.
    c. Kugelberg-Welander disease.
    d. Guillain-Barré syndrome (GBS).

16. To promote developmental care, nursing considerations for the infant with SMA should include:
    a. feeding by nasogastric tube.
    b. using an infant walker to develop muscle strength.
    c. incorporating verbal, tactile, and auditory stimulation.
    d. encouraging the parents to seek genetic counseling.

17. a. What are the most serious orthopedic problems associated with SMA?

    b. Describe the goal of treatment for nursing care for the child with SMA.

18. Which of the following is a true statement about GBS?
    a. GBS is an autosomal recessive inherited disease.
    b. GBS is more likely to affect children than adults, with children under the age of 4 years having the higher susceptibility.
    c. GBS is an acute demyelinating polyneuropathy with a progressive, usually ascending, flaccid paralysis.
    d. GBS is an autoimmune disorder associated with the attack of circulating antibodies on the acetylcholine receptors.

19. Which of the following results would be included in the diagnostic evaluation for the patient with GBS?
    a. Complete blood count elevated
    b. Cerebrospinal fluid high in protein
    c. Creatinine phosphokinase elevated
    d. Sensory nerve conduction time increased

20. The priority nursing consideration for the child in the acute phase of GBS is:
    a. careful observation for difficulty in swallowing and respiratory involvement.
    b. prevention of contractures.
    c. prevention of bowel and bladder complications.
    d. prevention of sensory impairment.

21. What are the characteristic symptoms of generalized tetanus?

22. a. Where are the spores of tetanus normally found?

    b. What is the incubation period for tetanus?

23. Terry, age 10 years, received his last tetanus toxoid immunization at the age of 4 years. He now comes to the clinic with a minor laceration sustained while working on his model airplanes. Is a dose of tetanus toxoid booster necessary at this time?
    a. Yes
    b. No

24. Maria, age 5, was born in South America and has been in the United States less than 1 year. While outside playing in the garden, she suffers a minor cut. Because Maria's mother does not think that Maria has ever received immunizations, which of the following actions would be most appropriate at this time to prevent tetanus?
    a. Have Maria go to the clinic tomorrow for the start of administration of all her needed immunizations.
    b. Administer tetanus immunoglobulin (TIG) now.
    c. Administer first injection of tetanus toxoid now.
    d. Administer both TIG and tetanus toxoid now.

25. Primary nursing implementations for the child with tetanus include:
    i. controlling or eliminating stimulation from sound, light, and touch.
    ii. placing the child in isolation.
    iii. arranging for the child not to be left alone, because these children are mentally alert.
    iv. realizing that the muscle relaxant vecuronium does not cause total paralysis.
    v. encouraging high intake of fluid.
    vi. implementing TIG therapy to neutralize toxins to be administered.

    a. i, ii, iii, and vi
    b. ii, iv, and v
    c. iii, v, and vi
    d. i, iii, and vi

26. Risk factors for infant botulism include:
    a. ingestion of honey.
    b. infants with diarrhea before the age of 3 months.
    c. infants living in urban areas.
    d. infants diagnosed with hypertonicity.

27. Infant botulism usually manifests with symptoms of:
    a. diarrhea and vomiting.
    b. constipation and generalized weakness.
    c. high fever and decrease in spontaneous movement.
    d. failure to thrive.

28. a. What is basis for the diagnosis of botulism?

    b. What is the treatment for botulism?

29. Nursing considerations aimed at parental support for the pediatric patient with botulism include:
    a. teaching the parents the importance of administering enemas and cathartics for bowel function after discharge.
    b. preparing the parents for the fact that the child will have muscular disability after the illness.
    c. teaching the parents the proper administration of antibiotics to continue treatment after discharge.
    d. teaching parents that the child will tire easily when muscular action is sustained and that timing of feedings after discharge is therefore important.

30. Tammy, age 13, is diagnosed with myasthenia gravis, which of the following priorities is included in the teaching plan for the family?
    a. Watching for signs of overmedication of anticholinesterase drugs, which include respiratory distress, choking, and aspiration
    b. Encouraging Tammy to be involved in strenuous activity and sports
    c. Suggesting to Tammy and her parents that they limit Tammy's scholastic activities in school to allow for adequate rest
    d. Reducing Tammy's weight to reduce symptom occurrence

31. Neonatal myasthenia gravis:
    a. occurs in approximately 30% to 50% of infants born to mothers with myasthenia gravis.
    b. produces elevated Moro reflex and shrill cry in the infant.
    c. may require administration of cholinesterase inhibitors to improve feeding ability.
    d. produces strength changes in the infant even after the maternal acetylcholine receptor antibodies have cleared the infant's system.

32. Spinal cord injuries are classified as either complete or incomplete. In a complete injury:
    a. there is loss of sensation, pain, and proprioception with normal cord function, including motor function.
    b. there is transient loss of neural function below the level of the acute spinal cord lesion, resulting in flaccid paralysis and loss of tendon autonomic and cutaneous reflex activity.
    c. there is no motor or sensory function more than three segments below the neurologic level of the injury.
    d. there is tetraplegia, commonly with sacral sparing, with patients gaining some motor recovery.

33. Diagnostic evaluation of the child who is seen with a spinal cord injury includes a complete neurologic examination. Motor system evaluation is done by:
    a. stimulating peripheral receptors by eliciting reflexes such as the patellar.
    b. observing gait; noting balance maintenance; and assessing the ability to lift, flex, and extend extremities.
    c. testing all 12 cranial nerves.
    d. using the blunt end of a safety pin and the sharp point to test each dermatome.

34. What is the general guideline used when determining whether a paraplegic person has the capacity for self-help in learning to walk?

35. Discuss the benefits of functional electrical stimulation (FES) for the child with spinal cord injury.

36. The nurse caring for the child with spinal cord injury and neurogenic bladder knows:
    a. to keep the patient's urine alkaline.
    b. that administration of dicyclomine (Bentyl) will relax the bladder musculature but will not promote increased bladder capacity or more adequate emptying.
    c. that the bladder that empties periodically by reflex action will not need intermittent catheterization.
    d. that pyelonephritis and renal failure are the most significant causes of death in longstanding paraplegic patients.

37. In discussing sexuality with the teenager who has a spinal injury, the nurse correctly includes information that:
    a. development of secondary sexual characteristics will be delayed.
    b. well-motivated young people can look forward to successful participation in marital and family activities.
    c. if injury occurs before onset of menstruation, ovulation and conception are not possible.
    d. females can easily experience vaginal or clitoral orgasms.

38. Clinical manifestations of juvenile dermatomyositis include:
    i. proximal limb and trunk muscle weakness.
    ii. stiff and sore muscles.
    iii. decreased ductal muscle strength and reflex response.
    iv. red rash over the malar areas and nose and violet discoloration of the eyelids.
    v. erythematous, scaly, atopic skin over extensor muscle surfaces.

    a. i, ii, iii, and iv
    b. i, ii, iv, and v
    c. iii, iv, and v
    d. ii, iii, and iv

39. Corticosteroid administration in muscular dystrophy has been shown to do all of the following except:
    a. increase muscle bulk and muscle power.
    b. improve pulmonary function.
    c. prolong ambulation.
    d. increase incidence of scoliosis.

40. What are the major complications of muscular dystrophy?

41. Major goals in the therapeutic management of children with muscular dystrophy include:
    a. promoting strenuous activity and exercise.
    b. promoting large caloric intake.
    c. promoting optimal function in all muscles for as long as possible.
    d. preventing cognitive impairment.

42. Diagnostic evaluation of muscular dystrophy includes:
    a. elevated EMG readings for amplitude and duration of motor unit potentials.
    b. absence of the polymerase chain reaction in the muscle biopsy.
    c. molecular genetic detection of deficient dystrophin by deoxyribonucleic acid analysis from peripheral blood or in muscle tissue obtained by biopsy.
    d. decreased serum creatine kinase levels.

CRITICAL THINKING—CASE STUDY

Kevin, age 4, has a history of premature delivery with CP diagnosed shortly after birth. Assessment findings include quadriplegia and deficient verbal communication skills but apparently normal level of intelligence. Kevin has been hospitalized several times in the past because of respiratory tract infection and gastric reflux. During Kevin's regular follow-up visit, his mother tells the nurse it is becoming harder to care for Kevin because of his needs. Because of Kevin's recent admission to the hospital for pneumonia, she worries that she is not giving Kevin the care he needs.

43. The nurse should explain to Kevin's mother that one of the complications associated with CP is respiratory problems. Which of the following assessment findings could most help explain why Kevin is having these problems?
    a. Constant drooling, which contributes to wet clothing and chilling
    b. Dietary imbalance with poor nutritional intake
    c. Nystagmus and amblyopia
    d. Coughing and choking, especially while eating, and history of gastric reflux

44. Kevin's mother asks the nurse how she can improve Kevin's communication skills, and a diagnosis of Impaired Verbal Communication is developed. Which of the following plans would be most appropriate for Kevin at this time to improve his communication skills?
    a. Purchase an electric typewriter or computer to facilitate communication skills.
    b. Enlist the services of a speech therapist.
    c. Teach Kevin the use of nonverbal communications skills such as sign language.
    d. Use audiotapes with Kevin to improve his speech abilities.

45. The nurse recognizes that an additional diagnosis is Altered Family Processes related to a child with a lifelong disability. Which of the following interventions should the nurse recognize as being important to include in the care plan?
    a. Explore potential for additional caregiving support.
    b. Refer the family to a support group of other parents of children with CP.
    c. Refer parents to social services for additional suggestions.
    d. All of the above.

46. Based on the information given about Kevin, identify the nursing goals that would assist him and his family.

47. While Kevin is in the hospital, the nurse should plan appropriate play activities that include:
    a. minimized speaking, because Kevin has difficulty with his speech.
    b. solitary play to allow Kevin's parents to be away from Kevin so that they can rest.
    c. helping Kevin relax muscles that are tense.
    d. those that require little intellectual functioning.

Answer Key

CHAPTER 1

1. d (p. 9)
2. b (p. 13)
3. c (pp. 9-10)
4. b (pp. 1-2; Box 1-1)
5. c (p. 7)
6. a (p. 7)
7. d (p. 7)
8. c (p. 8)
9. c (p. 8)
10. d (p. 8)
11. a (p. 8)
12. c (p. 8; Table 1-3)
13. b (p. 8)
14. d (p. 8)
15. Possible answers: Respiratory illnesses, infection, acute illness (p. 8)
16. Possible answers: Homelessness, poverty, low birth weight, chronic illnesses, adoption, day care centers (p. 8)
17. Childhood vaccination programs (p. 2)
18. a (p. 3)
19. b (p. 3)
20. d (p. 14)
21. Anticipatory guidance (p. 13)
22. e, g, h, c, b, i, d, a, f, j (p. 10)
23. Financial—no insurance; insurance that does not cover certain services; inability to pay for services
    System—need to travel great distances; state-to-state variations in benefits
    Information—lack of knowledge about prenatal or child health supervision; being unaware of available services (p. 10)
24. a. Diagnosis-related groups: a prospective payment system that allows for pretreatment billing for hospitals reimbursed by Medicare
    b. Health maintenance organizations: health services that use a network of specific providers for a set fee
    c. Managed care: a way to efficiently coordinate delivery of health services with the intent to provide an integrated approach to health care delivery (p. 13)
25. a (p. 11)
26. c (p. 11)
27. c (p. 11)
28. Evidence-based practice (p. 14)
29. c (p. 15)
30. e, b, g, f, i, d, c, h, a (pp. 12-15)
31. c (pp. 15-17)
32. a (pp. 15-17)
33. d (pp. 15-17)
34. c (pp. 15-17)
35. b (pp. 15-17)
36. a (pp. 15-17)

CHAPTER 2

1. j (p. 22), c (p. 21), a (p. 20), d (p. 21), g (p. 21), p (p. 29), f (p. 21), n (p. 28), k (p. 24), i (p. 22), b (p. 21), h (p. 22), l (p. 28), o (p. 28), r (p. 42), m (p. 28), q (p. 37), e (p. 21), s (p. 29)
2. d (p. 23), f (p. 23), c (p. 23), g (p. 30), b (p. 23), e (p. 23), a (p. 27)
3. f (p. 32), c (p. 32), e (p. 32), a (p. 32), k (pp. 34, 37; Table 2-1), g (p. 37; Table 2-1), m (p. 34), d (p. 32), j (pp. 34, 37; Table 2-1), n (p. 34), h (pp. 34, 37; Table 2-1), b (p. 32), l (pp. 34, 37; Table 2-1), i (pp. 34, 37; Table 2-1)
4. e, g, c, b, d, a, f (p. 35; Table 2-1)
5. b (p. 3)
6. a (p. 22)
7. d (p. 22)
8. g (p. 27), e (p. 29), a (p. 23), d (p. 26), b (p. 24), f (p. 30), h (p. 41), c (p. 25)
9. d (p. 22)
10. a (p. 22)
11. a (p. 25)
12. a (p. 23)
13. b (p. 23)
14. a (p. 23)
15. d (p. 39)
16. f, i, e, a, d, g, h, c, b (pp. 39-40; Box 2-4)
17. c (p. 40; Box 2-4)
18. d (p. 27)
19. c (p. 23)
20. a (p. 30)
21. d (p. 27), e (p. 32), b (p. 30), a (p. 32), c (p. 31)
22. c (p. 33)
23. d (p. 32)
24. d (p. 42; Box 2-5)
25. d (p. 42)
26. a (p. 34)
27. d (p. 30)
28. a (p. 35)
29. b (p. 35)
30. c (p. 36)
31. a (p. 36)
32. b (p. 36)
33. b (pp. 34, 37; Table 2-1)
34. d (p. 32)
35. a (p. 42; Table 2-2)
36. a (p. 37; Table 2-1)

CHAPTER 3

1. f, j, m, a, c, e, h, d, n, b, g, o, i, p, k, l, q (pp. 46-47, 49-51, 56-59, 63)
2. c (pp. 46-47)
3. b, a, a, b, c, c (pp. 47-48; Table 3-1)
4. b (pp. 48-49)
5. c (pp. 49-50)
6. Parental personality and mental well-being, systems of support, and child characteristics (pp. 51-52; Box 3-3)
7. T, F, T, T, F, T (pp. 51-52)
8. Birth order (p. 53)
9. c (p. 52)
10. a (pp. 52-53)
11. c (p. 54; Box 3-4)
12. b (p. 54; Box 3-5)
13. c (p. 55)
14. a (p. 55)
15. Promoting health and physical survival of children
Fostering the skills and abilities necessary for the children to be self-sustaining adults
Fostering behavioral capabilities to maximize cultural values and beliefs (p. 55)
16. b (p. 57)
17. F, T, F, F (pp. 55-57)
18. b (pp. 55-57)
19. b, a, c (p. 57)
20. a (p. 58; Family-Centered Care box)
21. a (p. 58)
22. a (p. 59)
23. b (pp. 58-60)
24. a (p. 60)
25. d (pp. 60-61)
26. c (pp. 60-61)
27. F, T, F, T, T, T, F, F (pp. 62-63; Box 3-7)
28. c (p. 62)
29. c (p. 63)
30. a, c, b (p. 64)
31. d (p. 49; Box 3-1)
32. a (pp. 48-49; Box 30-1; Table 3-1)
33. b (pp. 48-49, 55; Boxes 3-1, 3-2; Table 3-1)
34. d (pp. 47-48; Table 3-1)
35. Establish a healthy family unit. Seek support from extended family; seek parenting instruction. Attend support group for parents with twins. Identify community resources available for the family (pp. 48-49; Box 3-2; Table 3-1).
36. a. Occurs without any intervention; effective only when the consequences are meaningful; for example, forgetting ballet slippers results in the child having to dance in stocking feet
    b. Directly related to the rule; for example, child is not permitted to visit a friend's house for 1 day after coming home late from that friend's house
    c. Those that are imposed deliberately; for example, no watching TV until homework is finished (p. 59)
37. Corporal punishment usually takes the form of spanking and causes a dramatic short-term decrease in the behavior. However, the flaws include the following:
    a. It teaches children that violence is acceptable.
    b. It may physically harm the child if it is the result of parental rage.
    c. Children become "accustomed" to spanking, requiring more severe corporal punishment over time.
    d. It can result in severe physical and psychologic injury.
    e. It interferes with the parent-child interaction.
    f. When the parents are not around, the child is likely to misbehave, because the child has not learned to behave well for his or her own sake or what behavior is acceptable.
    g. It interferes with the child's development of moral reasoning (pp. 59-60).

CHAPTER 4

1. g, c, a, d, b, f, e (pp. 68-69)
2. b, m, d, i, e, c, q, g, k, h, l, f, j, p, o, n, a (pp. 70-72)
3. c, f, a, e, b, d (pp. 72-76)
4. d (p. 68)
5. "Healthy communities provide children not only with high-quality medical care, but also with a nurturing, safe place to live and grow. They provide a good infrastructure, which includes such structures as roads, sidewalks, schools, and playgrounds. Healthy communities address concerns through collaboration between and among citizens, businesses, and governmental and private agencies. They address the concerns using problem-solving strategies within the confines of the community's value system, thus increasing the community's own capacity to meet its needs.... The health of children and their families is greatly influenced by their community, and nurses can make a significant contribution by working with the community to promote children's health. Nurses working with pediatric populations need to understand the concepts and processes critical to addressing pediatric concerns from a community health perspective." (p. 68)
6. b (p. 70)
7. d (p. 69; Box 4-1)
8. a (p. 69; Box 4-2)
9. c (p. 69)
10. b (p. 70)
11. c (p. 70)
12. d (p. 71)
13. b (p. 71)
14. b (p. 72)
15. c (p. 72)
16. d (p. 72)
17. d (p. 73)
18. a (p. 73)
19. Health and social services, communication, recreation, physical environment, education, safety and

transportation, politics and government, and economics (p. 73)
20. b (p. 73)
21. c, a, b (p. 75)
22. c, a, a, b, c, b, c, b, a (pp. 71-74)
23. Prevention, preparedness and planning, response (pp. 69-70; Box 4-3)
24. b (pp. 69-70; Box 4-3)
25. Will nurses care for patients or their own family at the time of disaster? (pp. 69-70; Box 4-3)
26. d (pp. 69-70; Box 4-3)
27. c (p. 73)
28. a (p. 73)
29. c (p. 74)
30. c (p. 75)

CHAPTER 5

1. c (p. 82), e (p. 82), a (p. 79), f (p. 82), b (p. 80; Box 5-1), g (p. 82), d (p. 82), i (p. 87), k (p. 83), h (p. 102), j (p. 87), p (p. 80; Box 5-1), r (p. 80; Box 5-1), n (pp. 113-114), v (p. 95), m (p. 80; Box 5-1), t (p. 88), l (p. 80; Box 5-1), o (p. 80; Box 5-1), q (p. 80; Box 5-1), x (p. 98), s (p. 80; Box 5-1), z (p. 80; Box 5-1), u (p. 80; Box 5-1), w (p. 80; Box 5-1), y (p. 80; Box 5-1), bb (p. 85; Table 5-2), aa (p. 99), ii (p. 101), cc (pp. 85, 99; Table 5-2), gg (pp. 80, 102; Box 5-1), ee (pp. 79, 83, 88, 110), dd (p. 99), ff (p. 80; Box 5-1), hh (p. 102), jj (p. 101)
2. b (p. 105), d (p. 105), e (p. 106), g (p. 107), i (p. 107), c (p. 105), a (pp. 79, 104), f (p. 106), h (p. 107), j (p. 107), l (p. 107), k (p. 107), n (p. 111), m (p. 108)
3. d (p. 84)
4. c (pp. 85, 87-88; Table 5-2; Fig. 5-6)
5. a (p. 80; Box 5-1)
6. b, b, a, a, c, b, c, c, b, a, b, b, b, a, a, a, b, b (p. 95; Table 5-4)
7. d (p. 101)
8. c (p. 101)
9. a (p. 103)
10. a (p. 79)
11. d (p. 110; Box 5-8)
12. b (p. 105)
13. c (pp. 106-108)
14. c, b, d, a (pp. 80, 89, 99, 101, 106-107, 114-130; Boxes 5-1 and 5-3)
15. d (p. 107)
16. a (pp. 107-114)
17. d (p. 104)
18. a (p. 108)
19. b (p. 109)
20. c (p. 111)
21. d (p. 109; Box 5-7)
22. b (p. 111)
23. d (p. 107)
24. a (p. 80; Box 5-1)
25. a (pp. 107-109)
26. a (pp. 107-109)
27. c (pp. 107-109)

CHAPTER 6

1. d (p. 123), i (p. 138), g (p. 121), m (p. 131), c (p. 121), b (p. 120), e (p. 130), k (p. 144), a (p. 118), h (p. 130), l (p. 144), f (p. 119), j (p. 151)
2. c (pp. 118-120)
3. b (pp.118-120)
4. b (p. 120)
5. d (pp. 119-120)
6. d (p. 119; Box 6-1)
7. b (p. 121)
8. d (p. 121)
9. F, T, T, T, F (p. 122; Fig. 6-2; Nursing Care Guidelines box)
10. d (p. 121)
11. b, a, b, b, c, c, d (pp. 122-124)
12. d (pp. 125-126)
13. a. Storytelling
    b. "I" messages
    c. Bibliotherapy
    d. Drawing
    e. Directed play (pp. 125-126; Box 6-4)
14. Identifying information, chief complaint, present illness, past history, review of systems, family medical history, psychosocial history, sexual history, family history, nutritional assessment (p. 127; Box 6-5)
15. b (p. 127)
16. c (p. 127)
17. a (pp. 127-129; Box 6-5)
18. Approximate weight at 6 months, 1 year, 2 years, and 5 years of age; approximate length at 1 and 4 years; dentition, including age of onset, number of teeth, and symptoms during teething (p. 129)
19. Age of holding up head steadily; age of sitting alone without support; age of walking without assistance; age of saying first words with meaning; present grade in school; scholastic performance; whether the child has a best friend, and interaction with other children, peers, and adults (p. 129)
20. d (pp. 129-130)
21. Type, location, severity, duration, and influencing factors (pp. 127-128; Nursing Care Guidelines box)
22. a (p. 131; Nursing Care Guidelines box; Box 6-8)
23. c (pp. 130-131)
24. b (p. 131)
25. Family composition, home and community environment, occupation and education of family members, cultural and religious traditions (p. 131; Box 6-8)
26. c (pp. 133, 135, 138; Box 6-9)
27. b (p. 138)
28. a (pp. 138-140; Table 6-2)
29. d (p. 139; Nursing Care Guidelines box)
30. Body mass index for age; 3rd and 97th smoothed percentiles on all charts; 85th percentile for the weight-for-stature (pp. 139-140)
31. a (p. 142)
32. With the child in a supine position, fully extend the body by holding the head in midline position, grasping the knees together gently, and pushing down on the knees until the legs are fully extended and flat

against the table. Mark the end points of the tip of the head and the heel of the feet, and measure between the two spots (pp. 142-143).

33. T, F, T, T, F (pp. 139, 142, 144)
34. b (p. 142)
35. b (p. 144)
36. Apical; 1 full minute; abdominal; 1 full minute (pp. 148-149)
37. b (pp. 145, 147)
38. c (pp. 144-145)
39. c (p. 149; Tables 6-4 and 6-5)
40. d (pp. 151-152)
41. a (p. 152; Table 6-8), d (p. 152; Table 6-8), b (p. 152; Table 6-8), w (p. 173), c (p. 152; Table 6-8), d (p. 152; Table 6-8), e (p. 152; Table 6-8), f (p. 152; Table 6-8), k (p. 166), v (p. 173), l (p. 154), m (p. 164), i (p. 163), j (p. 163), g (p. 154), h (p. 152), p (p. 164), o (p. 173), n (p. 173), q (p. 166), r (p. 166), s (p. 168), u (p. 168), t (p. 168)
42. d (p. 152)
43. c (pp. 153-154)
44. a (p. 154)
45. Pupils equal, round, react to light, and accommodation (p. 155)
46. d (p. 155), j (p. 157), g (p. 155), c (p. 154), e (p. 155), b (p. 154), f (p. 155), i (p. 157), a (p. 154), h (p. 157)
47. b (p. 155)
48. a, b, c (pp. 156-157; Table 6-9)
49. d (p. 158; Table 6-9)
50. d (pp. 159-160)
51. d (p. 161)
52. a (p. 163)
53. a (pp. 163-164)
54. b (p. 166; Box 6-13)
55. a (p. 166)
56. a (p. 167; Fig. 6-32)
57. b (p. 168)
58. d (pp. 170-171)
59. c (p. 173)
60. Normal, abnormal, normal, normal, normal (p. 173)
61. Behavior, sensory testing, motor functioning, cerebellar functioning, reflexes, and cranial nerves (p. 174)
62. Corneal light reflex test—When light is shined directly into eyes from 16 inches, it is not reflected symmetrically within each pupil.
    Cover test—The uncovered eye moves (pp. 155-156).
63. d (pp. 118-121)
64. a (p. 127)
65. c (pp. 133, 135; Box 6-9)
66. a (pp. 136-137; Table 6-1)
67. d (p. 138)
68. Including the parent in the problem-solving process helps the nurse identify and eliminate solutions previously attempted. In addition, a parent who is included in the problem-solving process is more apt to follow through with a course of action (pp. 119-120).
69. b (pp. 124, 140; Nursing Care Guidelines box; Table 6-2)

70. d (pp. 169-170)
71. d (p. 169)
72. c (p. 121; Box 6-2)
73. b (p. 169)
74. S_1, apex; S_2, base (p. 167)
75. d (p. 167)

CHAPTER 7

1. Pain assessment, administration of analgesics at subtherapeutic levels, prolonged intervals in/between medications, and lack of systematic monitoring and evaluation of relief (p. 179)
2. b (p. 179)
3. T, T, F, T, F, F, T, T, T, F, T, F, T, T, T, F, T, F, T (pp. 180, 188, 191, 211, 214-215, 222; Box 7-1)
4. b (p. 202)
5. c (p. 180; Box 7-1)
6. a (pp. 180-181; Table 7-1)
7. d (p. 181; Table 7-1)
8. d (p. 209)
9. b (p. 182; Table 7-2)
10. a (p. 183; Table 7-2)
11. b (p. 186)
12. b (p. 188)
13. C: crying; R: requiring increased oxygen; I: increased vital signs: E: expression; S: sleeplessness (pp. 189-190)
14. d (p. 195; Nursing Care Guidelines box)
15. Possible answers: Distraction, relaxation, guided imagery, positive self-talk, thought stopping, cutaneous stimulation, behavioral contracting (pp. 220-221, Nursing Care Guidelines box)
16. c (pp. 194-195; Nursing Care Guidelines box)
17. b (p, 188; Box 7-2)
18. Nonopioids; opioids (pp. 198-199)
19. d (p. 199)
20. b (pp. 199, 202)
21. a (p. 202)
22. (1) Patient-administered boluses—can be infused according to the preset amount and lockout interval; (2) nurse-administered boluses—usually give an initial loading dose; (3) continuous basal infusion—delivers a constant amount of analgesic and is used when patient cannot control the infusion (p. 203)
23. d (p. 204)
24. c (p. 205)
25. b (p. 206)
26. c (p. 204; Box 7-3)
27. a (pp. 204, 221; Box 7-3)
28. d (p. 211)
29. b (pp. 207, 217)
30. d (pp. 186, 201, 211-222; Table 7-7; Box 7-4)
31. c (pp. 202, 213)
32. b (pp. 211, 219; Community Focus box)
33. Possible answers: Monitor and evaluate pain relief in a timely manner after administration of analgesics, titrate dosage to effect, make recommendations for alternate analgesics or addition of another analgesic or a combination of analgesics if therapy is not effective, use nonpharmacologic strategies (p. 214)

34. b (p. 216; Box 7-6)
35. d (p. 217)
36. a (p. 218)
37. Possible answers: Teaching patients self-control skills such as biofeedback and relaxation; modifying behavior patterns or techniques (p. 218)
38. c (p. 219)
39. c (p. 219)
40. T, F, T, T, F, T, T (pp. 220-222)
41. Need to acquire an understanding of the antecedents and consequences of headache pain. Explore with Beverly the fact that the headaches always occur in her first-period math class. Ask her to keep a headache diary in which she records the time of onset, activities before the onset, any worries or concerns as far back as 24 hours before the onset, severity and duration of the pain, pain medication taken and its effect, and activity pattern during headache episodes (p. 219).
42. Teach Beverly biofeedback techniques, relaxation training, and how to activate positive thoughts and engage in adaptive behavior appropriate to the situation (p. 247).
   Teach parents to focus attention on adaptive coping and maintenance of normal activity patterns (p. 219).
43. The nurse could expect an order of pentobarbital, usually administered rectally about 20 to 30 minutes before the examination. The medication usually lasts 1 to 2 hours after the initial dose. The dose the nurse would expect to administer is based on 2 to 5 mg/kg. Other options might be also used (p. 219; Table 7-10).
44. a (p. 222)
45. b (p. 222)

CHAPTER 8

1. Low oxygen, high carbon dioxide, low pH (p. 228)
2. The sudden chilling of the infant on entering a cooler environment from the warmer environment (p. 228)
3. c (p. 228)
4. b (p. 228)
5. a (p. 228)
6. T, F, T, F, T, F, F, T, F, F, F, T (pp. 228-230)
7. Rate of fluid exchange is seven times greater in infant; infant's rate of metabolism is twice as great in relation to body weight; infant's immature kidneys cannot sufficiently concentrate urine to conserve body water (p. 229).
8. b, a, c (p. 229; Box 8-1)
9. Maternal circulation; breast milk (p. 230)
10. d (p. 230)
11. a. 8 inches
   b. Yellow, green, pink, geometric shapes, checkerboards
   c. Low, high
   d. 20/100 and 20/400 (p. 231)
12. c (p. 231)
13. a, b, c (p. 232)

14. b (p. 232; Box 8-2)
15. a (pp. 235-236)
16. c (p. 238; Table 8-3)
17. d (p. 242)
18. g (p. 238; Table 8-3), a (pp. 230, 238; Table 8-3), c (p. 238; Table 8-3), i (p. 238; Table 8-3), b (p. 238; Table 8-3), d (p. 238; Table 8-3), j (p. 238; Table 8-3), e (p. 238; Table 8-3), h (p. 238; Table 8-3), f (p. 238; Table 8-3), l (p. 244), k (p. 230)
19. b (pp. 240-241)
20. a (p. 243)
21. d (p. 244)
22. a (p. 231)
23. d (p. 245)
24. a. Making a sharp, loud noise close to the infant's head should produce a startle reflex or other reaction, such as twitching of the eyelids (p. 246).
   b. Conduct auditory brainstem response or evoked otoacoustic emissions testing before discharge from the hospital (p. 254).
25. Obligatory nose breathers and are unable to breathe orally (p. 246)
26. c (pp. 246-248)
27. h (p. 246), c (p. 246), d (pp. 247, 249; Table 8-4), e (p. 247; Table 8-4), a (p. 249), g (pp. 247, 249; Table 8-4), b (p. 247), f (p. 247; Table 8-4)
28. a. Radiation
   b. Conduction
   c. Convection
   d. Evaporation (pp. 250-251)
29. d (p. 250)
30. a. Silver nitrate, erythromycin, or tetracycline ophthalmic drops or ointment (p. 252)
   b. Vitamin K (p. 252)
   c. Hepatitis B vaccine (p. 253)
31. a (p. 253)
32. a (pp. 255-256)
33. The medical benefits of male newborn circumcision are not sufficient to recommend it as a routine procedure. The policy stresses the need for parents to determine what is best for their child after they have been given accurate and unbiased information about the risks and benefits and alternatives to this elective procedure. It also advised that procedural analgesia be given to the infant during circumcision (p. 256).
34. d (pp. 259-260; Box 8-6)
35. a (pp. 259-260)
36. All statements are true (pp. 262, 265-266; Nursing Alert).
37. d (p. 264; Table 8-5)
38. d (p. 268)
39. d (p. 266)
40. c (pp. 231-232; Table 8-1)
41. Posture—full flexion of the arms and legs; square window—full flexion, hand lies flat on ventral surface of forearm; arm recoil—quick return to full flexion after arms released from full extension; popliteal angle—less angle/degree behind knee, less than 90 degrees; scarf sign—elbow does not reach midline with infant's arm pulled across the shoulder so that

infant's hand touches shoulder; heel to ear—knees flexed with a popliteal angle of less than 10 degrees when the infant's foot is pulled as far as possible up toward ear (p. 236; Box 8-3)

42. a (pp. 231-232)

43. Infant will maintain a patent airway. Infant will maintain a stable body temperature. Infant will experience no infection or injury. Infant will receive optimal nutrition (pp. 250-251, 259; Box 8-4).

44. Vital signs, daily weights, stool patterns, voiding patterns, feeding patterns and intake, cord condition and care (pp. 238, 240-242, 247, 250-251, 254-255, 259; Box 8-4)

45. c (pp. 261, 265; Box 8-7)

46. c (p. 262; Nursing Care Guidelines box)

47. a. Wet diapers: minimum of one for each day of life (day 2 = 2 wets; day 3 = 3 wets) until fifth or sixth day, at which time five or six per day to 14 days, then 6 to 10 per day

    b. Stools: at least two or three per day with breast-feeding

    c. Activity: has four or five wakeful periods per day; alerts to environmental sounds and voices

    d. Cord: keep above diaper line, nonodorous, drying

    e. Position for sleep: on back

    f. Safe transport home from hospital: use a federally approved infant care safety seat restraint, which should be a rear-facing safety seat with infant placed in the back seat; rolled blankets and towels may be needed between the crotch and legs to prevent slouching and can be placed along the sides to minimize lateral movement but should never be placed underneath or behind the infant (pp. 272-273; Community Focus box)

48. d (p. 246)

49. Adherent patches on the tongue and/or palate that cannot be wiped off may indicate an abnormal condition called *thrush* (candidiasis). If the patches can be wiped off, it is a normal finding, probably from the milk (pp. 239, 246; Table 8-3).

50. a. Wash hands before working with each infant and between infants (p. 251).

    b. Avoid long or artificial fingernails and contaminated hand lotions (p. 251).

    c. Use Standard Precautions of wearing gloves when handling infant until the blood and amniotic fluid are removed by bathing (p. 255).

CHAPTER 9

1. d (p. 285), m (p. 303), g (p. 291), o (p. 310), a (p. 280), h (p. 294), l (p. 286), c (p. 284), i (p. 304), b (p. 282), k (p. 285), j (p. 304), f (p. 295), n (p. 304), e (p. 287)

2. c (p. 279)

3. c (p. 280; Box 9-2)

4. d (p. 280)

5. c, b, a (pp. 280-281)

6. a (p. 282)

7. b, a, a, c, b, a, c, a (pp. 282-283)

8. c (p. 284)

9. T, T, F, T, T, F, F, F, F (p. 284)

10. c (p. 284)

11. d (p. 285)

12. a. Port-wine stains (p. 286)

    b. Infantile hemangiomas (p. 285)

    c. Café-au-lait spots (p. 285)

13. d (p. 287)

14. Hyperbilirubinemia, jaundice (p. 287)

15. Heme, globin, unconjugated bilirubin, conjugated bilirubin (p. 287)

16. c (p. 287)

17. a (p. 287)

18. a (p. 288; Table 9-1)

19. c (pp. 281, 287-290)

20. a (p. 292)

21. b (p. 289)

22. a (p. 290)

23. Gestational age 35 to 36 weeks, exclusive breastfeeding, maternal race (e.g., Asian or Asian American), significant bruising, blood group incompatibility or hemolytic disease, sibling with prior case of jaundice (p. 290)

24. d (pp. 291-292)

25. b (pp. 292-293)

26. a. Rh incompatibility (pp. 295-296)

    b. Rh negative, Rh positive, O, A, B (p. 297)

    c. Indirect Coombs, direct Coombs (p. 297)

    d. 72 hours, 26 to 28, intramuscular (p. 298)

    e. Isoimmunization (p. 295)

27. Documentation of blood volumes exchanged, the amount of blood withdrawn and infused, the time of each procedure, and the cumulative record of the total volume exchanged; vital signs monitored and evaluated frequently and correlated with the removal and infusion of blood; observation for signs of transfusion reaction, maintenance of adequate neonatal thermoregulation, blood glucose levels, and fluid balance (p. 299)

28. a (p. 299)

29. c (p. 300)

30. b (pp. 300-301)

31. a (p. 299)

32. c (pp. 300-301)

33. 125 mg/dl, 150 mg/dl (p. 301)

34. d (p. 301)

35. b (p. 302)

36. d (p. 302)

37. Administer 0.5 to 1 mg into the vastus lateralis muscle or ventrogluteal muscle during the first 24 hours of life (pp. 302-303).

38. d (pp. 309-310)

39. d (p. 305)

40. d (pp. 306-307)

41. a (pp. 308-309)

42. b (p. 309)

43. d (p. 310)

44. c (pp. 288-289; Table 9-1)
45. a (p. 289)
46. c (pp. 292-293; Nursing Care Plan)
47. d (pp. 292, 294)
48. d (p. 294)
49. Time phototherapy was started and stopped, proper shielding of eyes, type of fluorescent lamp by manufacturer, number of lamps, distance between lamp and infant (no less than 18 inches), used in combination with incubator or open bassinet, photometer measurement of light intensity, and occurrence of side effects (p. 294)
50. There is often an increase in the serum bilirubin level called "rebound effect"; this often resolves without resuming therapy (p. 294).
51. Teach to evaluate the number of voids and evidence of adequate breast-feeding; teach to bring infant to health care practitioner if indications of hyperbilirubinemia occur and for follow-up visit in 2 or 3 days for evaluation of feeding and elimination patterns (p. 295).

CHAPTER 10

1. a. Low-birth-weight infant (p. 317; Box 10-1)
    b. Extremely low–birth-weight infant (p. 317; Box 10-1)
    c. Small-for-gestational-age infant (p. 317; Box 10-1)
    d. Large-for-gestational-age infant (p. 317; Box 10-1)
    e. Preterm (premature) infant (p. 317; Box 10-1)
    f. Full-term infant (p. 317; Box 10-1)
    g. Postterm (postmature) infant (p. 317; Box 10-1)
    h. Fetal death (p. 317; Box 10-1)
    i. Neonatal death (p. 317; Box 10-1)
    j. Perinatal mortality (p. 317; Box 10-1)
    k. Late-preterm infant (p. 317; Box 10-1)
    l. Thermal stability (p. 321)
    m. Neutral thermal (or thermoneutral) environment (p. 321)
    n. Convective heat loss (p. 321)
    o. Radiant heat loss (p. 321)
    p. Conductive heat loss (p. 322)
2. d (pp. 315-317; Box 10-1)
3. c (p. 317)
4. c (p. 318)
5. Feeding behavior, activity, color, oxygen saturation (Spo$_2$), vital signs (p. 318)
6. a (p. 318)
7. T, F, F, T, T, F, F (pp. 318-320)
8. Infant will exhibit adequate oxygenation; infant will maintain stable body temperature (p. 320).
9. Nonshivering thermogenesis (p. 320)
10. a (p. 320)
11. Hypoxia, metabolic acidosis, hypoglycemia (p. 320)
12. a (p. 321), b (p. 321), d (p. 321), c (p. 321), f (p. 321), e (p. 322)
13. b (pp. 321, 322)

14. Describe shape of chest (barrel, concave), symmetry, presence of incisions, chest tubes, or other deviation. Describe use of accessory muscles: nasal flaring or substernal, intercostal, or subclavicular retractions. Determine respiratory rate and regularity. Auscultate and describe breath sounds: stridor, crackles, wheezing, diminished sounds, areas of absence of sound, grunting, diminished air entry, equality of breath sounds. Determine whether suctioning is needed. Describe ambient oxygen and method of delivery; if intubated, describe size of tube, type of ventilator and settings, and method of securing tube. Determine oxygen saturation by pulse oximetry and partial pressure of oxygen and carbon dioxide by transcutaneous oxygen (tcPo$_2$) and transcutaneous carbon dioxide (tcPco$_2$) (p. 319; Nursing Care Guidelines box).
15. a (p. 322)
16. a. Peripheral veins on the dorsal surfaces of the hands or feet (pp. 322-323)
    b. Percutaneous central venous catheter (PCVC), also called the "peripherally inserted central venous catheter" (PICC) (p. 323)
    c. Redness, edema, or color change at site; blanching at site (p. 323)
17. b (p. 323)
18. c (p. 324)
19. T, F, F, T, F, T, T, T, F, F, F, T, T (pp. 323-326)
20. a (p. 326)
21. b (p. 327; Box 10-3)
22. d (p. 326)
23. c (p. 326)
24. Nonnutritive sucking (p. 326)
25. d (pp. 329-330)
26. d (pp. 330-331; Nursing Care Guidelines box)
27. Benzyl alcohol, hyperosmolar (p. 331)
28. T, T, F, T, F, T, F, T, T, T, F, T (pp. 333-337; Box 10-5)
29. Supine (p. 336)
30. a (pp. 338-339)
31. Vulnerable child syndrome (p. 342)
32. a (p. 341)
33. c (pp. 342-343)
34. b (p. 344)
35. d (p. 346)
36. c (pp. 354-355)
37. b (p. 346)
38. a (p. 350)
39. a (p. 355)
40. Deficient surfactant production causes unequal inflation of alveoli on inspiration and the collapse of alveoli on end expiration; infants are unable to keep their lungs inflated and therefore exert a great deal of effort to reexpand the alveoli with each breath (p. 348).
41. c (p. 352), j (p. 351), d (p. 352), a (p. 349), e (p. 352), b (p. 349), g (p. 350), f (p. 350), h (p. 352), i (pp. 352, 353)
42. c (pp. 351-352)

43. a (p. 355)
44. b (p. 355)
45. d (p. 359)
46. a (p. 361)
47. Because of the infant's poor response to pathogenic agents, there is often no local inflammatory response at the portal of entry to indicate an infection (p. 362).
48. d (p. 364)
49. d (p. 365)
50. c (p. 366)
51. b (p. 366)
52. c (p. 359)
53. a (p. 367)
54. Hematocrit of 65% or greater; the small-for-gestational-age infant (p. 367)
55. Cryotherapy, laser therapy (p. 368)
56. Infant may be stuporous or comatose; seizures may begin after 6 to 12 hours and become more frequent and severe. Between 24 and 72 hours, deterioration in the level of consciousness may occur. After 72 hours, stupor and disturbances of sucking and swallowing are seen. Muscular weakness of the hips and shoulders in the full-term infant and lower limb weakness in the preterm infant occur. Apneic episodes may occur (p. 369).
57. d (pp. 370-371)
58. c (p. 371)
59. c (p. 371)
60. c (p. 372)
61. b (p. 373)
62. c (pp. 374-375)
63. d (p. 376)
64. F, T, F, T, T, F, T, T, T, F, T, T, T (pp. 376-379)
65. d (p. 379; Box 10-13)
66. d (p. 380)
67. Toxoplasmosis; Other agents such as hepatitis B, parvovirus, human immunodeficiency virus; Rubella; Cytomegalovirus infection; Herpes simplex; Syphilis (p. 380)
68. Transplacental, during vaginal delivery, or in breast milk (p. 381; Table 10-10)
69. c (p. 317; Box 10-1)
70. b (p. 316)
71. b (p. 354)
72. c (pp. 338-339)
73. a (pp. 352, 356: Nursing Care Plan)
74. Number of apneic spells; the appearance of the infant during and after attacks, whether the infant self-recovers or whether tactile stimulation is needed to restore breathing (p. 347)
75. Strong, vigorous suck; coordination of sucking and swallowing; a gag reflex; sucking on the gavage tube, hands, or pacifier; rooting and wakefulness before and sleeping after feedings (pp. 326-327)
76. The nurse should use therapeutic positioning to reduce the potential for acquired positional deformities and to accommodate necessary medical equipment and medical needs. On discharge the nurse instructs the parents to place the infant in the supine sleeping position (p. 336).

CHAPTER 11

1. f, g, e, a, b, c, d (p. 391)
2. b (p. 393)
3. c (p. 395)
4. d (pp. 393-394)
5. All are true (pp. 395, 398).
6. d (pp. 395-396; Table 11-1)
7. a (pp. 400, 402; Box 11-2)
8. a (p. 399)
9. c (p. 400; Box 11-1), k (p. 417), d (p. 401), a (p. 400; Box 11-1), b (p. 400), i (p. 411), g (p. 400; Box 11-1), f (p. 400; Box 11-1), j (p. 400; Box 11-1), h (p. 400; Box 11-1), e (p. 400; Box 11-1)
10. Hydrocephalus (p. 401)
11. a. Ultrasound of the uterus and elevated maternal concentrations of a-fetoprotein (AFP) (p. 402)
    b. 16 to 18 weeks of gestation (p. 402)
12. b (p. 402)
13. a. Preserve renal function (p. 403).
    b. Preserve renal function and achieve maximum urinary continence (p. 403).
14. d (p. 404)
15. c (p. 401)
16. b (p. 406)
17. c (p. 408)
18. a (p. 412)
19. a (p. 412)
20. c (p. 414)
21. Infection, malfunction (p. 413)
22. 2 months, 18 months, 10 to 12 years (p. 415)
23. F, T, T, F, T, T (p. 415)
24. c (p. 417)
25. a (p. 417)
26. d (p. 417)
27. Infants should be placed prone on a firm surface during awake time. Thirty minutes of supervised tummy time per day in infants younger than 6 months of age is recommended. The supine sleeping position is still recommended, but alternating the infant's head position for sleep can prevent unilateral moldings (p. 418).
28. A helmet is used that fits the largest diameter of the head. The helmet is worn 23 hours a day, usually for 3 months (p. 418).
29. b, a, c (p. 420; Box 11-5)
30. b (p. 420)
31. c, a, b (p. 422)
32. It worsens hip development by promoting hip extension (p. 422).
33. c (p. 423)
34. c, e, a, d, f, b, k, i, h, g, j (p. 419; Table 11-4)
35. b, a, c, d (p. 424; Box 11-6)
36. d (p. 424)
37. d (p. 426), b (p. 426), a (p. 425), c (p. 426), e (p. 426)
38. c (p. 428)
39. Speech impairments that require speech therapy; improper drainage from the middle ear, resulting in recurrent otitis media, which can lead to hearing impairment and insertion of pressure equalizer tubes

for prevention; extensive malposition of teeth and maxillary arches, requiring extensive orthodontics and dental prosthesis (pp. 428, 430)
40. c (pp. 430-431)
41. d (p. 431)
42. b (p. 430)
43. c (p. 431)
44. a (p. 435)
45. Look for physical findings of an absent anal opening; identify infants not passing stool within the first 24 hours after birth or infants who have meconium that appears at a location other than the anal opening; watch for other symptoms, including abdominal distention, vomiting, flat perineum, and absence of midline intergluteal groove (p. 441).
46. b (p. 441)
47. Incarcerated (pp. 445-446)
48. All statements are true (pp. 447-448).
49. d (pp. 446-447)
50. c (p. 449), b (p. 443), a (p. 444), j (p. 453), d (p. 448), e (p. 449), l (p. 449), i (p. 450), f (p. 450), g (p. 452), h (p. 453), k (p. 455)
51. Evaluation of prenatal and postnatal influences, karyotype, anatomic features, surgical possibilities, future fertility, and sexual function (pp. 457-458)
52. c (pp. 402, 406)
53. b (p. 407)
54. b (pp. 406-407)
55. Infant will not experience complications. Infant will not receive damage to the spinal lesion or surgical site. Family will receive support and education (pp. 406-407).
56. c (p. 406)
57. Urinary retention (p. 407)
58. a (p. 407)

CHAPTER 12

1. i (p. 467), b (p. 466), t (p. 468), d (pp. 466-467), f (p. 467), a (p. 465), g (p. 467), c (p. 477), h (p. 467), e (p. 467), j (p. 467), p (p. 467), n (p. 467), bb (p. 465), l (p. 467), k (p. 467), m (p. 467), o (p. 467), r (p. 468), z (p. 469), q (p. 467), x (p. 468), v (p. 468), s (p. 468), w (p. 468), aa (p. 469), u (p. 468), y (p. 468)
2. l (p. 473), a (p. 471), u (p. 493), c (p. 468), b (p. 472), e (p. 473), i (p. 473), d (p. 473), g (p. 473), f (p. 473), k (p. 473), h (p. 473), j (p. 473), p (p. 473), m (p. 474), r (p. 478), n (p. 478), t (p. 485), o (p. 474), q (p. 476), v (p. 494), s (p. 476)
3. e (p. 486), c (p. 486), a (p. 485), d (p. 486), b (p. 486)
4. c (p. 501), e (p. 495), a (p. 496; Box 12-5), d (p. 501), f (p. 502), h (p. 496; Box 12-5), g (p. 496; Box 12-5), b (p. 501)
5. g (p. 516), e (p. 511; Box 12-6), a (p. 511; Box 12-6), b (p. 511; Box 12-6), c (p. 511; Box 12-6), d (p. 512), f (p. 512)
6. c (p. 565)
7. b (p. 565)
8. a (p. 565)
9. Expected behavioral response: f, d, c, e, b, a (p. 465; Box 12-1)
   Age of appearance: d, c, a, e, f, b (p. 465; Box 12-1)
10. d (p. 465)
11. c (p. 465; Box 12-2)
12. b (p. 467)
13. c (p. 475)
14. a (p. 467)
15. d (p. 467)
16. Liver (p. 467)
17. a (p. 467)
18. a (p. 468)
19. b (p. 468)
20. b (p. 468)
21. a (p. 468)
22. d (p. 468)
23. 1.008 to 1.012 (p. 468)
24. c (p. 468)
25. b (p. 469)
26. d (p. 469)
27. b (p. 471)
28. a (p. 471)
29. a (pp. 472-473)
30. b (p. 473)
31. c (p. 475)
32. b (p. 475)
33. b (p. 476)
34. c (p. 476)
35. d (pp. 478-479; Table 12-2)
36. c (p. 480)
37. b (pp. 480-481)
38. d (p. 485)
39. c (pp. 485, 517)
40. c (p. 486)
41. b (p. 487)
42. c (pp. 484, 488; Table 12-3)
43. a (p. 493)
44. d (p. 489)
45. c (p. 490)
46. d (p. 493)
47. c (p. 491)
48. c (p. 491)
49. a (p. 490)
50. b (p. 492)
51. a (pp. 504-505)
52. c, e, b, d, a (p. 499; Table 12-5)
53. b (p. 510; Box 12-6)
54. c (p. 512)
55. c (p. 512)
56. a (p. 512)
57. The following should be checked: Nutrition, sleep and activity, number and condition of teeth, immunization status, safety precautions used in the home (p. 516).
58. c (p. 516)
59. b (p. 517)
60. d (p. 509)

CHAPTER 13

1. g (p. 524), f (p. 524), a (p. 531), h (p. 525), e (p. 524), i (p. 522), l (p. 525), n (p. 528), k (p. 531), o (p. 528), b (p. 531), m (p. 532), p (p. 528), j (p. 532), d (p. 528), c (p. 531)
2. Nursing Child Assessment Satellite Training (NCAST) Feeding Scale (p. 536)
3. b (p. 522)
4. b (p. 522)
5. c (p. 522)
6. a (p. 523)
7. c, d, a, b, e (p. 524)
8. Iron deficiency anemia, zinc deficiency, and rickets (p. 524)
9. Estimated average requirements, tolerable upper-limit nutrient intakes, nutrient intakes associated with a low risk for adverse effects, adequate intakes (p. 524)
10. c (p. 524)
11. c (p. 525)
12. b (p. 525)
13. d (p. 526)
14. c (p. 527)
15. c (p. 527)
16. d (p. 528)
17. d (pp. 529-531, 584; Box 13-3)
18. c (p. 530)
19. c (p. 530)
20. b (p. 530)
21. a (p. 531)
22. c (p. 531)
23. b (p. 532)
24. a (p. 532)
25. a (p. 533)
26. c (p. 532)
27. a (p. 535)
28. Possible answers: infant organic disease, dysfunctional parenting behaviors, subtle neurologic problems, subtle behavioral problems, and disturbed parent-child interactions (p. 535)
29. d (p. 535)
30. a (p. 535)
31. c (p. 537)
32. c (p. 537)
33. b (p. 538)
34. d (p. 539)
35. a (pp. 539-540)
36. c (p. 542)
37. F, T, F, F, T (pp. 542-546)
38. d (pp. 528-532)
39. a (pp. 528-532)
40. c (pp. 528-532)
41. b (pp. 528-532)

CHAPTER 14

1. n (pp. 557, 558; Table 14-1), c (p. 554), a (p. 554), e (p. 554), g (p. 554), b (p. 554), f (pp. 556, 557), h (pp. 556, 571), j (p. 556), l (pp. 556-557; Table 14-1), i (p. 556), k (p. 556), d (p. 554), m (pp. 556, 558; Table 14-1), o (pp. 557-559; Box 14-1; Table 14-1), q (p. 558), u (p. 558), p (p. 558), x (p. 560), w (p. 560), y (p. 562), r (p. 558), aa (pp. 561, 567), cc (p. 569), t (pp. 558-559; Box 14-1), bb (p. 569), s (p. 558), z (p. 563), v (p. 559)
2. a (p. 576), i (p. 575), k (p. 576), g (p. 573), j (p. 576), h (p. 574), e (p.572), f (p. 576), c (p. 575), d (p. 572), b (p. 572)
3. c (p. 554)
4. a (p. 555)
5. b (p. 555)
6. c (p. 556)
7. c (p. 556)
8. a (p. 557)
9. b (p. 558)
10. d, a, f, e, b, h, g, c (p. 559; Box 14-1)
11. d (p. 559)
12. c (p. 560)
13. b (p. 561)
14. c (p. 565; Table 14-2)
15. c (p. 561)
16. a (p. 562)
17. Physical characteristics—Voluntary control of anal and urethral sphincters; ability to stay dry for 2 hours; regular bowel movements; gross motor skills of sitting, walking, and squatting; fine motor skills to remove clothing
    Mental characteristics—Recognizes urge to defecate or urinate; communicative skills to indicate needs; cognitive skills to imitate behavior and follow directions
    Psychologic characteristics—Expresses willingness to please parent; able to sit for 5 to 10 minutes; demonstrates curiosity about toilet habits; impatient with soiled or wet diapers (p. 564)
18. a (p. 566)
19. a (p. 565)
20. c (p. 567)
21. d (p. 568)
22. c (p. 569)
23. d (p. 569)
24. Possible answers: Negativism—toddlers do not like to take orders; regression—they fear losing new skills; rigidity—upset when rituals are disrupted; self-centeredness—believe the world revolves around them; stranger anxiety; toilet training; security object lost; overstimulation; fears (p. 569; Box 14-2)
25. d (p. 569)
26. b (p. 570)
27. a (p. 570)
28. c (p. 570)
29. d (p. 570)
30. b (p. 571)
31. c (p. 572)
32. b (p. 572)
33. a (p. 572)
34. a (p. 572)
35. b (p. 572)
36. d (p. 573)
37. c (p. 573)

38. b (p. 573)
39. d (p. 574)
40. c (pp. 574-575)
41. d, e, c, f, a, b (pp. 575-582)
42. Motor vehicle (p. 576)
43. a (p. 576)
44. c (p. 576)
45. b (p. 577)
46. b (p. 579)
47. b (p. 579)
48. a (p. 580)
49. b (p. 581)
50. c (p. 581)
51. Foods: Hot dogs, nuts, dried beans, pits from fruit, bones, gum
    Play objects: Anything with small parts
    Household objects: Drawstring jackets or hoods, thumbtacks, nails, screws, coins, jewelry, old refrigerators, storage chests
    Electric: Outlets, garage doors, car windows (pp. 582-583)
52. Temperament, psychosocial development, nutrition, sleep and activity, dental health, injury prevention (pp. 553, 563-564)
53. a (pp. 568-569, 582)
54. d (pp. 568-569, 582)
55. b (pp. 568-569, 582)

CHAPTER 15

1. m (p. 587), i (p. 587), a (p. 585), k (p. 587), c (p. 586), q (p. 588), j (p. 587), b (p. 586), e (p. 586), n (p. 587), f (p. 586), l (p. 587), g (p. 586), p (p. 588), h (p. 587), o (p. 588), d (p. 586)
2. ee (p. 591), h (p. 589), x (p. 599), k (p. 590), g (p. 588), c (p. 588), e (p. 588), a (p. 588), f (p. 588), b (p. 588), i (p. 589), l (p. 590), d (p. 588), r (p. 598), u (p. 598), m (p. 591), v (p. 599), n (p. 592), cc (p. 600), p (p. 597), y (p. 599), w (p. 599), aa (p. 599), o (p. 597), j (p. 590), s (p. 598), z (p. 599), bb (p. 600), q (p. 597), t (p. 598), ff (p. 599), dd (p. 599)
3. 3, 5 (p. 585)
4. 2 to 3 kg (4.5 to 6.5 lb) (p. 585)
5. b (p. 586)
6. d (p. 587)
7. c (p. 587)
8. a (p. 587)
9. b (p. 588)
10. c (p. 588)
11. d (p. 588)
12. c (p. 589)
13. c (p. 589)
14. a (p. 590)
15. c (p. 589)
16. d (p. 593; Table 15-1)
17. b (p. 598)
18. b (p. 592)
19. Present ideas as exciting; talk to the child about activities he or she will be involved with; behave confidently on the first day (p. 596).

20. b (p. 596)
21. a (p. 596)
22. c (pp. 597-598; Box 15-1)
23. d (p. 599)
24. b (p. 599)
25. c (p. 600; Box 15-2)
26. d (p. 599)
27. b (p. 600)
28. T, T, F, F (p. 603; Table 15-2)
29. d (p. 604)
30. a (pp. 596-597)
31. c (pp. 596-597)
32. b (pp. 596-597)
33. d (pp. 596-597)

CHAPTER 16

1. c (p. 609; Table 16-1; Fig. 16-2)
2. Child will not spread infection to others; child will not experience complications; child will have minimal discomfort; child and family will receive adequate emotional support (pp. 615-616).
3. c (p. 609; Table 16-1), a (p. 608; Table 16-1), b (p. 609; Table 16-1), d (p. 610; Table 16-1), g (p. 612; Table 16-1), f (p. 611; Table 16-1), e (p. 610; Table 16-1), h (p. 613; Table 16-1), j (p. 612; Table 16-1), i (p. 614; Table 16-1)
4. d (p. 615)
5. a (p. 615)
6. d (p. 615)
7. b (p. 615)
8. Varicella (chickenpox) and zoster (herpes zoster or shingles) (p. 615)
9. Varicella-zoster immune globulin (VarZIG) or immune globulin intravenous (IGIV) (p. 615)
10. b (p. 616)
11. a (p. 616)
12. c (p. 616)
13. c (p. 616)
14. d (p. 608)
15. a (pp. 616-617; Box 16-1)
16. d (p. 617)
17. T, T, T, T, F, F, F, T, F (pp. 617-618)
18. c (p. 619; Box 16-2)
19. a (p. 620)
20. d (p. 621)
21. a (pp. 620-621; Box 16-3)
22. d (p. 621)
23. d (p. 621)
24. b (p. 621)
25. c (p. 621)
26. a (p. 625)
27. Assess the victim; terminate exposure to the poison; identify the poison; call poison control center for immediate advice (p. 622).
28. b (p. 624)
29. a (p. 625)
30. b (p. 625)
31. c (p. 625)
32. Lead; mercury; iron (pp. 626-627)

33. c (p. 627)
34. T, T, T, F, T, F, T, T, T, T, F, F, T (pp. 626-630)
35. b (p. 630)
36. a (p. 628)
37. d (pp. 629-630)
38. a (p. 630)
39. d (p. 632), g (p. 632), c (p. 632), b (p. 632), a (p. 631), e (p. 632), f (p. 632)
40. a (p. 633)
41. b (p. 633)
42. a (p. 633)
43. e (p. 633), d (p. 634), a (p. 633), b (p. 633), c (p. 634)
44. F, T, T, F, F, F, T (p. 634)
45. c (pp. 636-637)
46. d (p. 637)
47. d (p. 637)
48. d (p. 635)
49. a (p. 637)
50. c (pp. 637-638)
51. d (pp. 638-639)
52. a (pp. 616-617)
53. b (p. 617)
54. b (p. 617)
55. a (p. 617)
56. b (p. 617)
57. a (p. 617)
58. c (p. 621)

CHAPTER 17

1. c (p. 645)
2. Begins with shedding of the first deciduous tooth; ends at puberty with the acquisition of final permanent teeth (with the exception of the wisdom teeth) (p. 645)
3. a (p. 645)
4. T, F, T, F, T, F, T, F, T, T (pp. 645-646)
5. b (p. 646)
6. b (p. 646)
7. d (p. 646)
8. d (p. 646)
9. a (p. 648)
10. c (p. 646)
11. 10 years, 12 years (p. 646)
12. a (p. 647)
13. c (p. 648)
14. b (p. 648)
15. c (p. 648)
16. f (p. 650), g (p. 650), e (p. 650), c (pp. 648-649), d (p. 648), b (p. 648), a (p. 628), h (p. 651), j (p. 648), i (p. 648)
17. c (p. 650)
18. b (p. 651)
19. b (p. 652)
20. d (p. 652)
21. d (p. 653)
22. c (p. 653; Community Focus box)
23. Their own self-assessment and what they interpret as the opinion of family members and outside social contacts (p. 654)

24. a (p. 655)
25. c (p. 654)
26. Children learn to subordinate personal goals to group goals. Children learn that division of labor is an effective strategy for the attainment of a goal. Children learn about the nature of competition and importance of winning. Children will work hard to develop skills needed to become members of a team, thus improving their social, intellectual, and skill growth (p. 657).
27. d (p. 657)
28. F (p. 658), T (p. 658), T (p. 658), T (p. 658), F (p. 658), T (p. 660), F (p. 660), T (p. 660), T (p. 660), F (p. 661), T (p. 662)
29. c (p. 661)
30. To help the child interrupt or inhibit forbidden actions; to help child identify an acceptable form of behavior so that he or she can identify what is right in future situations; to provide understandable reasons as to why one action is appropriate and another action is not; to stimulate child's ability to empathize with the victim (p. 661)
31. a (p. 662)
32. b (p. 664)
33. b (p. 664)
34. Children in elementary school who are left to care for themselves without adult supervision before or after school (p. 664)
35. Hygiene, nutrition, exercise, recreation, sleep, safety (p. 665)
36. Balance food and physical activity by having a lifestyle that combines sensible eating with regular physical activity; choose a diet with plenty of nutrient-dense foods such as grain products, vegetables, and fruits; choose a diet low in fat, saturated fat, and cholesterol; choose protein foods that are lean; eat a variety of foods; choose a diet moderate in salt and sugar; choose calcium-rich foods (p. 667).
37. a (p. 668)
38. a (p. 668)
39. c (p. 668)
40. T (p. 667), F (p. 667), F (p. 668), F (p. 668), T (p. 668), T (p. 671), T (p. 672), T (p. 672), T (p. 669), T (p. 669), T (p. 669), F (p. 670), F (p. 676), T (p. 676), F (p. 677), T (p. 678)
41. Limit playing time, monitor game selection and content, and increase access to games and information that are educational (p. 671)
42. Health appraisal, health promotion, emergency care and safety, communicable disease control, counseling and guidance, adjustment to individual student needs (p. 673; Box 17-7)
43. c (p. 676)
44. c (pp. 645, 677, 678; Family-Centered Care box)
45. a (p. 669)
46. a (p. 667)
47. b (p. 647)
48. b (p. 666)
49. The bike should be sized to fit the child. The child should be able to stand with the balls of both feet on

the ground when seated on the bike, to place both feet flat on the ground when straddling the center bar, and to grasp the brake lever easily and comfortably. The helmet should be hard shelled and lined with Styrofoam; it should be adjusted to the child's head and fit securely without limiting the child's vision or hearing; it should be brightly colored for better visibility and carry the U.S. Consumer Product Safety Commission seal (p. 677).

CHAPTER 18

1. d (p. 685)
2. Contact with agents that cause injury to the skin as a chemical, physical trauma, or infectious organism; hereditary factors; allergens; systemic disease where the lesions are a cutaneous manifestation (p. 685)
3. c, b, e, a, d (p. 685)
4. j (p. 686), f (p. 686), h (p. 686), a (p. 686), b (p. 686), d (p. 686), c (p. 686), e (p. 686), i (p. 686), g (p. 686), k (p. 687)
5. d (p. 690; Nursing Alert)
6. c (p. 686)
7. b (p. 690)
8. c (p. 687)
9. a (p. 687)
10. c (p. 688)
11. a (pp. 688-689)
12. d (p. 690)
13. a (p. 690)
14. b (p. 689)
15. c (p. 690)
16. Increased erythema, especially beyond the wound margin; edema; purulent exudate; odor; pain; increased temperature (p. 690; Nursing Alert)
17. d (p. 691)
18. b (p. 692)
19. c (p. 693)
20. b (p. 694; Table 18-3)
21. a (p. 697; Table 18-5)
22. c (p. 695)
23. a (pp. 695, 697; Table 18-5)
24. d (p. 698)
25. a. Observation of the white eggs (nits) firmly attached to the hair shafts that do not dislodge easily when removal is attempted; scratch marks and/or inflammatory papules caused by secondary infection may be found on the scalp (p. 698)
    b. That the no-nit policies in schools are detrimental, causing lost time in the classroom and inappropriate allocation of the school nurse's time, and that such a response is not warranted because pediculosis is not a serious medical condition (p. 701)
26. a (p. 700)
27. b (p. 699)
28. d (p. 699)
29. b (p. 701)
30. d (p. 703)
31. e, d, f, a, c, b (p. 702; Tables 18-6 and 18-7)
32. b (pp. 703-704)

33. a (p. 703)
34. d (p. 706)
35. a (p. 707)
36. c (p. 707)
37. d (p. 707), c (p. 707), h (p. 704), f (p. 706), e (p. 706), b (p. 708), a (p. 708), g (p. 708)
38. b (p. 708)
39. 7 days; almost immediately (p. 709)
40. b (p. 710)
41. d (pp. 711, 713; Box 18-1)
42. c (p. 710)
43. a (p. 712; Table 18-9)
44. b (p. 713; Table 18-10)
45. a (pp. 714-715; Table 18-10)
46. b (p. 715)
47. b (p. 716)
48. c (p. 716; Nursing Alert)
49. d (p. 716)
50. b (p. 717)
51. c (p. 718)
52. d (p. 719)
53. b (p. 722)
54. d (p. 723)
55. a (p. 726)
56. T, F, T, F (p. 728)
57. c (p. 729)
58. d (p. 730)
59. T (p. 730), F (p. 731), F (pp. 731-732), T (p. 731), T (p. 731), T (p. 732), T (p. 732), F (p. 733), T (p. 734), T (p. 734)
60. b (pp. 686, 690, 704)
61. c (pp. 704-705)
62. a (p. 706)
63. d (pp. 690-691, 705-706)
64. b (pp. 691-692)

CHAPTER 19

1. d (p. 739)
2. a (p. 740)
3. T (p. 741), T (p. 739), T (p. 741; Box 19-1), F (p. 739), T (pp. 741-742), F (p. 742), F (p. 743), F (p. 742), T (p. 739)
4. f (p. 739), d (p. 739), a (pp. 741, 742), e (p. 744), b (p. 742), c (p. 742), g (p. 739)
5. c (p. 742)
6. pubertal delay (p. 742), precocious puberty (p. 742)
7. b (p. 743)
8. a (p. 744)
9. Pubertal growth spurt (p. 744), genetic endowment (p. 744)
10. b (p. 743; Fig. 19-4)
11. d (p. 744; Fig. 19-6)
12. b (pp. 744-745)
13. 2 to 8; 15.5 to 55; 4 to 12; 15.5 to 66 (p. 745)
14. c (pp. 745-746)
15. d (pp. 746-747, 756-757)
16. b (p. 746)
17. b (p. 746)
18. b (p. 747)

19. c (p. 747)
20. c (p. 747)
21. a (p. 748)
22. d (p. 748)
23. d (pp. 749, 750)
24. c (p. 8750)
25. Realization of romantic or erotic attractions; erotic daydreaming; romantic partners or dates without sexual activity; sexual activity with others; self-identification of the orientation that best fits one's current circumstances and understanding; publicly self-identifying sexual orientation; intimate committed sexual relationship (p. 751)
26. b (p. 751)
27. a (p. 752)
28. d (p. 753)
29. Authoritative parenting is characterized by parental expectations of mature behavior on the part of the adolescent and setting and enforcing reasonable limits for behavior; this type of parenting is related to greater psychosocial maturity and school performance and less substance abuse among adolescents (p. 753).
30. a (p. 755)
31. d (p. 747)
32. a (p. 753)
33. b (p. 754)
34. d (p. 754)
35. Injuries, homicide, suicide (p. 756)
36. a (p. 756)
37. c (p. 756)
38. d (p. 757)
39. T (pp. 763-764), T (pp. 756-757), F (p. 758), T (p. 757), T (p. 769), F (p. 757), T (p. 759), T (p. 759), F (p. 758), F (p. 770), F (p. 765), T (p. 754), T (p. 754), T (p. 7547), T (p. 754), F (p. 754), T (p. 762), T (p. 763), T (p. 762), T (p. 757), F (pp. 770-771), F (p. 771)
40. Accessible, appropriate (p. 758)
41. Giving adolescents written materials during "teachable moments"; directing the adolescent to health resources in the community and on the Internet; teaching adolescents how the health care system works and how to keep their own personal health information (p. 759)
42. Active listening; responding to an adolescent's emotions; ensuring confidentiality and privacy (p. 759)
43. c (p. 762)
44. b (pp. 762-763)
45. c (p. 763)
46. d (p. 763)
47. b (p. 763)
48. obese; overweight (p. 763)
49. b (pp. 764-765)
50. The adolescent has a specific plan (p. 766).
51. a (p. 766)
52. a (p. 768)
53. c (pp. 768-769)
54. c (p. 769)
55. c (pp. 749, 764)

56. c (pp. 764, 767-768)
57. d (p. 740; Table 19-1)
58. c (pp. 767-768)
59. c (pp. 750-751, 770)

CHAPTER 20

1. c (p. 776)
2. d (pp. 776-777)
3. a (pp. 776-777)
4. d (p. 777)
5. b (p. 777)
6. c (pp. 777-778)
7. d (p. 779)
8. c (p. 779)
9. a (p. 779)
10. d (p. 780; Box 20-1)
11. d (p. 780), a (p. 779), d (p. 780), e (p. 778), b (p. 779), g (p. 778), c (p. 780), b (p. 779), f (pp. 778, 779), c (p. 780), a (p. 779)
12. Primary amenorrhea (p. 781), secondary amenorrhea (p. 781), oligomenorrhea (p. 781), dysmenorrhea (p. 782)
13. Oral contraceptive pills will protect the endometrium and provide sufficient estrogen for bone density. Unopposed estrogen can lead to endometrial hyperplasia and risk for endometrial adenocarcinoma (pp. 781-782).
14. c (p. 782)
15. d (pp. 781-782)
16. b (p. 783), c (p. 783), d (p. 783), h (p. 785), i (p. 799), a (p. 784), e (p. 784), f (p. 784), g (p. 784)
17. c (p. 783)
18. b (pp. 784-785)
19. Wipe from the front to the back after toileting. Avoid tight-fitting clothes and nylon underpants. Avoid douching because it leads to changes in the normal vaginal microflora. Discuss sexual transmission of disease and use of condoms for prevention (p. 785).
20. T (p. 785), T (p. 785), F (p. 786), F (p. 786), T (p. 786), T (p. 785), F (p. 786), F (p. 787), F (p. 786), T (p. 787), T (p. 787), T (p. 785), F (p. 786)
21. a (p. 787)
22. d (p. 786)
23. c (pp. 787-788)
24. b (p. 788)
25. Preventing subsequent pregnancies and enhancing life outcomes for the adolescents and infant (p. 789)
26. a (pp. 789-790)
27. c (p. 790)
28. d (pp. 791-792, 797; Table 20-1)
29. c (p. 790)
30. c (p. 793)
31. a (p. 793; Table 20-1)
32. d (p. 793)
33. Allowing adolescents to role-play refusal skills (for sexual activity) in a safe environment (p. 794)
34. d (p. 795)
35. a (pp. 795-796)

36. T (p. 796), F (p. 796), F (p. 796), T (p. 797), T (p. 797), T (p. 797), T (p. 798), F (p. 797), F (pp. 797-798), T (p. 798), T (p. 799)
37. b (p. 798)
38. d (p. 798)
39. b (p. 799)
40. Human papillomavirus, anogenital warts, cervical dysplasia, carcinoma (p. 799)
41. d (pp. 799-800)
42. Recommendations include Pap screening in adolescents 3 years after initiation of sexual intercourse or by age 21; thereafter it is recommended women have annual screening with traditional Pap smears or every 2 years with liquid-based cervical cytologic screening (pp. 799-800).
43. a (p. 799)
44. b (p. 800)
45. a (pp. 800-801)
46. b (p. 776)
47. a (p. 776)
48. a (p. 778)
49. c (pp. 776, 778)
50. d (p. 788)
51. d (pp. 787-788)
52. a (p. 785)

CHAPTER 21

1. T (p. 806), T (p. 815), T (p. 806), F (p. 811; Box 21-1), F (p. 806), F (p. 807), T (p. 807), T (p. 806), T (p. 808), T (p. 806), T (p. 808), T (p. 806), T (p. 808), T (p. 808)
2. d (p. 808)
3. d (p. 808)
4. c (p. 809)
5. a (p. 810)
6. d (pp. 810-811)
7. b (p. 811)
8. c (p. 807)
9. c (p. 814)
10. b (pp. 814-815)
11. Reduce the quantity eaten by purchasing, preparing, and serving smaller portions; alter the quality consumed by substituting low-calorie, low-fat foods for high-calorie foods, especially for snacks; eating regular meals and snacks, particularly breakfast; severing the association between eating and other stimuli such as eating while watching television (p. 814)
12. a (p. 811)
13. a (p. 814)
14. b (p. 815)
15. A strong fear of becoming fat, a distorted body image, and progressive weight loss (p. 815)
16. Repeated episodes of binge eating followed by inappropriate compensatory behaviors, such as self-induced vomiting; misuse of laxatives, diuretics or other medications; fasting; or excessive exercise (p. 815)
17. d (p. 817)
18. d (p. 817)
19. a (pp. 817-818)
20. b (pp. 818-819; Box 21-8)
21. c (p. 818)
22. c (p. 816)
23. Reinstitution of normal nutrition or reversal of the malnutrition; resolution of disturbed patterns of family interaction; individual psychotherapy to correct deficits and distortions in psychologic functioning (p. 818)
24. c (p. 819)
25. b (p. 819)
26. a (pp. 820, 822-823)
27. d (p. 819)
28. T (p. 824), T (p. 824), F (p. 824), F (p. 824), T (p. 823), F (p. 824), T (pp. 823, 830), T (p. 825), T (p. 825)
29. a (pp. 826-827)
30. b (p. 827)
31. c (p. 828)
32. b (p. 828)
33. a (pp. 828-829)
34. Cohesive family, peer models for conventional behavior, connectedness to school and community organizations, social support in the form of perceptions that adults outside the family care about the youth, and the availability of people to talk to about problems (p. 829)
35. b (p. 833)
36. a. Crack (or rock) (p. 830)
    b. Injection (p. 830)
    c. Antifatigue agent; long periods of sleep (p. 830)
    d. Constricted pupils, respiratory depression, cyanosis, and needle marks seen on extremities of chronic users (p. 831)
    e. Rohypnol (flunitrazepam) (p. 831)
    f. Methamphetamine (p. 831)
    g. Rapid loss of consciousness, respiratory arrest, fatal cardiac arrhythmias (p. 831)
    h. Dissolving instantly in water or other drinks, including alcohol (p. 831)
    i. Exhaustion, dehydration (p. 831)
    j. Hallucinogens (p. 832)
37. c (p. 834)
38. d (p. 834)
39. d (pp. 836-838; Box 21-11)
40. a (p. 832)
41. c, d, b, a, e (p. 834)
42. b (p. 835)
43. d (pp. 834-837; Box 21-10)
44. c (p. 839)
45. a (p. 839)
46. c (pp. 839-840)

CHAPTER 22

1. f, b, h, a, d, i, c (p. 845; Box 22-1), j (p. 847), g, e (p. 845; Box 22-1)
2. b (p. 848), f (p. 852), c (p. 848), e (p. 847), a (p. 847), d (p. 847)

3. b (pp. 850, 854), n (p. 870), c (pp. 855, 857-858), a (p. 846), d (p. 867), f (pp. 867-868), h (pp. 867-869), o (p. 870); Box 22-6), i (p. 949), l (p. 949), g (p. 947), j (p. 869), e (p. 867), k (pp. 855, 869-870), p (pp. 869, 872), m (p. 870)
4. a (p. 845)
5. d (p. 845)
6. b (p. 846)
7. d (p. 847)
8. a (p. 848)
9. d (p. 849)
10. e, c, a, b, d (pp. 849-851; Table 22-1)
11. b (p. 855)
12. b (p. 855)
13. b (p. 848)
14. c (p. 857)
15. a (p. 857)
16. d (p. 858)
17. c (pp. 858-860)
18. b (p. 859)
19. Possible responses: Share complete information. Share information in manageable doses. Be sensitive to parents' reactions. Listen carefully. Provide technical information in understandable terms. Offer to share information. Provide information about resources (p. 859).
20. a (p. 861)
21. Home, school (p. 861)
22. a (p. 863)
23. c (p. 864)
24. d (p. 865)
25. b (p. 869)
26. False reassurance; assuring parents that the child will grow out of the problem when the parents are struggling to accept reality (p. 871)
27. Approach behaviors: a, c, e, f, g
    Avoidance behaviors: b, d (p. 867)
28. b (p. 867)
29. d (p. 868)
30. c (pp. 868-869)
31. d (p. 869)
32. a (p. 866)
33. Possible answers: Facilitate support from professionals; encourage expression of emotions; describe the behavior; give evidence of understanding; give evidence of caring; help parents focus on feelings; facilitate parent-to-parent support (pp. 858-859)
34. b (pp. 859-860)
35. d (pp. 869-870)
36. c (p. 859)
37. Possible answers: Makes many sacrifices; helps the child even when the child is capable; provides inconsistent discipline; is dictatorial; hovers and overdoes praise; protects the child from every discomfort; restricts play; denies the child opportunities for growth; sets goals too high or too low; monopolizes the child's time (p. 870; Box 22-5)
38. a (p. 872)
39. d (p. 870)
40. d (p. 962; Box 22-4)

41. a (p. 870)
42. a (p. 871)
43. b (p. 871)
44. a (p. 872)
45. a (p. 872)
46. a (pp. 850-851, 855; Tables 22-1 and 22-2)
47. c (pp. 849-855)
48. c (pp. 849-855)
49. b (pp. 850-851, 855; Tables 22-1 and 22-2)
50. a (pp. 850-851, 855; Tables 22-1 and 22-2)

CHAPTER 23

1. b (p. 879), d (p. 887), e (p. 886), a (p. 879), c (p. 887), j (p. 903), f (p. 886), i (p. 903), g (p. 880), h (p. 901)
2. b (p. 887)
3. c (p. 880)
4. Possible answers: Listen for an "invitation" to talk about the situation; use open-ended, nonjudgmental questions to explore the family's wishes; answer questions honestly; address fantasies or misunderstandings; remain neutral (p. 881; Box 23-2).
5. c (p. 881; Table 23-2)
6. d (p. 881; Table 23-2)
7. a (p. 881)
8. c (p. 885)
9. a (p. 883)
10. b (p. 884)
11. d (p. 885)
12. c (p. 885)
13. Children who are dying are allowed the opportunity to remain with those they love and with whom they feel secure. Many children who were thought to be in imminent danger of death have gone home and lived longer than expected. Siblings can feel more involved in the care and often have a more positive perception of the death. Parental adaptation is often more favorable, as is shown by their perceptions of how the experience at home affected their marriage, social reorientation, religious beliefs, and views on the meaning of life and death. Parents who have used home hospice feel significantly less guilt after the child's death than those whose child died in the hospital (p. 886).
14. d (p. 887)
15. b (p. 887)
16. d (pp. 888-891; Table 23-4)
17. d (pp. 889-890)
18. Possible answers: Loss of senses; confusion; muscle weakness; loss of bowel and bladder control; difficulty swallowing; change in respiratory pattern; weak, slow pulse (pp. 891-892; Box 23-7)
19. d (pp. 894-895)
20. Possible responses: Recall events that were important with their family; draw pictures or leave messages for important friends and family; reassure parents and others that they are not afraid and are ready to die; experience visions of "angels"; mention that someone is waiting for them (pp. 891-892).

21. c (p. 891)
22. a (p. 891)
23. a (pp. 894-895)
24. All statements are false (pp. 896-897).
25. d (p. 897)
26. a (p. 897)
27. c (p. 898)
28. c (p. 898)
29. d (p. 899)
30. d (p. 899)
31. d (p. 901)
32. Possible answers: Denial, anger, depression, guilt, ambivalence (pp. 902-903)
33. b (p. 903)
34. a (pp. 892-894; Nursing Care Plan)
35. c (pp. 892-894; Nursing Care Plan)
36. d (pp. 892-894; Nursing Care Plan)
37. a (pp. 892-894; Nursing Care Plan)

CHAPTER 24

1. h (p. 910), a (p. 908), c (p. 909), b (p. 909), e (p. 909), d (p. 909), f (p. 910), i (p. 910), g (p. 901), m (p. 918), j (p. 911), l (p. 918), k (pp. 917-918), n (pp. 918, 920), o (p. 922)
2. a (p. 923), c (p. 923), b (p. 923), f (p. 924), d (p. 924), e (p. 924), g (p. 924), k (p. 924), h (p. 924), m (p. 924), i (p. 924), j (p. 924), l (p. 924), n (p. 924), q (p. 927), o (p. 927), p (p. 926), r (p. 927)
3. g (p. 930), n (p. 932), j (p. 932), c (p. 929), e (p. 929), l (p. 932), f (p. 929), h (p. 929), p (p. 934), b (p. 929), i (p. 932), d (p. 929), k (p. 932), m (p. 932), r (p. 034), o (p. 934), a (pp. 928-929), q (p. 934)
4. o (p. 941), l (p. 941), c (p. 935), e (p. 935), b (p. 935), g (p. 936), a (p. 935), d (p. 935), h (p. 936), f (p. 935), k (p. 913), q (p. 942), n (p. 941), i (p. 936), p (p. 942), j (p. 936; Box 24-11), m (p. 941)
5. b, d, c, a (p. 909; Table 24-1)
6. b (p. 908)
7. Possible answers: Nonresponsiveness to contact; poor eye contact during feeding; diminished spontaneous activity; decreased alertness to voice or movement; irritability; slow feeding (p. 911; Box 24-2)
8. a (p. 911)
9. *Fading* means to take the child physically through each sequence of the desired activity and gradually fade out physical assistance so that the child becomes more independent (p. 911).
10. *Shaping* means to wait for the child to give a response that approximates the desired behavior, then reinforce the child by gestures of social approval, such as touching or talking to him or her (pp. 911-912).
11. d (p. 913)
12. Pros: Marriage could help the couple achieve a mutually satisfying and supportive relationship, meaningful companionship, and a more normal sociosexual adjustment.
Cons: Concerns include suitable living accommodations and contraceptive methods to prevent pregnancy. Parenting would require specialized assistance

to help the couple learn to meet the needs of their offspring (p. 913).
13. c (p. 913)
14. b (p. 913)
15. *Task analysis* means to break the process of a skill into its components. It is used when teaching a cognitively impaired child to help the child master one step of a skill at a time, building on the parts that the child has mastered already (pp. 911-912, 915-916; Box 24-4).
16. d (p. 916)
17. The child should be able to sit quietly for 3 to 5 minutes; to watch what he or she is doing while working on a task; to follow physical gestures or cues; to follow verbal commands; to relate clothing with the appropriate body part; and to be willing to participate (pp. 916-917).
18. b (p. 917)
19. c (p. 918)
20. b (p. 918)
21. Possible answers: Separated sagittal suture; oblique palpebral fissures (upward, outward slant); small nose; depressed nasal bridge (saddle nose); high, arched narrow palate; excess and lax neck skin; wide space between big and second toes; plantar crease between big and second toes; hyperflexibility; muscle weakness (p. 919; Box 24-5)
22. b (p. 920)
23. c (p. 921)
24. a (p. 922)
25. b (p. 922)
26. c (p. 923)
27. d (p. 923)
28. d (p. 924; Table 24-5)
29. b (p. 926; Box 24-8)
30. a (pp. 925-926, 936; Boxes 24-8 and 24-11)
31. d (p. 926)
32. d (p. 927)
33. a (pp. 927-928)
34. b (p. 931)
35. d (p. 931)
36. f, d, b, a, e, c (p. 929; Box 24-9)
37. Possible answers: Talk to the child about everything that is occurring. Emphasize aspects of procedures that are felt and/or heard. Approach the child with identifying information. Explain unfamiliar sounds. Encourage rooming-in for parents. Encourage parents to participate in the care. Bring familiar objects from home. Orient the child to the immediate surroundings. If the child has sight on admission, use this opportunity to point out significant aspects of the room and to have the child practice ambulating with the eyes closed (pp. 927-933).
38. b (p. 933)
39. a (p. 934)
40. b (p. 934)
41. b (p. 936; Box 24-11)
42. c (pp. 935-936)
43. a (pp. 935-936)
44. d (pp. 938-939; Box 24-12)

45. c (pp. 939-940)
46. b (pp. 935-936)
47. A situated approach shifts the emphasis from correcting the disabilities to supporting those with disabilities so that they can achieve more (p. 936).
48. c (p. 942)
49. c (p. 942)
50. a (p. 942)
51. d (p. 942; Appendix B: Denver Developmental Screening Test)
52. d (pp. 917-922)
53. b (p. 920)
54. c (pp. 916, 935)

CHAPTER 25

1. j (p. 954), i (p. 952), g (p. 951), a (p. 946), c (p. 948), h (p. 952), b (pp. 946-947), d (p. 947), f (p. 951), e (p. 950)
2. Possible responses: Advances in medical technology, parents' desire, cost considerations, improving quality of life, cost of care, and recognition of families' valuable contributions (p. 947)
3. c (pp. 948-949; Box 25-1)
4. c (pp. 947-948)
5. d (p. 948)
6. b (p. 959)
7. The child's medical, nursing, education, and other therapeutic needs; family members' (including siblings') education and training, coping skills, and adjustment needs; community readiness in areas such as availability of equipment, appropriate nursing and other personnel, education and developmental services, respite care, and emergency plans; financial arrangements (pp. 941, 950; Box 25-4)
8. Fully trained pediatric staff; 24-hour availability; family-centered care; continuing education; certification; accreditation such as by The Joint Commission or Community Health Accreditation Program (p. 949; Box 25-3)
9. c (pp. 949-950)
10. d (p. 951)
11. d (p. 951)
12. Facilitate timely access to services, promote continuity of care, enhance family well-being, reduce complexity of care for the child, reduce fragmentation of care, prevent duplication of services, decrease burden of care for the family, improve outcomes, maximize use of resources (p. 951)
13. a (p. 952)
14. b (p. 952)
15. c (pp. 954, 956)
16. Possible responses: Encouraging activities to develop self-confidence and self-esteem; displaying increased awareness of and respect for family caregivers; recognizing that families vary in defining their role; demonstrating an ability to understand the family's approach to caregiving; sharing perspectives, not just tasks and functions; supporting family in their primary, irreplaceable role as caregiver; exchanging expertise in providing care to the child; assisting family in recognizing their contributions as worthwhile; identifying strengths and resources of child and family; negotiating options, priorities, and preferences; assisting with coping by allowing family to find meaning in caring for child at home; communicating with the family (pp. 954-955)
17. c (p. 955)
18. c (p. 955)
19. c (p. 955)
20. d (pp. 951, 957)
21. d (p. 955)
22. b (p. 958)
23. Possible answers: Respect the family's choices even when the nurse's approach is different from the family's. Parental preferences should be respected unless risk or harm is posed to the child or the written medical orders are not followed. Negotiate changes in written orders. Communicate honestly and respectfully. Document carefully. Use agency policy as a guide. Contact the case manager or nursing supervisor to help negotiate (p. 955).
24. b (p. 958)
25. c (pp. 958-959)
26. c (p. 959)
27. b (p. 960)
28. a (p. 960)
29. c (pp. 956, 962)
30. b (p. 957)
31. c (p. 957)

CHAPTER 26

1. k (p. 977), j (p. 974), i (p. 973), h (p. 973), g (p. 983), f (p. 981), e (p. 966), d (p. 966), c (p. 966), b (p. 965), a (p. 986)
2. b (p. 981), d (p. 994), a (p. 981), c (p. 979; Box 26-5)
3. b (p. 965)
4. b, c, a (pp. 965-966; Box 26-1)
5. b (p. 971)
6. a (p. 972)
7. b (p. 966)
8. c (p. 969; Table 26-1)
9. c (pp. 969-970; Fig. 26-3)
10. d (p. 971)
11. d (p. 972)
12. a (p. 972)
13. Possible answers: Opportunities to master stress and feel competent in their coping abilities; new socialization experiences; broadened interpersonal relationships (pp. 972-973)
14. b (p. 972)
15. c (pp. 974-975)
16. Possible answers: Include family in care planning; observe for negative effects of continuous visiting by parents (encourage the parents to leave for brief periods; arrange for sleeping quarters on the unit but outside the child's room; plan a schedule of alternating visits with the other parent or with another family member); provide information; provide a therapeutic

presence; complement and augment the parents' caregiving responsibilities (pp. 975-976).

17. c (p. 975)
18. d (p. 976)
19. b (p. 977)
20. b (p. 978)
21. c (p. 978)
22. c (p. 978)
23. b (p. 978)
24. c (p. 978)
25. Possible answers: Provides diversion; brings about relaxation; helps child feel secure; helps lessen stress; provides a means for tension release; encourages interaction; helps develop positive attitudes; acts as an expressive outlet; provides a means for accomplishing therapeutic goals; places child in active role; gives more control and choices to the child (p. 979; Box 26-6)
26. a (p. 980)
27. Possible answers: Allows for creative expression; allows nurse to assess adjustment and coping; serves as a springboard for discussion; provides distraction, diversion (p. 981)
28. c (p. 982)
29. d (p. 984)
30. The child life specialist is a health care professional with extensive knowledge of child growth and development and the special psychosocial needs of children who are hospitalized and their families. These professionals help prepare children for hospitalization, surgery, and procedures. It is a collaborative role that is designed to help ensure the best possible hospital experience for the child and family (pp. 978-979; Box 26-5).
31. d (p. 986)
32. Possible answers: Encourage parents to stay with their child. Provide information about child's condition in understandable language. Establish a routine that maintains some similarity to daily events in child's life whenever possible. Schedule undisturbed times. Reduce stimulation (p. 987).
33. d (p. 988; Box 26-7)
34. c (p. 988; Box 26-7)
35. c (p. 991)
36. d (pp. 990-991)
37. d (p. 991)
38. c (p. 991)
39. The process involves evaluating children's thoughts regarding admission and related procedures. It is similar to precounseling techniques; however, instead of supplying information, the nurse listens to the child's explanations. Projective techniques such as drawing, doll play, or storytelling are especially effective. The nurse then bases additional teaching on what has already been learned (p. 992).
40. a (p. 993)
41. c (p. 994)
42. d (p. 994)
43. a (pp. 984-986)
44. d (pp. 984-986)
45. d (pp. 984-986)
46. a (pp. 984-986)

CHAPTER 27

1. i (p. 1010), c (p. 999), b (p. 1000), a (p. 1000), h (p. 1010), g (p. 1010), f (p. 1010), e (p. 1009)
2. m (p. 1011), h (p. 1015), j (p. 1016), k (p. 1016), a (p. 1010), e (p. 1011), b (p. 1011), d (p. 1011), c (p. 1011), i (p. 1015), l (p. 1016), f (pp. 1011, 1013), g (pp. 1015-1017)
3. l (p. 1031), e (pp. 1019-1020; Box 27-3), f (pp. 1019-1020; Box 27-3), b (pp. 1019-1020; Box 27-3), i (p. 1026), a (p. 1019), g (p. 1020), c (pp. 1019, 1050), h (p. 1020), j (p. 1028), m (p. 1031), k (p. 1030), d (pp. 1019-1020; Box 27-3)
4. j (pp. 1044, 1046), e (pp. 1037-1038), a (p. 1031), h (pp. 1039, 1041), g (p. 1041), b (p. 1032), k (p. 1049), c (p. 1037), f (pp. 1039, 1042-1044), d (p. 1037), i (p. 1041)
5. d (pp. 999-1000)
6. a (p. 1000)
7. c (p. 1000)
8. d (p. 1000)
9. b (p. 1001)
10. c (p. 1003)
11. a (p. 1002)
12. b (p. 1004)
13. d (p. 1004)
14. Possible answers: Expect success. Have extra supplies handy. Involve the child. Provide distraction. Allow expression of feelings. Provide positive reinforcement. Use play in preparation and postprocedure (pp. 1004-1005).
15. Examples of appropriate responses:
    a. Ambulation: Give a toddler a push-pull toy.
    b. Range-of-motion exercises: Touch or kick balloons.
    c. Injections: Make creative objects out of syringes.
    d. Deep breathing: Practice band instruments.
    e. Extending the environment: Move the patient's bed to the playroom.
    f. Soaks: Put marbles or coins at the bottom of bath container.
    g. Fluid intake: Make freezer pops using the child's favorite juice (pp. 1005-1006; Box 27-1).
16. b (p. 1006)
17. c (p. 1005)
18. a (p. 1007; Table 27-1)
19. b (p. 1007)
20. c (p. 1008)
21. c (pp. 1007-1008)
22. d (p. 1008)
23. c (p. 1009)
24. c (p. 1010)
25. c (p. 1010)
26. c (p. 1011)
27. a (pp. 1012-1013; Box 27-4)
28. b (p. 1011)
29. c (p. 1014)
30. a (p. 1014)
31. a (p. 1014)
32. a (p. 1015)
33. a (p. 1016)

34. d (p. 1016)
35. a (pp. 1016, 1017)
36. c (p. 1016; Box 27-3)
37. d (p. 1019)
38. d (p. 1020)
39. Possible answers: Horizontal position with the back supported and the thigh grasped firmly by the carrying arm; the football hold; the upright position with the buttocks on the nurse's forearm and the front of the body resting against the nurse's chest; transport in their crib, on a stretcher, wheelchair with a safety belt, wagon with raised sides, or stretcher with high sides up and safety belt in place (p. 1021; Fig. 27-5)
40. Possible answers: Remove and reapply restraints periodically. Secure restraints to the frame—not the side rails—of the bed or crib. Leave one fingerbreadth between skin and the device. Tie quick-release knots. Ensure that the restraint does not tighten as the child moves (pp. 1021-1022; Fig. 27-6).
41. b (pp. 1022-1023; Table 27-5; Fig. 27-9)
42. d (p. 1024; Fig. 27-11)
43. c (p. 1024; Fig. 27-12, *A*)
44. d (p. 1025)
45. a (p. 1025)
46. b (p. 1025)
47. b (p. 1028)
48. b (p. 1028)
49. a (p. 1030)
50. c (p. 1031)
51. b (p. 1030)
52. d (p. 1031)
53. a (pp. 1031-1032)
54. d (p. 1033)
55. b (pp. 1033-1034; Fig. 27-16)
56. a (p. 1034)
57. c (pp. 1035-1036; Table 27-7)
58. d (p. 1038)
59. a (p. 1038)
60. d (p. 1039)
61. a (p. 1039)
62. b (pp. 1039-1040)
63. c (p. 1041)
64. b (p. 1042)
65. c (p. 1048)
66. a (p. 1049)
67. b (pp. 1005-1007)
68. b (pp. 1005-1007)
69. a (p. 1002)
70. d (p. 1009)

CHAPTER 28

1. c (pp. 1052-1053), b (p. 1052), a (p. 1052), t (p. 1077), u (p. 1077), f (p. 1055; Box 28-1), g (p. 1055; Box 28-1), d (p. 1055; Box 28-1), e (pp. 1057-1058), k (p. 1053), l (p. 1053), m (p. 1063), p (p. 1061), i (p. 1053), n (p. 1063), j (p. 1053), o (p. 1063), h (p. 1053), s (p. 1064), r (p. 1064), q (p. 1064)

2. d (p. 1053)
3. a (p. 1053)
4. d (pp. 1053-1054)
5. b (p. 1055)
6. Isotonic (pp. 1058-1059)
7. Hypotonic, less (p. 1059)
8. Hypertonic, loss, intake, more (p. 1059)
9. b (p. 1059)
10. c (p. 1059; Tables 28-3 and 28-4)
11. c (p. 1060)
12. d (p. 1061)
13. c (p. 1062)
14. c (p. 1062)
15. b (p. 1062)
16. Anasarca (p. 1062)
17. b (p. 1063)
18. c (p. 1063; Fig. 28-4)
19. d (p. 1067), c (p. 1066), a (pp. 1065-1066), b (p. 1066; Box 28-4)
20. b (p. 1065; Table 28-7)
21. a (p. 1068)
22. 1 g wet diaper weight equals 1 ml urine (p. 1068).
23. b (p. 1058; Table 28-2)
24. d (pp. 1067-1068)
25. Oral rehydration solution (containing 75 to 90 mmol sodium and 111 to 139 mmol glucose; Pedialyte RS, Rehydralyte) for the first 4 to 6 hours; if this is tolerated, then fluids (containing 30 to 60 mmol sodium and 111 to 139 mmol glucose; Pedialyte, Lytren, Resol, or Infalyte) for the next 18 to 24 hours at 1 to 2 oz/lb divided into frequent feedings (p. 1069)
26. a (p. 1069)
27. a (pp. 1069-1070)
28. c (pp. 1070, 1072)
29. F (p. 1070), T (p. 1070), T (p. 1070), T (p. 1070), F (p. 1071), F (p. 1071), T (p. 1070), T (p. 1071), F (p. 1082), F (pp. 1071, 1077), T (p. 1075), F (p. 1077), T (p. 1078), T (p. 1077), T (p. 1071), F (p. 1077)
30. Infusions of systemic fluids with a large-bore needle inserted into the medullary cavity of a long bone that provides a safe and rapid alternate route for administration of fluids; used when systemic access is vital and venous access cannot be obtained quickly (p. 1072)
31. b (p. 1072)
32. c (p. 1073)
33. a (pp. 1073-1074)
34. d (pp. 1074-1075)
35. c (pp. 1073, 1075)
36. a (pp. 1076-1077)
37. Date and time of insertion; manufacturer, gauge, and length of catheter; site of insertions; number of attempts; if any blood samples were drawn and sent to laboratory; how the IV catheter was secured and what junction securement devices (Luer-Lok) were used; appearance of the site after insertion and fluid infusing; what flushing solution was used

and amount; what IV solution was used and amount in bag when started; how the patient tolerated the procedure; the name of the nurse starting the IV and completing documentation (p. 1076; Box 28-8)

38. Date and time of fluid initiation; type of IV solution used and the amount in the bag; type of delivery system used (e.g., Baxter Pump) and the rate of infusion; any additives (type and dose) in the solution (p. 1076; Box 28-8)

39. Reason for discontinuing IV (fluid completed and physician orders to stop after completion); confirmation that the IV device was not damaged when inspected after removal; appearance of site; type of dressing applied; patient tolerance of procedure (p. 1076; Box 28-8)

40. b (p. 1077; Nursing Care Guidelines box)

41. The three types of phlebitis are (1) mechanical, caused by rapid infusion rate or manipulation of the IV; (2) chemical, caused by medications such as naficillin; and (3) bacterial, caused by staphylococcal infection. The initial sign of phlebitis is erythema or redness at the insertion site; pain may not be present (p. 1077).

42. b (pp. 1077-1078; Community Focus box)

43. a. IV tubing and solution administration set is changed every 72 hours or per hospital policy (pp. 1077-1078).
    b. The Centers for Disease Control and Prevention guidelines recommend lipid-containing parenteral nutrition fluids be changed after 24 hours (p. 1078).
    c. The Centers for Disease Control and Prevention guidelines recommend pure intralipid infusions be changed after 12 hours (p. 1078).

44. d, c, b, a, c, d (pp. 1078, 1080-1081)

45. The turbulent-flow flush is successful in preventing clot formation. This is accomplished by forward flushing motion on the syringe with a flush-stop-flush-stop technique. This creates a swirling and vigorous fluid movement that clears the catheter better than the continuous flush motion. This technique is combined with the positive pressure technique, which includes holding the syringe stopped down once the flush is completed, and clamping the catheter and then removing the syringe. This prevents the blood from backing into the tip of the catheter (p. 1078).

46. Using maximum barrier techniques during insertion, practicing good hand washing, performing skin antisepsis with 2% chlorhexidine, using antimicrobial-impregnated catheter, promptly removing catheters when they are not in use (p. 1082)

47. d (p. 1082)

48. b (p. 1081; Nursing Care Guidelines box)

49. c (p. 1084)

50. b (p. 1084; Nursing Alert)

51. d (pp. 1084-1085)

52. c (p. 1085)

53. a (p. 1085)

54. b (p. 1085)

55. Parents' ability to perform the procedure and adapt to the changes within the home; psychosocial readiness of the family and existence of family support system; availability of a pharmacy that can prepare the solution; a practitioner to handle day-to-day emergency needs; insurance coverage (pp. 1085-1086)

56. c (pp. 1058-1059)

57. c (pp. 1066-1067)

58. d (p. 1068)

59. d (p. 1068)

60. c (p. 1061)

61. c (p. 1061)

62. a (pp. 1063-1064, 1067)

63. c (p. 1071)

CHAPTER 29

1. c (pp. 1090-1092; Box 29-2)

2. b (p. 1090)

3. Intractable diarrhea of infancy (p. 1090)

4. c (p. 1090; Box 29-2)

5. a (p. 1090)

6. T (p. 1093), T (p. 1090; Box 29-2), T (p. 1090), F (p. 1090; Box 29-2), F (p. 1093), T (p. 1090), T (p. 1095; Box 29-2)

7. d (pp. 1090, 1093)

8. b (p. 1093)

9. a. *Clostridium difficile* (p. 1093)
   b. Bacterial gastroenteritis or inflammatory bowel disease (p. 1094)
   c. Glucose intolerance (p. 1094)
   d. Fat malabsorption (p. 1094)
   e. Parasitic infection or protein intolerance (p. 1094)

10. a (p. 1094)

11. Assessment of fluid and electrolyte imbalance; rehydration; maintenance fluid therapy; reintroduction of adequate diet (p. 1094)

12. a (pp. 1094-1095; Box 29-5; Table 29-3)

13. d (p. 1095)

14. d (p. 1095)

15. c (p. 1097)

16. c (pp. 1097-1098)

17. d (p. 1098)

18. d (p. 1099)

19. a. Hypovolemic (p. 1100)
    b. Cardiogenic (p. 1100)
    c. Vasogenic (p. 1100)
    d. Anaphylactic (p. 1101)
    e. Septic (p. 1101)
    f. Neurogenic (p. 1101)

20. g (p. 1103), e (p. 1103), f (p. 1103), b (p. 1102), i (p. 1103), d (p. 1103), h (p. 1103), a (p. 1102), j (p. 1103), c (p. 1102)

21. b (p. 1102)

22. c (p. 1103)

23. Ventilation, fluid administration, improvement of the pumping action of the heart (vasopressor support) (p. 1104; Emergency Treatment box)

24. c, a, b (p. 1105)

25. a (p. 1107)
26. d (p. 1108)
27. Wash hands before inserting the tampon; do not use a soiled or dropped tampon; insert carefully to avoid vaginal abrasion; alternate use with sanitary napkins (e.g., use tampons during the day and sanitary napkins during the night); do not use superabsorbent tampons; do not leave tampon in the body longer than 4 to 6 hours; remove the tampon immediately with development of sudden fever, rash, vomiting, diarrhea, muscle pain, dizziness, or feeling of near-fainting (p. 1109).
28. Extreme heat sources, exposure to cold, electricity; chemicals, radiation (p. 1109)
29. Scald, contact (p. 1109)
30. All statements are true (pp. 1109-1110, 1112).
31. a (p. 1110)
32. b (p. 1111; Fig. 29-2)
33. d (p. 1112)
34. a (p. 1111)
35. c (p. 1112)
36. c (p. 1114)
37. b (p. 1114)
38. d (p. 1114)
39. b (p. 1114)
40. d (p. 1115)
41. Airway compromise, shock, infection (p. 1115)
42. b (pp. 1114-1115)
43. a (p. 1116)
44. b (p. 1116)
45. c (p. 1117)
46. c (p. 1118)
47. b (p. 1119)
48. a (p. 1119)
49. a (p. 1127)
50. a (p. 1121)
51. b (p. 1121)
52. b (p. 1123)
53. d (p. 1122)
54. d (p. 1131)
55. b (p. 1112)
56. a (p. 1115)
57. b (pp. 1113-1114, 1120)
58. c (p. 1128)
59. d (pp. 1116, 1124)
60. c (p. 1131)
61. The history provides valuable information about the duration, severity, associated symptoms, and potential cause of the diarrhea. Has the patient been exposed to infectious agents, traveled to an area of high susceptibility, been introduced to new foods, had contact with foods that may be contaminated, or been exposed to animals or birds? What drugs is the child currently taking? Any possible ingestions? Family history of recent illness? Specific questions include the onset and duration of diarrhea, presence of fever and other symptoms, frequency and character of the stools, urinary output, vomiting, and recent intake of food and fluids (p. 1093).

CHAPTER 30

1. F (p. 1135), T (p. 1136), T (p. 1136), F (p. 1136), F (p. 1137), T (p. 1137), T (p. 1137), T (p. 1137), T (p. 1137), T (p. 1137), T (p. 1138), T (p. 1144), T (p. 1144), F (p. 1145), F (p. 1142; Box 30-2)
2. Anatomic integrity of the lower urinary tract, detrusor control, and competence of the urethral sphincter mechanism (p. 1139)
3. A, N, A, A, N, N, A (p. 1141; Table 30-1)
4. c (p. 1138), f (p. 1143; Box 30-2), h (p. 1143; Box 30-2), j (p. 1149), k (pp. 1152, 1156, 1163), b (p. 1138), d (p. 1139), i (p. 1143; Box 30-2), e (p. 1140), g (p. 1143; Box 30-2), a (p. 1143; Box 30-2), m (p. 1163), l (p. 1167), o (p. 1172), n (p. 1172), p (p. 1172), q (p. 1156)
5. a (p. 1143; Table 30-2)
6. d (p. 1143; Table 30-2)
7. a (p. 1140)
8. d (p. 1144)
9. d (p. 1145)
10. b (p. 1145)
11. a. Eliminate the current infection.
    b. Identify contributing factors to reduce the risk for recurrence.
    c. Prevent systemic spread of the infection.
    d. Preserve renal function (p. 1147).
12. a (p. 1145)
13. d (pp. 1145-1146)
14. d (p. 1147)
15. a (p. 1147; Table 30-4)
16. b (p. 1148)
17. c (p. 1149)
18. During cystoscopy a gel-like bulking agent is injected into the mucous membrane where the affected ureter enters the bladder. This results in elongation of the tunnel and passive closure of the ureteral orifice, making the retrograde flow of bladder urine more difficult. It eliminates the need for daily antibiotics and requires no incision. It can be performed as an outpatient procedure requiring only brief anesthetic (pp. 1149-1150).
19. b (pp. 1150-1151)
20. b (p. 1151)
21. Hypertensive encephalopathy, acute cardiac decompensation, acute renal failure (p. 1152)
22. b (p. 1153)
23. a (p. 1154)
24. b (p. 1154)
25. a (p. 1154)
26. a (p. 1154)
27. c (pp. 1156, 1158)
28. c (p. 1156)
29. a (p. 1157)
30. c (p. 1157)
31. F (p. 1159), F (p. 1159), F (p. 1159), T (p. 1159), T (p. 1159), T (p. 1160), F (p. 1160), T (p. 1160), T (p. 1161), F (pp. 1161-1162)
32. c (p. 1160)
33. a (p. 1161)

34. a (p. 1162)
35. c (p. 1163)
36. b (pp. 1163-1164)
37. a (pp. 1164-1165; Table 30-7)
38. c (p. 1165)
39. Monitoring and assessing fluid and electrolyte balance (p. 1166)
40. b (pp. 1168, 1170)
41. b (p. 1169)
42. c (p. 1170)
43. c (pp. 1168-1169)
44. a. Hemodialysis; peritoneal dialysis; hemofiltration (p. 1172)
    b. Hemodialysis (p. 1173)
    c. Protein loss (p. 1173)
    d. Hemodialysis (p. 1173)
    e. Peritonitis (p. 1175)
    f. Growth rate, skeletal maturation, normal growth (p. 1173)
    g. Fluid overload, surgical procedures (p. 1176)
45. b (p. 1173)
46. a (p. 1177)
47. d (p. 1177)
48. b (pp. 1154-1156)
49. d (pp. 1156-1157)
50. c (p. 1157)
51. d (pp. 1157-1158)
52. Teach the family to recognize signs of relapse and to bring the child for treatment at the earliest indications of relapse; provide instruction about testing urine for albumin, administration of medications, side effects of medications, and prevention of infection; emphasize the importance of restricting salt (e.g., no additional salt during relapse and steroid therapy), followed by a regular diet for the child in remission (p. 1158).
53. Teach the family and Darlene about the disease, its implications, and the therapeutic plan; the possible psychologic effects of the disease and the treatment; the technical aspects of the procedure, including possible complications and changes to observe for. (p. 1175).
54. Provide dietary instructions for foods that reduce excretory demands on kidneys and provide sufficient calories and protein for growth. Encourage intake of carbohydrates to provide calories for growth and foods high in calcium to prevent bone demineralization. Recommend foods that are rich in folic acid and iron because anemia is a complication of chronic renal failure. Limit phosphorus, salt, and potassium as needed and prescribed. Teach parents and Darlene how to read food labels carefully for content and to modify meals. Arrange for renal dietitian to meet with Darlene and her family to help them understand dietary needs and to assist Darlene in independent formulation of dietary allowances when she is away from home (pp. 1169-1171).
55. Serum creatinine is the best predictor of renal function because the BUN can be elevated from dehydration, hemorrhage, high protein intake, and corticosteroid therapy. The serum creatinine is an indicator of the end product of protein metabolism in muscle and is thus a more stable and better indicator of renal function (pp. 1143, 1167; Table 30-3).

CHAPTER 31

1. g (p. 1182), b (p. 1182), i (p. 1182), a (p. 1182), e (p. 1182), j (p. 1182), d (p. 1182), k (p. 1182), c (p. 1182), aa (p. 1184), l (p. 1183), t (p. 1183), m (p. 1183), x (p. 1183), u (p. 1183), n (p. 1183), h (p. 1182), w (p. 1182), v (p. 1183), o (p. 1183), f (p. 1182), y (p. 1182), p (p. 1183), q (p. 1183), z (p. 1184), r (p. 1183), s (p. 1183)
2. h (p. 1185), b (p. 1185), i (p. 1185), c (p. 1185), j (p. 1185), n (p. 1185), a (p. 1184), k (p. 1182), f (p. 1187), o (p. 1186), d (p. 1185), l (p. 1185), g (p. 1279), m (p. 1185), p (pp. 1186-1187), t (p. 1187), e (p. 1200), v (p. 1187), q (pp. 1187, 1193; Fig. 31-10), w (p. 1187), u (p. 1187), s (p. 1187), r (p. 1187)
3. f, a, e, g, d, b, h, c (p. 1187)
4. q, k, d, e, l, h, n, b, p, f, a, c, g, o, i, m, j (pp. 1188-1189)
5. g (p. 1194), c (p. 1194), a (p. 1191), e (p. 1193), f (p. 1194), b (p. 1192), d (pp. 1192, 1193)
6. c (p. 1195; Table 31-5), e (p. 1195; Table 31-5), a (p. 1195), g (p. 1196), i (p. 1197), f (p. 1196), h (pp. 1196-1197), u (p. 1207), j (p. 1197), n (p. 1198), q (p. 1199), t (p. 1201), m (p. 1198), k (p. 1197), o (p. 1199), s (p. 1200), p (p. 1199), l (p. 1198), b (p. 1195; Table 31-5), r (p. 1200), d (p. 1195; Table 31-5)
7. e (p. 1208), b (p. 1208), f (p. 1208), h (p. 1208), d (p. 1208), i (p. 1208), a (p. 1208), j (p. 1208), l (pp. 1208-1209), c (pp. 1208-1209), m (p. 1209), r (p. 1215), g (p. 1208), q (pp. 1215-1216), o (p. 1213), s (p. 1216), n (p. 1214), k (p. 1208), p (p. 1213)
8. b (p. 1183)
9. a (p. 1182)
10. c (p. 1182)
11. b (p. 1182)
12. c (p. 1183)
13. Fewer number of alveoli, smaller size of the alveoli, more shallow air sacks, decreased surface area for gas exchange (p. 1184)
14. d (p. 1184)
15. b (p. 1185)
16. a (p. 1185)
17. c (p. 1185)
18. b (p. 1186)
19. d (p. 1186)
20. a (p. 1188)
21. c (p. 1189)
22. Capacity is the combination of two or more lung volumes. This includes inspiratory capacity (IC), functional residual capacity (FRC), and vital capacity (VC) (p. 1191; Fig. 31-8).
23. b, c, a, c, b, a (p. 1190; Table 31-1)

24. b, f, a, e, d, c (pp. 1191-1192; Table 31-2)
25. c (pp. 1191-1192)
26. b (p. 1194)
27. a (p. 1192; Table 31-4)
28. b (p. 1195; Table 31-5)
29. c (p. 1195; Table 31-5)
30. b (p. 1195; Table 31-5)
31. c (p. 1196)
32. b (p. 1197)
33. a (p. 1197)
34. d (p. 1198)
35. c (p. 1199)
36. c (p. 1198)
37. c (p. 1199)
38. b (p. 1199)
39. b (p. 1201)
40. d (p. 1202)
41. c (p. 1204)
42. a (p. 1204)
43. b (p. 1204)
44. c (p. 1205)
45. b (p. 1205)
46. Possible answers: Avoid toys, blankets, clothing, and pets that shed fine hair or lint. Avoid aerosols, powder, dust, and smoke. Eliminate toys with small removable parts. Clothing should have loose-fitting collars that do not cover the tracheostomy tube opening. When the child is outside, the artificial nose or a thin cloth is used to prevent cold air, dust, dirt, or sand from entering the tube. Bathe the child in a tub filled with shallow water; no water or soap should enter the tube (pp. 1206-1207).
47. a (pp. 1207-1208)
48. Possible responses: Obstructive lung disease—tracheomalacia; choanal atresia; vocal paralysis; meconium aspiration; aspiration of a foreign body, mucus, or vomitus; epiglottitis; pneumonia; pertussis; severe tonsillitis; tumors; anaphylaxis; laryngospasm

    Restrictive lung disease—respiratory distress syndrome, cystic fibrosis, pneumothorax, pulmonary edema, pleural effusion and abdominal distention, muscular dystrophy, paralytic conditions

    Respiratory center depression—cerebral trauma at birth, intracranial tumors, central nervous system infection, drug overdose (p. 1208)
49. d (p. 1208; Box 31-8)
50. b (pp. 1211-1210)
51. c (p. 1210)
52. b (p. 1210)
53. a (p. 1196)
54. a (p. 1214)
55. c (p. 1215)
56. i, h, c, b, e, f, g, d, a (p. 1216; Table 31-6)
57. d (pp. 1216-1217b)
58. b (p. 1189)
59. c (p. 1189)
60. a (p. 1208; Box 31-8)
61. d (pp. 1198-1199)

CHAPTER 32

1. d (p. 1226), i (p. 1228), e (p. 1226), m (p. 1228), g (p. 1228), b (p. 1241), h (p. 1228), p (p. 1230), a (p. 1220), l (p. 1228), f (p. 1228), q (p. 1231), n (p. 1230), c (p. 1230), j (p. 1228), r (p. 1231), o (p. 1230), k (p. 1228)
2. j (p. 1234), o (p. 1234), b (p. 1233; Box 32-4), k (p. 1234), n (p. 1234), a (p. 1233; Box 32-4), g (p. 1234), l (p. 1234), e (p. 1234), i (p. 1234), m (p. 1234), h (p. 1234), f (p. 1233), p (p. 1234), c (p. 1233; Box 32-4), d (p. 1237)
3. o (p. 1251), d (p. 1242), p (p. 1251), u (p. 1244; Box 32-8), b (p. 1238; Table 32-1), g (p. 1246), a (p. 1221), q (p. 1241), h (p. 1249), t (p. 1244; Box 32-7), e (p. 1243), v (p. 1242), l (p. 1250), i (p. 1249), n (p. 1251), s (p. 1244; Box 32-7), f (p. 1243), c (pp. 1239-1240), r (p. 1244), j (p. 1249), m (p. 1250), k (p. 1250)
4. c (p. 1259), b (p. 1259), e (p. 1260), d (p. 1260), a (pp. 1255-1256)
5. o (p. 1271), f (p. 1243), i (pp. 1276-1277), a (p. 1261, j (p. 1269), c (pp. 1265, 1268; Box 32-7), k (p. 1280), e (p. 1269), b (pp. 1265, 1268; Box 32-10), h (pp. 1272, 1274-1279), l (p. 1282), q (p. 1284), p (p. 1284), g (p. 1272), n (pp. 1282, 1286), d (p. 1269), s (pp. 1285-1286), m (p. 1282), r (p. 1284), w (pp. 1269-1277), aa (p. 1281), t (p. 1266), x (p. 1271), u (pp. 1275-1277), z (p. 1281), v (pp. 1272, 1275-1279; Box 32-2), y (pp. 1272-1275), bb (p. 1283)
6. b (p. 1220)
7. c (p. 1220)
8. c (pp. 1221, 1248; Box 32-1)
9. c (p. 1222)
10. b (pp. 1278, 1287)
11. b (p. 1222)
12. a (p. 1225)
13. b (p. 1226)
14. c (p. 1226)
15. d (p. 1227)
16. b (p. 1228)
17. c (p. 1228)
18. c (p. 1229)
19. d (p. 1229)
20. c (p. 1229)
21. c (p. 1229)
22. a (p. 1229)
23. c (pp. 1230-1231)
24. c (p. 1230)
25. b (p. 1230)
26. a (p. 1232)
27. a (p. 1233; Box 32-5, Fig. 32-3)
28. Possible answers: Tympanic membrane retraction, tympanosclerosis, tympanic perforation, adhesive otitis media, chronic suppurative otitis media, labyrinthitis, mastoiditis, meningitis, cholesteatoma (pp. 1233-1234)
29. d (p. 1234)
30. c (p. 1234)
31. b (p. 1234)

32. a (p. 1235)
33. d (p. 1235)
34. b (p. 1235)
35. c (p. 1237)
36. c (pp. 1237-1241)
37. d (p. 1241)
38. c (pp. 1238-1239)
39. a (p. 1239)
40. b (p. 1239)
41. a (pp. 1237-1241)
42. a (pp. 1237-1241)
43. b (p. 1238)
44. d (p. 1237)
45. a (p. 1243)
46. c (p. 1239)
47. c, a, b (p. 1245; Box 32-8)
48. d (pp. 1246-1247)
49. Possible answers: Perform respiratory assessment, administer oxygen, administer antibiotics, institute isolation procedures, promote rest and conservation of energy, administer antitussives, administer fluids, use mist tent, prevent chilling, position the child comfortably, control fever, suction to maintain patent airway, promote postural drainage, involve the family (p. 1248)
50. c (p. 1248)
51. b (p. 1250)
52. d (p. 1252)
53. a (p. 1251; Box 32-13)
54. c (p. 1253)
55. c (p. 1254)
56. a (p. 1254)
57. c (pp. 1255-1256)
58. Possible answers: Treat infection (or the precipitating cause), maintenance of adequate cardiac output and vascular volume, hydration, adequate nutritional support, comfort measures, prevention of complications such as gastrointestinal ulceration and aspiration, and psychologic support. Prone positioning may be used to improve oxygenation, but studies have not demonstrated prone positioning to decrease the total number of days on mechanical ventilation; in addition, this requires close communication and coordination among the health care team (p. 1257).
59. c (pp. 1258-1259)
60. b (p. 1259)
61. Cotinine (p. 1260)
62. Possible answers: Allergic "shiners," obligatory mouth breathing, nasal crease, facial tics and mannerisms to avoid scratching the nose, open mouth caused by chronic nasal obstruction (allergic gape), extra wrinkles below the lower eyelids (Dennie lines) (pp. 1261-1262)
63. b (pp. 1261-1262)
64. c (p. 1264; Box 32-16)
65. c (pp. 1263-1276)
66. d (pp. 1263-1276)
67. b (pp. 1263-1276)
68. a (pp. 1263-1276)
69. b (pp. 1263-1276)
70. b (pp. 1263-1276)
71. d (pp. 1263-1276)
72. c (pp. 1263-1276)
73. c (pp. 1263-1276)
74. b (pp. 1263-1276)
75. c (pp. 1263-1276)
76. d (pp. 1263-1276)
77. b (pp. 1280-1289)
78. c (pp. 1280-1289)
79. d (pp. 1280-1289)
80. b (pp. 1280-1289)
81. a (pp. 1280-1289)
82. d (p. 1380)

CHAPTER 33

1. b (p. 1295; Box 33-1)
2. F, T, T, T, T, F (p. 1295)
3. a. Digestion, absorption, metabolism (p. 1295)
   b. Enzymes, hormones, hydrochloric acid, mucus, water, and electrolytes (p. 1296)
   c. Small intestine (p. 1296)
4. Measurement of intake and output, measurement of height, measurement of weight, abdominal examination, laboratory studies of urine and stool (p. 1298)
5. a (p. 1300; Table 33-1)
6. b (p. 1299; Table 33-1)
7. n (p. 1310), p (p. 1325), j (p. 1299; Table 33-1), f (p. 1299; Box 33-2), g (p. 1298; Box 33-2), h (p. 1298; Box 33-2), m (p. 1307), a (p. 1298), l (pp. 1298, 1303; Box 33-2), o (p. 1303), d (p. 1298; Box 33-2), e (p. 1298; Box 33-2), b (p. 1298; Box 33-2), i (p. 1298; Box 33-2), k (p. 1299; Table 33-1), c (p. 1298; Box 33-2)
8. b (pp. 1298, 1301)
9. d (p. 1301)
10. "Although the blood test does determine whether you have antibodies to the *H. pylori* germ, it does not tell whether you still have it or whether it is an old infection. Looking into your stomach allows your doctor to actually view your stomach for signs of change from the disease and allows for biopsy of your stomach to determine whether the germ is still present and active in your stomach" (p. 1299; Table 33-1).
11. b (p. 1303)
12. b (p. 1304)
13. d (p. 1304)
14. b (p. 1304)
15. d (p. 1305)
16. c (p. 1306)
17. d (p. 1305; Box 33-5)
18. Absence of ganglion cells in the affected areas of the intestine produces a loss of the rectosphincteric reflex and an abnormal microenvironment of the cells of the affected intestine. The absence of the ganglion cells results in a lack of enteric nervous system stimulation, which decreases the ability of the internal sphincter to relax and increases intestinal tone and decreases peristalsis (p. 1305).

19. b (p. 1306)
20. d (p. 1307)
21. b (p. 1307)
22. b (p. 1309)
23. b (p. 1309)
24. a (p. 1309)
25. Periumbilical pain, followed by nausea, right-sided lower quadrant pain, and then later vomiting with fever (p. 1310)
26. d (pp. 1310-1311)
27. a. McBurney point (p. 1310)
    b. Midway between the right anterosuperior iliac crest and the umbilicus (p. 1310)
    c. Rebound tenderness (p. 1310)
28. c (p. 1314; Box 33-8)
29. a (p. 1315)
30. In CD the chronic inflammatory process may involve any part of the GI tract, from the mouth to the anus, but most commonly affects the terminal ileum. It can affect segments of the intestine with intact mucosa in between. CD involves all layers of the wall. The inflammation may result in ulcerations, fibrosis, adhesions, stiffening of the bowel wall, and obstruction. In UC the inflammation is limited to the colon and rectum, with the distal colon and rectum often the most severely affected. UC involves the mucosa and submucosa; it also involves continuous segments with varying degrees of ulceration, bleeding, and edema. Long-standing UC can cause shortening of the colon and strictures (p. 1315).
31. c (p. 1316)
32. c (p. 1317)
33. b (pp. 1317-1318)
34. a (pp. 1319-1320)
35. c (p. 1319)
36. c (p. 1319)
37. (1) Bismuth, clarithromycin, and metronidazole; (2) lansoprazole, amoxicillin, and clarithromycin; (3) metronidazole, clarithromycin, and omeprazole (p. 1321)
38. b (pp. 1320-1321)
39. d (p. 1321)
40. b (p. 1322)
41. d (p. 1323)
42. c (p. 1323)
43. a (p. 1324)
44. a (p. 1324; Box 33-12)
45. a (p. 1325).
46. c (p. 1325)
47. Malrotation, volvulus (p. 1325)
48. a (p. 1325)
49. c (p. 1326)
50. d (p. 1327)
51. a (p. 1330)
52. a (p. 1330; Table 33-3), a (p. 1330; Table 33-3), e (p. 1332), a (p. 1330; Table 33-3), d (p. 1332), c (p. 1330), b (p. 1332), b (p. 1334), f (p. 1332)
53. a (p. 1333)

54. a (p. 1333)
55. c (p. 1334)
56. Early detection, support and monitoring of the disease, recognition of chronic liver disease, and prevention of spread of the disease (p. 1333)
57. c (p. 1335)
58. c (p. 1335)
59. Questions about the patient's pain: When did the pain start? Has it been constant or intermittent? What were you doing when the pain started? Where did the pain start, and does the pain radiate or move to other areas? How would you describe the pain intensity and quality? What makes the pain better? What makes it worse? How have you tried to treat the pain? Has there been change in normal activities because of the pain?
    Questions about related symptoms or review of associated symptoms: Is there nausea or vomiting? If there is, did it start before or after the pain? Is there diarrhea or constipation? How would you describe your last stool? When did it occur? Are there urinary tract signs and symptoms such as frequency, difficulty with flow, burning? Is there fever? If so, how much fever? How long has the fever been present? Have you taken medications for the fever? If so, when was the last dose taken? Is there hunger or lack of hunger?
    Questions about the reproductive system: For females—When was your last menstrual period? For males and females—Are you sexually active? Do you have any genital discharge? (pp. 1310-1311; Box 33-7)
60. b (p. 1311; Nursing Alert)
61. d (p. 1312)
62. A white blood cell count with a differential elevated greater than $10,000/mm^3$, with an elevated number of bands indicating a shift to the left; C-reactive protein elevation that rises within 12 hours of the onset of infection (p. 1311)
63. a (pp. 1312-1314)
64. a (pp. 1312-1314; Nursing Care Plan)
65. Nursing assessment would include the history of normal bowel habits for Jose, including the consistency, color, frequency, and any pain or bleeding noted with previous bowel movements. How long has the mother noted Jose to be constipated? Is this the first episode, or has he had other episodes? If he has had other episodes, how long did they last? What was his age at onset? Does he have any tendency toward withholding behaviors? Does he not want to stop and go to the bathroom, or does he usually have a regular time that he goes to the bathroom? Is he toilet-trained, or is he still soiling himself? What is his diet like? How much fluid does he drink and what kinds? Did his diet and activities change while the family was up north working? Did they change when he came back home? Is Jose taking any medications? Is he taking over-the-counter vitamins with iron for children? (p. 1304)

66. a. The major task is to educate the parents regarding normal bowel patterns and to participate in the education and treatment of the child (p. 1304).

   b. Explain that sometimes constipation is due to environmental changes, stresses, and changes in toileting patterns. Sometimes children do not like to interrupt play to go to the bathroom, or sometimes previously passing a stool that caused pain may trigger stool-withholding. Sometimes adding more fiber and water to the diet can correct the problem. Review with Jose's mother foods high in fiber that are appropriate for Jose's age and amounts she should expect him to eat. Make sure to address the cultural factors and financial abilities of the family in stressing high-fiber foods. Stress the need for Jose's snacks to include more fresh fruits to expand fiber sources that also contain less sugar. Can bran be incorporated into cereals? Incorporate the use of beans found in Mexican dishes into soups or salads for Jose. Ask his mother to establish a time for Jose to go to the bathroom, preferably after a meal for about 5 to 10 minutes, that is unhurried and private and does not interrupt his playtime (pp. 1303-1304).

CHAPTER 34

1. p, h, m, j, f, d, b, k, a, l, e, i, c, n, o, g (p. 1341)
2. d (p. 1341), k (p. 1342), a (p. 1342), l (p. 1342), c (p. 1341), j (p. 1341), n (p. 1343), e (p. 1341), b (p. 1341), h (p. 1341), g (p. 1341), i (p. 1341), m (p. 1343), f (p. 1341)
3. j (p. 1344), e (p. 1344), o (p. 1344), m (p. 1344), a (p. 1344), l (p. 1345), d (p. 1344), q (p. 1344), g (p. 1344), b (p. 1344), i (p. 1344), c (p. 1344), f (p. 1344), p (p. 1344), k (p. 1344), r (p. 1344), h (p. 1344), n (p. 1344)
4. d, a, e, b, f, c (p. 1346; Fig. 34-4)
5. t, v, q, g, u, f, l, b, i, m, d, j, o, s, n, a, e, h, r, c, k, p (pp. 1345-1349; Table 34-1)
6. f (p. 1351), d (p. 1351), b (p. 1365), e (p. 1351), a (p. 1350), g (p. 1352), c (p. 1365)
7. h (p. 1352), c (p. 1352), l (p. 1354), a (p. 1352), f (p. 1353), m (p. 1354), g (p. 1353j), j (p. 1354), r (p. 1405), n (p. 1351), d (p. 1353), i (p. 1354), o (p. 1351), k (p. 1354), e (p. 1353), p (p. 1354), b (p. 1352), q (p. 1354)
8. g (p. 1355), f (p. 1356; Table 34-3), e (p. 1356; Table 34-3), b (p. 1354), d (p. 1356; Table 34-3), a (pp. 1344, 1354), c (p. 1393)
9. h (p. 1363), i (p. 1371), f (p. 1361), b (p. 1360), l (p. 1371), d (p. 1362), j (p. 1362), a (p. 1360), g (p. 1362; Fig. 34-9), k (p. 1362), e (p. 1401), c (p. 1360)
10. p (p. 1394), h (p. 1385), q (pp. 1394-1395), b (p. 1384), i (p. 1386), c (p. 1384), r (p. 1395; Box 34-13), k (p. 1392), d (p. 1384), v (p. 1395; Box 34-13), f (p. 1384), a (p. 1384), w (p. 1395; Box 34-13), n (p. 1394), g (p. 1384), s (p. 1395), j (p. 1395), e (p. 1384), t (p. 1395; Box 34-13), l (p. 1395), m (p. 1395), y (p. 1395), o (p. 1394), u (p. 1395; Box 34-13), x (p. 1395)
11. e (p. 1380), h (p. 1380), g (p. 1380), a (p. 1379), f (p. 1380), c (p. 1377), i (p. 1380), d (p. 1378), b (p. 1379)
12. g (p. 1400), o (p. 1404), c (p. 1400), d (p. 1399), j (p. 1399), k (p. 1400), e (p. 1399), h (p. 1400), l (p. 1400), f (p. 1399), a (p. 1399), i (p. 1400), m (p. 1400), n (p. 1404), b (p. 1400)
13. a (p. 1341)
14. a (p. 1341)
15. b (p. 1341)
16. c (p. 1342)
17. a (p. 1342)
18. b (p. 1345)
19. d (p. 1345)
20. a (p. 1345)
21. b (p. 1345)
22. c (p. 1347)
23. c (pp. 1347-1348)
24. b (p. 1348)
25. Possible answers: Pulses, especially below the catheterization site, for equality and symmetry (pulse distal to the site may be weaker for the first few hours after catheterization but should gradually increase in strength); temperature and color of the affected extremity, since coolness or blanching may indicate arterial obstruction; vital signs, which may be taken as frequently as every 15 minutes, with special emphasis on the heart rate, which is counted for 1 full minute for evidence of dysrhythmias or bradycardia; blood pressure, especially for hypotension, which may indicate hemorrhage from cardiac perforation or bleeding at the site of initial catheterization; dressing for evidence of bleeding or hematoma formation in the femoral or antecubital area; fluid intake, both intravenous and oral, to ensure adequate hydration (blood loss in the catheterization laboratory, the child's preprocedure NPO status, and diuretic actions of contrast material used during the procedure put the child at risk for hypovolemia and dehydration) (p. 1349)
26. d (p. 1349)
27. d (pp. 1351-1352)
28. c (p. 1400)
29. d (p. 1353)
30. b (p. 1354)
31. c (p. 1354)
32. a (p. 1357)
33. b (p. 1393)
34. c (p. 1359)
35. d (p. 1359)
36. c (p. 1359)
37. d (pp. 1361-1362)
38. b (p. 1362)
39. b (p. 1362)
40. a (p. 1365)
41. c, d, c, d, b, c, d, a, d, a, d, b, c, b, b (defects with increased pulmonary blood flow: pp. 1367-1368, Box 34-4; obstructive defects: pp. 1369-1370, Box 34-5; defects with decreased pulmonary blood flow: pp. 1371-1372, Box 36-6; mixed defects: pp. 1372-1373, Box 34-7)
42. c (pp. 1367, 1371-1372, 1374)

43. d (pp. 1367, 1371-1372, 1374)
44. b (pp. 1370-1375)
45. c (p. 1372; Box 34-7)
46. a (p. 1374)
47. c (p. 1375)
48. d (p. 1353)
49. Possible answers: Signs of congestive heart failure, activity restrictions and/or guidance, nutritional guidelines, medications (p. 1381)
50. c (p. 1377)
51. a (p. 1377)
52. a (p. 1377)
53. d (p. 1378)
54. d (p. 1378)
55. Possible answers: Tachypnea, bradycardia, laryngospasm, dysrhythmias, use of accessory muscles, skin color of the face, the child's tolerance of the procedure (p. 1378)
56. d (p. 1378)
57. a (p. 1378)
58. a (p. 1379)
59. b (p. 1379)
60. d (p. 1379)
61. d (p. 1379)
62. d (p. 1379)
63. d (p. 1379)
64. c (p. 1379)
65. Hematologic—hemolysis, clotting abnormalities, renal tubular necrosis, anemia, hemorrhage, fat emboli, thromboemboli, and infection
Cardiac—heart failure, low cardiac output syndrome, decreased peripheral perfusion, dysrhythmias, hypokalemia, and cardiac tamponade
Pulmonary—atelectasis, pneumothorax, pulmonary edema, and pleural effusion
Neurologic—cerebral edema, brain damage, and seizure activity
Other—bacterial endocarditis, postpericardiotomy syndrome (pp. 1380-1381)
66. c (p. 1381)
67. b (p. 1383)
68. a (p. 1383)
69. a (p. 1384)
70. d (p. 1385)
71. d (p. 1385)
72. b (p. 1386)
73. c (p. 1388)
74. a (pp. 1386-1387)
75. c (p. 1390)
76. b (p. 1390)
77. c (p. 1393)
78. d (p. 1393)
79. c (p. 1396)
80. b (p. 1396)
81. a (p. 1402)
82. a (p. 1404)
83. c (p. 1400)
84. c (pp. 1351-1364)
85. a (pp. 1351-1364)
86. d (pp. 1351-1364)

CHAPTER 35

1. F (p. 1410), F (p. 1415), F (p. 1412), T (p. 1412), T (p. 1410), T (p. 1410), T (p. 1410), F (p. 1410), T (p. 1415), F (pp. 1412-1414), T (p. 1415), F (p. 1415), T (p. 1413; Table 35-1), F (p. 1412), T (p. 1412), T (p. 1412), T (p. 1410), T (p. 1424)
2. c (pp. 1414, 1417; Fig. 35-2)
3. Inadequate production of RBCs or RBC components, increased destruction of RBCs, excessive loss of RBCs (p. 1416)
4. Decrease in the oxygen-carrying capacity of blood and consequently a reduction in the amount of oxygen available to the cells (p. 1416)
5. k (p. 1412), h (p. 1412), f (p. 1416; Box 35-1), j (p. 1412), l (p. 1415), i (p. 1415), o (p. 1412), p (p. 1412), q (pp. 1412, 1413), b (p. 1416; Box 35-1), c (p. 1416; Box 35-1), a (p. 1416; Box 35-1), g (p. 1412; Box 35-1), n (p. 1412), m (p. 1412), d (p. 1412; Box 35-1), e (p. 1416, Box 35-1)
6. Can result from any tissue destruction such as bacterial or viral infections, hemorrhage, neoplastic disease, toxicity, operative procedures, burns, or tissue ischemia (p. 1415)
7. a (p. 1417)
8. a. Leukemia, hyperplastic (p. 1417)
   b. Aplastic anemia, hypoplastic, aplastic (p. 1417)
9. b (p. 1416)
10. b (pp. 1417-1418)
11. c (p. 1419)
12. b (p. 1420; Table 35-2)
13. a (p. 1422)
14. a (p. 1423)
15. b (pp. 1417, 1424)
16. d (p. 1423)
17. a (pp. 1423-1424; Drug Alert and Nursing Alert)
18. "This is a normally expected change and usually means that an adequate dosage of iron has been reached" (p. 1424).
19. b (p. 1425)
20. d (pp. 1426, 1434)
21. c (p. 1426)
22. Dehydration, acidosis, hypoxia, temperature elevation (p. 1426)
23. c (p. 1426)
24. b (pp. 1426, 1432)
25. c (pp. 1428-1429)
26. d (p. 1429)
27. d (pp. 1429, 1431)
28. b (p. 1431)
29. d (p. 1433; Drug Alert)
30. a (p. 1432)
31. c (pp. 1436-1437)
32. d (p. 1438)
33. a (p. 1439)
34. Primary, or congenital; secondary, or acquired (pp. 1439-1440)
35. a. Bone marrow aspiration, which demonstrates the conversion of red bone marrow to yellow, fatty bone marrow (p. 1440)

b. Anemia; leukopenia; low platelet counts (p. 1440)

c. Immunosuppressive therapy; bone marrow transplant (p. 1440)

36. d (p. 1440)
37. d (p. 1442; Table 35-5), i (p. 1441), e (p. 1441; Table 35-4), a (p. 1442; Table 35-5), b (p. 1442; Table 35-5), c (pp. 1441-1442; Table 35-5), g (p. 1441), f (p. 1441), h (p. 1441)
38. a (p. 1443)
39. a (p. 1443)
40. b (p. 1443; Drug Alert)
41. d (pp.1443-1445; Table 35-7)
42. a (p. 1446)
43. c (p. 1446)
44. a (pp. 1446, 1447)
45. d (p. 1447; Drug Alert)
46. a (p. 1448)
47. b (p. 1448; Box 35-7)
48. a (pp.1448-1450)
49. Nonthrombocytopenic purpura, arthritis, nephritis, abdominal pain (p. 1450)
50. d (p. 1452)
51. Lymphadenopathy, hepatosplenomegaly, oral candidiasis, chronic or recurrent diarrhea, failure to thrive, developmental delay, parotitis (p. 1453; Box 35-8)
52. Slowing growth of the virus, promoting or restoring normal growth and development, preventing complicating infections and cancers, improving quality of life and prolonging survival (p. 1454)
53. T, T, F, T, F (pp. 1454-1455)
54. c (p. 1455)
55. ELISA and Western blot will be positive because of presence of maternal antibodies derived transplacentally. Maternal antibodies may persist in the infant up to 18 months of age (p. 1454).
56. d (p. 1456)
57. b (p. 1455)
58. a (p. 1456)
59. a (p. 1457)
60. c (p. 1428)
61. Plan preventive schedule of medication around the clock, not only when needed to prevent pain; prevent resistance to administration by reassuring child and family that analgesics, including opioids, are medically indicated, that high doses may be needed, and that children rarely become addicted (pp. 1432-1433).
62. d (p. 1432)
63. a (p. 1433)
64. Implement Standard Precautions to prevent the spread of virus, including the following: wear gloves when in contact with any body fluid; wash hands carefully; wear gowns, masks, and eye protection; use needle precautions and precautions with trash and linen. Instruct family in appropriate precautions. Clarify any misconceptions about communicability of virus among the family and community. Assess home situation and implement protective measures. Place restrictions on behaviors and contact for affected children who bite or who do not have control of their bodily secretions (p. 1455; see also Infection Control, Chapter 27).
65. Cindy will experience minimized risk for infection; will not spread disease to others; will have education concerning the transmission and control of infectious diseases as she gets older; will receive optimal nourishment; growth and development will be promoted; will adhere to antiretroviral therapy; will have prolonged survival and no cancer development; will participate in family and peer-group activities; will exhibit minimal or no evidence of pain or irritability. Family will receive adequate support and will be able to meet needs of the infant (pp. 1454-1455).

CHAPTER 36

1. e (p. 1463), i (p. 1463), g (p. 1465), a (p. 1463), h (p. 1477), b (p. 1463), c (p. 1480), f (p. 1468), d (p. 1473)
2. o (p. 1468), f (p. 1465), t (p. 1469), n (p. 1468), b (p. 1481), g (p. 1466), d (p. 1465), h (p. 1467), a (p. 1463), i (p. 1467), c (p. 1465), j (p. 1467), e (p. 1465), k (p. 1468), p (p. 1478), r (p. 1468), v (p. 1469), l (p. 1468), x (p. 1469), m (p. 1468), w (p. 1469), q (p. 1468), y (p. 1469), s (pp. 1468-1469), u (p. 1469)
3. g, f, e, d, c, b, a (p. 1464; Box 36-1)
4. c (p. 1473), f (p. 1477), e (p. 1477), a (p. 1473), d (p. 1477), b (p. 1473)
5. t (p. 1490), c (p. 1483), e (p. 1483), u (p. 1490), g (p. 1500), a (p. 1501), d (p. 1483), b (p. 1483), i (p. 1486), f (p. 1485; Box 36-3), k (p. 1486), l (p. 1487), h (p. 1486), m (pp. 1487-1490), j (p. 1486), n (p. 1493), v (p. 1496), o (p. 1487), w (p. 1499), p (p. 1487), x (p. 1501), q (p. 1488), y (p. 1501), r (p. 1488), s (p. 1490)
6. c (p. 1462)
7. a (p. 1463)
8. b (p. 1482)
9. d (p. 1562)
10. b (p. 1562)
11. c (p. 1568)
12. c, a, d, b, e (pp. 1562-1568; Table 36-2)
13. a (p. 1466)
14. Gastrointestinal tract—Nausea and vomiting; give antiemetic around the clock.
Skin—Alopecia; introduce idea of wig; stress necessity of scalp hygiene.
Head—Xerostomia (dry mouth); stress oral hygiene and liquid diet.
Urinary bladder—Cystitis; encourage liberal fluid intake and frequent voiding (pp. 1466-1467; Table 36-2).
15. b (p. 1468)
16. Possible answers: Unusual mass or swelling; unexplained paleness and loss of energy; sudden tendency to bruise; persistent, localized pain or limping; prolonged, unexplained fever or illness; frequent headaches, often with vomiting; sudden eye or vision

changes; excessive, rapid weight loss (pp. 1463-1464; Box 36-1)

17. Colony-stimulating factor (p. 1469)
18. c (p. 1474)
19. a (p. 1476)
20. Possible answers: Liberal oral and/or parenteral fluid intake; frequent voiding immediately after feeling the urge, including immediately before bed and after arising; administration of drug early in the day to allow for sufficient fluid and frequent voiding; administration of mesna, a drug that inhibits the urotoxicity of cyclophosphamide and ifosfamide (p. 1477)
21. d (p. 1477)
22. a (p. 1478)
23. d (p. 1478)
24. d (p. 1479)
25. c (p. 1479)
26. d (p. 1481)
27. Possible answers: Anemia, infection, and bleeding (p. 1481)
28. d (p. 1482; Table 36-3)
29. b (p. 1484)
30. c (p. 1482; Table 36-3)
31. c (p. 1483)
32. b (p. 1484)
33. d (p. 1485)
34. a (p. 1485)
35. b (p. 1485; Box 36-3)
36. d (p. 1486)
37. c (p. 1486)
38. b (p. 1487)
39. b (p. 1488)
40. e, c, d, b, a (p. 1488; Fig. 36-5)
41. d (p. 1490)
42. d (p. 1489; Table 36-4)
43. Possible answers: Braid the hair if it is long; then cut it and save the braid. Show child how he or she looks at each stage of the process. Give the child a cap or scarf to wear. Ensure privacy during the procedure. Emphasize that the hair will begin to grow back after surgery. Introduce the idea of wearing a wig (p. 1490).
44. d (p. 1492)
45. c (p. 1491)
46. a (p. 1494)
47. c (p. 1494-1495)
48. d (p. 1495)
49. b (p. 1495)
50. c (p. 1497)
51. d (p. 1498)
52. d (p. 1499)
53. a (p. 1500)
54. b (p. 1501)
55. c (p. 1573)
56. d (p. 1573)
57. b (p. 1573)
58. a (p. 1573, 1574)

CHAPTER 37

1. r (p. 1509), j (p. 1509), c (p. 1508), l (p. 1509), e (pp. 1508-1509), n (p. 1509), g (p. 1509), s (p. 1509), h (p. 1509), b (p. 1508), i (p. 1509), f (p. 1509), k (p. 1509), m (p. 1509), t (p. 1510), o (p. 1509), d (p. 1508), p (p. 1509), a (p. 1508), q (p. 1509)
2. b (p. 1512; Box 37-2), d (p. 1512), a (p. 1512), f (p. 1512), l (p. 1514), e (p. 1512), h (p. 1513), c (p. 1512), n (p. 1515), i (p. 1513), r (p. 1516), j (p. 1514), t (p. 1516), m (p. 1515), o (p. 1516), k (p. 1514), p (p. 1516), g (pp. 1512-1513; Box 37-4), q (p. 1516), s (p. 1516)
3. k (p. 1526), c (p. 1525), a (p. 1525), q (p. 1528), o (p. 1528), m (p. 1527), i (p. 1526), e (p. 1525), b (p. 1525), r (p. 1529), n (p. 1527), f (p. 1528), d (p. 1525), g (p. 1528), s (p. 1529), h (p. 1525), l (p. 1526), j (p. 1526), p (p. 1528)
4. i (p. 1538), b (p. 1535), j (p. 1543), d (p. 1535), c (p. 1543), e (p. 1541), g (p. 1535), a (p. 1535), h (p. 1538), f (p. 1541)
5. b, f, l, g, k, c, i, e, d, h, j, a (p. 1518; Table 37-1)
6. a (p. 1508)
7. b (p. 1545), i (p. 1546; Box 37-10), a (p. 1545), k (p. 1546; Box 37-10), s (p. 1546; Box 37-10), p (p. 1548), m (p. 1546), f (p. 1546; Box 37-10), h (p. 1546; Box 37-10), dd (p. 1553), c (p. 1545), d (p. 1547), e (pp. 1546-1548; Box 37-10), j (p. 1546; Box 37-10), l (pp. 1545-1546; Box 37-10), n (pp. 1546, 1548; Box 37-10), r (p. 1548), t (pp. 1546, 1549; Box 37-10), v (p. 1547; Box 37-10), g (p. 1546; Box 37-10), w (p. 1547; Box 37-10), cc (p. 1553), q (p. 1546; Box 37-10), x (pp. 1547, 1549; Box 37-10), bb (p. 1553), u (pp. 1546, 1553; Box 37-10), z (p. 1550), aa (p. 1549), o (p. 1548), y (pp. 1546, 1548; Box 37-10)
8. d (p. 1510)
9. c (p. 1511)
10. b (p. 1513)
11. Function of the cerebral cortex is permanently lost; eyes follow objects only by reflex or when attracted to the direction of loud sounds; all four limbs are spastic but can withdraw from painful stimuli; hands show reflexive grasping and groping; the face can grimace; some food may be swallowed; the child may groan or cry but utters no words (p. 1513; Box 37-4).
12. a (p. 1514; Nursing Care Guidelines box)
13. d (p. 1515)
14. c (p. 1516)
15. c (p. 1517)
16. c (p. 1512; Box 37-3)
17. a (pp. 1517-1518; Table 37-1)
18. c (p. 1517; Table 37-1)
19. b (p. 1519)
20. d (p. 1519)
21. b (p. 1520)
22. c (p. 1521)
23. a (p. 1522)
24. d (p. 1524)

25. a (p. 1525)
26. c (pp. 1525-1526; Fig. 37-8)
27. c (p. 1526)
28. a (p. 1527)
29. c (p. 1528; Table 37-3)
30. c (p. 1532)
31. a (pp. 1529-1531)
32. b (p. 1529; Box 37-5)
33. d (p. 1531)
34. d (p. 1533)
35. The need for adequate supervision (p. 1533)
36. a (p. 1534)
37. d (p. 1534)
38. c (p. 1535)
39. a (p. 1537)
40. b (p. 1539; Nursing Alert)
41. b (p. 1540)
42. d (p. 1541)
43. a (p. 1542)
44. a (p. 1543)
45. b (p. 1543)
46. c (p. 1544)
47. a (p. 1543)
48. b (p. 1544)
49. Birth injuries and acute infections (p. 1545)
50. a (pp. 1547-1548; Table 37-5)
51. b (pp. 1547-1548)
52. b (p. 1549)
53. a (p. 1550)
54. d (p. 1550)
55. c (p. 1551)
56. a (p. 1553; Nursing Alert)
57. a (p. 1553)
58. d (p. 1555)
59. c (p. 1557)
60. d (p. 1558)
61. b (p. 1559)
62. c (p. 1561)
63. a (p. 1561)
64. d (p. 1563)
65. c (p. 1563)
66. d (p. 1519)
67. b (pp. 1523-1524, 1531-1533)
68. c (pp. 1524, 1533)
69. b (pp. 1523-1524, 1533)

CHAPTER 38

1. g (p. 1568), e (p. 1568), a (p. 1615), n (p. 1569), h (p. 1568), c (p. 1567), k (p. 1569), f (p. 1568), i (p. 1569), b (p. 1567), j (p. 1569), l (p. 1569), d (p. 1568), m (p. 1569)
2. j (p. 1576), n (pp. 1577-1578), c (p. 1571), e (p. 1574), l (p. 1576), f (p. 1575), h (p. 1576), a (p. 1570), i (p. 1576), d (p. 1574), k (p. 1578), g (p. 1575), m (p. 1577), b (p. 1571)
3. u (pp. 1591-1592), b (p. 1579), d (p. 1580), c (p. 1579), e (p. 1581), g (p. 1584), f (p. 1583), o (p. 1586), l (pp. 1585, 1586), m (p. 1569), h (p. 1584), j (p. 1585), q (p. 1586), i (p. 1585), k (p. 1585), n (p. 1585), p (p. 1586), r (p. 1586), s (p. 1590), a (p. 1579), t (p. 1591)
4. j (p. 1596), c (p. 1594), g (p. 1598), b (p. 1594), q (p. 1596), d (p. 1596), m (p. 1596), n (p. 1596), f (p. 1596), i (p. 1596), e (p. 1594), k (p. 1596), u (p. 1597), a (p. 1594), p (p. 1596), h (p. 1596), t (p. 1597), l (p. 1596), s (p. 1597), o (p. 1598), r (p. 1597)
5. b (p. 1599), d (p. 1600), a (p. 1599), f (p. 1600), e (p. 1600), h (p. 1603), j (p. 1610), g (p. 1603), i (p. 1603), c (p. 1612), k (p. 1610)
6. Target tissues:
   a. Thyroid gland
   b. Ovaries, testes
   c. Bones
   d. Gonads
   e. Skin
   f. Adrenal cortex
   g. Renal tubules
   h. Ovaries, testes
   i. Uterus, breasts
   j. Ovaries, breasts
   Hormone's effect: g, c, f, h, a, j, e, i, d, b (pp. 1568-1569; Fig. 38-2)
7. Tropic (p. 1570)
8. d (p. 1570)
9. c (p. 1570)
10. d (p. 1571; Box 38-3)
11. c (pp. 1571, 1574; Box 38-3)
12. a (p. 1574)
13. c (p. 1574)
14. c (p. 1574)
15. Acromegaly results from hypersecretion of growth hormone that occurs after epiphyseal closure. Hyperfunction of the pituitary that occurs before the epiphyseal closure is not considered acromegaly (p. 1575).
16. c (p. 1577)
17. b (p. 1578)
18. c (p. 1578)
19. a (p. 1580)
20. d (p. 1581)
21. c (p. 1583)
22. c (p. 1584)
23. b (p. 1584)
24. a (p. 1586)
25. b (p. 1587)
26. d (p. 1588)
27. b (p. 1591)
28. a (p. 1593)
29. c (p. 1593)
30. d (p. 1596)
31. d (pp. 1595-1596)
32. a (p. 1597)
33. c (p. 1598)
34. To maintain near-normal blood glucose values while avoiding too-frequent episodes of hypoglycemia (pp. 1598-1599)
35. b (p. 1600)
36. c (p. 1602)

37. Give 10 to 15 g of simple carbohydrate, such as a tablespoon of table sugar, fruit juice, 8 oz of milk, Insta-Glucose (cherry-flavored glucose), carbonated sugar-containing drinks (not sugarless), sherbet, gelatin, cake icing, sugar-containing candy (LifeSavers, Charms), or glucose tablets (pp. 1602-1603).
38. c (p. 1603)
39. c (p. 1604)
40. a (p. 1604)
41. d (p. 1608)
42. c (p. 1609)
43. d (p. 1609)
44. a (p. 1610)
45. c (p. 1610)
46. b (p. 1612)
47. d (p. 1613)
48. b (p. 1614)
49. Possible answers: Feelings of guilt as with any chronic disease; overprotectiveness; neglect; fear of the unknown; may block feelings that give pain; may feel threatened by independent development; may feel left out (pp. 1614-1615)
50. b (pp. 1606-1607)
51. c (pp. 1606-1607)
52. c (pp. 1606-1607)
53. d (pp. 1606-1607)

CHAPTER 39

1. a. Falls; being struck by or against an object; motor vehicle accidents; fires and burns; drowning; pedestrian-vehicle accidents; bicycle injuries; firearm injuries; sports injuries, especially for school-age children and adolescents; poisonings, especially for young children (p. 1621)
   b. Become active in legislative efforts, assist with public awareness campaigns, provide individual prevention counseling for children and family, implement home visits to identify potential sources of danger in the home, administer screening questions about safety issues on admission and discharge from the hospital or health clinic visits (p. 1621).
2. b (p. 1621)
3. b (pp. 1621-1622)
4. The cervical spine is immobilized by holding the head in a neutral position and not allowing movement of the head or body in any direction (p. 1622).
5. a (p. 1624)
6. Orthostatic hypotension, increased workload of the heart, thrombus formation (p. 1625)
7. Numbness, tingling, changes in sensation, loss of motion (p. 1627)
8. a (pp. 1629-1631; Table 39-1)
9. c (p. 1630), a (p. 1630), f (p. 1630), b (p. 1630), j (p. 1633), e (p. 1630), h (p. 1630), i (p. 1633), g (p. 1630), d (p. 1630), l (p. 1634), k (p. 1634), m (p. 1634)
10. a (p. 1629)

11. c (pp. 1633-1634)
12. Financial strains decrease or eliminate family resources; focus of attention is placed on the affected child and other family members' needs may not be met; family members may have difficulty accepting child's altered body image; family members may be unable to express feelings and may have difficulty coping with crises; parents often experience guilt and have the perception of failing to protect the child (p. 1628).
13. d (p. 1642)
14. b (p. 1640; Box 39-5)
15. h (p. 1638), s (p. 1638; Box 39-4), a (p. 1635), d (p. 1637), e (p. 1638), b (p. 1636), c (p. 1636), f (p. 1638), o (p. 1635), p (p. 1636), j (p. 1638), i (p. 1638), r (p. 1638), n (p. 1625), l (p. 1638; Box 39-4), m (p. 1638; Box 39-4), k (p. 1638; Box 39-4), g (p. 1638), q (p. 1638)
16. Pain, pallor, pulselessness, paresthesia, and paralysis (p. 1639)
17. b (p. 1639)
18. To regain alignment and length of the bony fragments by reduction; to retain alignment and length by immobilization; to restore function to the injured parts; to prevent further injury (p. 1640)
19. a (p. 1642)
20. d (p. 1644)
21. c (p. 1645)
22. c (pp. 1644-1645; Family-Centered Care box)
23. To fatigue the involved muscle and reduce muscle spasm so that bones can be realigned; to position the distal and proximal bone ends in desired realignment to promote satisfactory bone healing; to immobilize the fracture site until realignment has been achieved and sufficient healing has taken place to permit casting or splinting (p. 1646)
24. b (p. 1648; Nursing Alert)
25. a (pp. 1648-1650)
26. b (pp. 1650-1651)
27. b (p. 1652, Nursing Alert)
28. l (p. 1647, Box 39-8), o (p. 1650), j (p. 1647; Box 39-8), k (p. 1647; Box 39-8), a (pp. 1627, 1650), b (p. 1638), n (p. 1652), p (p. 1651), q (pp. 1651-1652), d (p. 1647), c (p. 1647), e (p. 1647), f (p. 1647), m (p. 1648), i (pp. 1647-1648), h (p. 1647), g (p. 1647)
29. c (pp. 1652-1653)
30. c (p. 1652)
31. a (p. 1653)
32. c (p. 1656), g (p. 1658), a (p. 1656), e (p. 1657), h (p. 1653), f (p. 1656), b (p. 1656), d (p. 1657)
33. d (p. 1656)
34. a (p. 1657)
35. Ligaments, epiphysis, growth plate (p. 1658)
36. g (p. 1659; Table 39-4), i (p. 1659; Table 39-4), e (p. 1659; Table 39-4), d (p. 1658), h (p. 1656; Table 39-4), c (p. 1658), j (p. 1659; Table 39-4), a (p. 1658), b (p. 1658), f (p. 1659; Table 39-4)
37. c (pp. 1659-1660)

38. b (pp. 1660-1661)
39. b (p. 1660)
40. a (p. 1662)
41. a (p. 1663)
42. a (p. 1665)
43. d (p. 1666)
44. a (p. 1667)
45. Lordosis, kyphosis, spondylolisthesis (pp. 1667-1668)
46. d (p. 1669)
47. Realignment and straightening with internal fixation and instrumentation, along with bony fusion of the realigned spine (p. 1670)
48. b (p. 1669)
49. a (p. 1670)
50. a (p. 1673)
51. b (p. 1674)
52. d (p. 1674)
53. b (p. 1675)
54. b (p. 1676)
55. a (p. 1678)
56. a. Methotrexate: Significant potential adverse effects including potential for increased infection, malignancy, liver and lung toxicity, and birth defects (p. 1684)
    b. Diet: Eat a well-balanced diet without exceeding caloric expenditure and maintain appropriate weight on corticosteroids. A low-salt diet may be required if the patient becomes nephritic or hypertensive. A low-fat diet is indicated in children with dyslipidemia. Maximizing peak bone mass in adolescent SLE is essential with a diet rich in calcium and vitamin D (p. 1685).
    c. Sun exposure: Avoid excessive exposure; use sunscreen (with a sun protection factor of at least 30), hat, and protective clothing; schedule outdoor activities in morning and evening (p. 1686).
    d. Birth control medications: Pregnancy is a potential trigger for disease flare; because estrogen can trigger disease flare, low-dose estrogen or progesterone-only contraceptives are preferred (p. 1685).
57. To minimize disease activity with appropriate medications; to help child and family cope with the complications of the disease and treatment (p. 1684)
58. Corticosteroids (p. 1684)
59. Fostering adaptation and self-advocacy skills (p. 1686)
60. d (p. 1677)
61. c (p. 1678)
62. a (pp. 1679-1680)
63. c (p. 1682)
64. Liver enzymes and complete blood count with differential and platelet counts (p. 1678)
65. A well-balanced diet without the problems of weight control that often result from potential for more than body requirements related to decreased mobility (p. 1679)

CHAPTER 40

1. T (p. 1690), F (p. 1690), T (p. 1690), F (p. 1690), T (p. 1690), T (p. 1690), T (p. 1690), T (p. 1690), T (p. 1693)
2. d, c, b, a (p. 1691)
3. a (p. 1691)
4. b (p. 1693)
5. f (p. 1693; Box 40-3), e (p. 1693; Box 40-3), l (p. 1694), d (p. 1692; Box 40-3), c (p. 1693; Box 40-3), a (p. 1693; Box 40-3), g (p. 1693; Box 40-3), b (p. 1693; Box 40-3), i (pp. 1693; Box 40-2), j (p. 1693; Box 40-2), k (p. 1693; Box 40-2), h (p. 1693; Box 40-2)
6. a (p. 1694)
7. d (p. 1694)
8. d (pp. 1694-1695; Box 40-4)
9. a (p. 1695)
10. b (p. 1695)
11. The nature of the physical disability, defects associated with the disorder, and interpersonal and social influences encountered by the affected child (pp. 1695, 1699)
12. T (p. 1695), F (p. 1696), T (p. 1696), F (p. 1697), T (p. 1697), T (p. 1697), T (p. 1698), T (p. 1698), F (p. 1698), F (p. 1698), T (p. 1699), T (p. 1699), T (p. 1699), T (p. 1699)
13. c (p. 1701)
14. a (p. 1703)
15. a (p. 1703)
16. c (p. 1705)
17. a. Scoliosis; hip subluxation and dislocation (p. 1704)
    b. To assist the child and family in dealing with the illness while progressing toward a life of normalization within the child's capabilities (p. 1704)
18. c (p. 1705)
19. b (p. 1706)
20. a (p. 1706)
21. Progressive stiffness and tenderness of the muscles in the neck and jaw, with difficulty opening the mouth and spasms of facial muscles (pp. 1707-1708)
22. a. Spores are found in soil, dust, and the intestinal tracts of humans and animals, especially herbivorous animals; they are most prevalent in rural areas but readily carried to urban areas by wind (p. 1707).
    b. Incubation period is 3 days to 3 weeks (p. 1708).
23. b (p. 1707)
24. d (pp. 1707-1708)
25. d (pp. 1708-1709)
26. a (p. 1709)
27. b (p. 1709)
28. a. History, physical examination, and laboratory detection of the toxin or organism in the patient's stool and, less commonly, blood (pp. 1709-1710)
    b. Immediate administration of human botulism immune globulin intravenously (BIG-IV) without waiting for laboratory diagnosis (p. 1710)

29. d (p. 1710)
30. a (pp. 1710-1711)
31. c (p. 1711)
32. c (p. 1715)
33. b (p. 1716)
34. The paraplegic patient who has function down to and including the quadriceps muscle or who has muscle function below the L3 level will have little difficulty learning to walk with or without braces and crutches (p. 1716).
35. FES may enable the child to sit, stand, and walk with the aid of crutches, a walker, etc.; can be used to elicit grasp and release from the hand; helps cardiovascular conditioning; decreases pressure ulcers and increases blood flow; helps to reduce complications due to bladder and bowel incontinence; assists males in achieving penile erection (p. 1718).
36. d (pp. 1720-1721)
37. b (p. 1723)
38. b (p. 1724)
39. d (p. 1727)
40. Contractures, scoliosis, disuse atrophy, infections, obesity, and respiratory and cardiopulmonary problems (p. 1726)
41. c (p. 1727)
42. c (p. 1727)
43. d (p. 1694)
44. b (p. 1698)
45. d (p. 1701)
46. Kevin will acquire mobility within personal capabilities, acquire communication skills or use appropriate assistive devices, engage in self-help activities, receive appropriate education, develop a positive self-image, and receive appropriate nutrition and feeding assistance. The family members will receive appropriate education and support in their efforts to meet Kevin's needs. Kevin will receive appropriate care if hospitalized or in the community (pp. 1693, 1701).
47. c (p. 1698)